SLOW DEATH
BY RUBBER DUCK

SLOW DEATH
BY RUBBER DUCK

HOW THE TOXICITY
OF EVERYDAY LIFE
AFFECTS OUR HEALTH

RICK SMITH / BRUCE LOURIE

ALFRED A. KNOPF CANADA

PUBLISHED BY ALFRED A. KNOPF CANADA

www.penguinrandomhouse.ca

Knopf Canada and colophon are registered trademarks.

LIBRARY AND ARCHIVES CANADA CATALOGUING IN PUBLICATION

Smith, Rick, 1968–, author
Slow death by rubber duck : how the toxicity of everyday
life affects our health / Rick Smith and Bruce Lourie. — 10th
anniversary edition.
"Fully expanded and updated".

Issued in print and electronic formats.

ISBN 978-0-7352-7570-6
eBook ISBN 978-0-7352-7571-3

1. Environmental toxicology—Popular works. 2. Pollution—Health aspects. 3. Pollution. 4. Industries—Environmental aspects. 5. Business enterprises—Environmental aspects. 6. Pollution—Government policy.
I. Lourie, Bruce, author II. Title.

RA1213.S62 2019   615.9'02   C2018-902707-X
C2018-902708-8

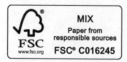

Book design by Leah Springate
Cover image © Lawrence Manning / Corbis Collection / Getty Images

Printed and bound in Canada

2 4 6 8 9 7 5 3 1

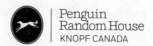

For our families

CONTENTS

INTRODUCTION TO THE
TENTH-ANNIVERSARY EDITION

You live your life like a canary in a coalmine
You get so dizzy even walking in a straight line

—THE POLICE, "CANARY IN A COALMINE,"
Zenyatta Mondatta, 1980

WHAT BETTER WAY TO CELEBRATE an anniversary than to poison ourselves all over again?

Ten years ago, we set out to write a very different kind of book
about pollution. One that shed light on the toxic chemicals in common
consumer products that touch the lives of everybody on this planet.
Not an obvious kind of pollution, like the smog of the Industrial
Revolution or the acid rain of the 1980s, but rather a subtle—though
no less harmful—pollution that invades our bodies every day and is
linked to such modern epidemics as breast cancer and diabetes.

To tell the story of this pollution, to make it real, to illustrate its
danger and the ways we can all protect ourselves, we experimented
with these chemicals on ourselves (and a few intrepid volunteers).
Over the course of writing our first book, *Slow Death by Rubber Duck*
(2009) and our second, *Toxin Toxout* (2013), we conducted a series of a
dozen experiments to see if we could raise and lower the levels of these
chemicals in our bodies in real time: a kind of huge multi-year science
fair project with ourselves as the guinea pigs.

Our two books struck a chord around the world. Both were best-
sellers at home in Canada and abroad and took us as far as Australia's
Sydney Writers' Festival (twice!). *Slow Death* has been featured by the

Washington Post (which called it "hard-hitting in a way that turns your stomach and yet also instills hope"), Dr. Oz, Fox News, and *Oprah* magazine, and translated into seven languages. It turns out that wherever consumers are in the world, they are united in their exposure to toxic chemicals and hungry for information on how to protect themselves and their families from this danger.

A decade later, we decided to commemorate the tenth anniversary of *Slow Death by Rubber Duck* with the definitive volume on toxic pollution. The book in your hand has all the groundbreaking experiments from both *Slow Death by Rubber Duck* and *Toxin Toxout*, and it has been completely overhauled and updated.

As an added bonus, and to rekindle that old-time toxic feeling, we undertook a brand-new experiment on ourselves for good measure.

Quick Refresher

Before we get toxic all over again, let's take a step back and remind ourselves why we should be concerned about the synthetic chemicals that surround us. It's simple: the scientific evidence linking these chemicals to human disease is even more convincing than it was when *Slow Death* was first released in 2009. Exposure to these many substances— and the resulting hazards—remains widespread.

Of the eighty thousand or so chemicals in commerce (the building blocks of all the consumer products we surround ourselves with every day), a great many have now also been found in the human body. This chemical exposure is estimated to contribute to health costs that may exceed an astonishing 10 percent of global gross domestic product (GDP).[1] How prevalent is this personal toxicity?

In the United States, studies by the Environmental Working Group (EWG) found 553 different industrial chemicals, pollutants and pesticides in 550 individuals across forty states. In one recent study, EWG found 232 toxic chemicals in the umbilical cord blood of ten babies, demonstrating that kids these days are being born "pre-polluted."[2] In Europe, widespread exposure to chemicals in food and consumer products used in homes, schools and offices has been linked to problems with brain development in children.[3]

In Canada, Environmental Defence Canada's groundbreaking Toxic Nation project, launched in 2005, continues to expose the dangers of pollution through testing Canadians for measurable levels of toxic chemicals soaked up by their bodies. Like efforts in the United States and Europe, the Toxic Nation project applies scientific testing techniques—previously restricted to the pages of obscure scientific journals—to the raging public debate about what pollutants we are exposed to, in what amounts and from which sources—and tells us what we can do about it. Over the past fifteen years Environmental Defence Canada has tested a wide range of consumer and personal care products for more than 130 pollutants. They also tested the blood and urine of more than fifty Canadians from all walks of life. People of all ages. Men, women and kids from different parts of the country and different ethnic backgrounds. They all turned out to be polluted to some degree.

To date, less research has been conducted in developing countries, but we can reasonably assume that to the extent people are exposed to the same chemicals in those areas, the results would be similar.[4]

The results are even more alarming when we consider the cases of very specific chemicals. For instance, phthalates—an ingredient in many plastics used to keep the material pliable—have been convincingly linked to asthma, attention-deficit hyperactivity disorder, breast cancer, obesity and type 2 diabetes, low IQ, neurodevelopmental issues, behavioural issues, autism spectrum disorders, altered reproductive development and male fertility issues.[5] The presence of triclosan, that ubiquitous "antibacterial" ingredient in everything from personal-care products to footwear, is increasing dramatically in the bodies of people, and in lakes and rivers, and has been linked to increasing rates of allergies.[6] The evidence of harm from mercury exposure continues to accumulate, with recent experiments revealing effects as varied as autoimmune diseases in adult women and hormone alterations in kids.[7]

Exposure to one synthetic chemical is worrisome enough, but the mixture of a large number of toxic chemicals in our bodies, *all at once*, has a more profound effect than the chemical industry would like us to believe. Individual chemicals are tested in isolation to determine a "safe" level, which presumes that so long as the concentration of that chemical in your body is below that level, you'll be good to go, with no ill effect.

This rationalization falls apart, of course, when we have hundreds or thousands of synthetic chemicals in us at the same time: these chemicals can actually *amplify* each other's individual impacts.[8]

The most recent wrinkle in the story is the stunning new science now coming to light indicating widespread plastic pollution in the environment and in common products. It turns out that plastic never really breaks down. It just gets pounded into smaller and smaller bits by the passage of time, sunlight and the action of waves. These microscopic particles then enter the food chain, air and soil. In the past couple of years, scientists have started to find them in a disturbing range of products, including table salt, honey, shellfish and . . . beer. In one recent study, 83 percent of tap water in seven countries was found to contain plastic micro-fibres. It seems certain that a steady diet of this plastic residue is one reason for humanity's elevated levels of plasticizing chemicals—like phthalates—described above.

A Kind of Progress

As we noted in the original introduction to *Slow Death*, surging public engagement in the debates about environment and health was an exciting consequence of strong scientific evidence linking toxic chemicals to serious human disease. The public's everyday behaviour was undergoing a marked and positive change.

If anything, this trend has only accelerated.

As one example, the organic food and beverage industry has grown rapidly worldwide, an increase driven largely by the desire of people everywhere to avoid consuming toxins. In 2015, the global market for certified organic food and drink (produced without the use of chemical inputs) was estimated to be US$92 billion, which represents a 70 percent increase over the $54.1 billion in sales in 2009.[9] Traditionally, the organic food industry was based mainly on fresh produce, and while organic fruits and vegetables retain the highest sales growth, the industry has expanded to include many processed foods and meats.[10]

Other trends reflect an increasing desire on the part of consumers to avoid everyday exposure to toxins. In the cleaning products aisle, toxin-conscious brands such as Method and Seventh Generation now compete for market share with the likes of traditional brands such as Clorox and Procter & Gamble. That has led to the surest sign of market success—namely, the big companies getting into the game with products like Clorox's Green Works. Even Martha Stewart's line of cleaning products is made with non-toxic ingredients: surely a cultural bell-wether if ever there was one.[11]

Eco-friendly products and "green consumerism" continue to gain ground and are consistently an area where opportunities exist for creative brands and entrepreneurs to respond to changing consumer needs. In a 2011 global survey of executives from commercial companies around the world, 70 percent of respondents had placed sustainability permanently on their management agendas, all within the past six years.[12] Over two-thirds of respondents say their organization's dedication to sustainability has increased and will continue to do so.[13]

As a result of the accumulating science and consumer awareness in this area, governments are acting. Not quickly, but they are moving. The laws governing bisphenol A (BPA) present a good example of this progress. Following the Canadian ban on BPA in baby bottles in 2008 (Canada was the first country in the world to do this), the European Union followed suit in 2010, and in early 2011 China did as well. Effective in 2013, France has further outlawed the use of BPA in plastic food containers. After a dozen U.S. states followed Canada's lead, the U.S. Food and Drug Administration (FDA) banned BPA in baby bottles and sippy cups in 2012. Perhaps most significantly, in April 2013 the state of California added BPA to its Proposition 65 list of toxic chemicals that cause cancer or birth defects, resulting in BPA warnings being posted at point of sale in retail locations, with warning labels directly on BPA-containing products imminent.

Thanks to the work of Environmental Defence Canada and others, the Canadian government has classified the antibacterial triclosan as "toxic" under the country's pollution law, and both the Canadian and American Medical Associations have called for restrictions on the household use of this chemical.[14, 15] In 2017 the FDA banned triclosan in consumer soaps and hand washes.

Rubber Duck Wars

Appropriately, there is no finer example of our reduced daily exposure to toxic chemicals than the fact that rubber ducks are now much safer than when *Slow Death* was first published. What has happened with phthalates in kids' toys is a textbook example of what can be achieved in short order when good ideas get around.

In both Europe and the United States the discussion about phthalates in children's toys began in 1998. Europe moved quickly. On the heels of a variety of studies linking phthalates with human health problems, the European Union proposed an emergency ban of six phthalates (phthalates are a family of chemicals) in toys likely to be placed in the mouths of kids three years of age and younger. The ban, though temporary, was significant. It was the first time the E.U. had enacted an immediate prohibition under its new General Product Safety Directive (GPSD, 2002).

After many twists and turns, and despite millions of euros in chemical industry lobbying, in 2005 the temporary action was made permanent. DEHP (diethylhexyl phthalate), DBP (dibutyl phthalate) and BBP (benzyl butyl phthalate) were banned outright, and DINP (diisononyl phthalate), DIDP (diisodecyl phthalate) and DNOP (di-n-octyl phthalate) were prohibited in toys and childcare articles designed to be sucked or chewed by children under three years old.

In the United States events took a very different course. In 1998, twelve consumer and environmental groups filed a petition urging the U.S. Consumer Product Safety Commission (CPSC) to ban toys containing phthalates that were intended for children five years of age and under. The CPSC responded by calling for further study to assess phthalate toxicity to humans. Review led to review, process was heaped on more process, until finally the CPSC ruled that "there is no demonstrated health risk" posed by the chemicals and thus no justification for banning them in children's products.[16]

And so the Rubber Duck Wars were joined. In denying the anti-phthalate petition at the federal level, the CPSC pushed advocates to continue their fight in the courts of more local jurisdictions. Less frequently targeted by lobbyists and corporate influencers, lower courts sometimes take a bolder stance in favour of common sense. In this case, anti-phthalate advocates turned specifically to California (which, if it were a nation, would have the tenth-largest economy in the world). California environmentalists and public health advocates were up to the challenge. And as one of the most charismatic phthalates sources around, the yellow bath-time icon, beloved by *Sesame Street* alumni everywhere, took centre stage in America's ongoing phthalates debate.

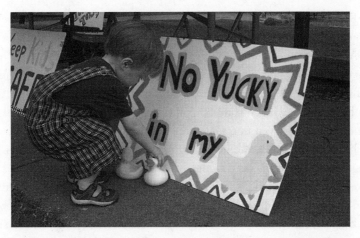

One hundred smiling rubber ducks and toddlers put pressure on Congress to ban phthalates in toys. Rally organized by Ann Arbor Ecology Center, Clean Water Action and the Breast Cancer Fund in Ann Arbor, Michigan, June 2008.

Janet Nudelman is the director of programme and policy for the San Francisco–based Breast Cancer Prevention Partners (BCPP). She and her organization focus on identifying and eliminating environmental links to the disease. "Only one in ten breast cancers can be explained by a genetic history for the disease," she explained. "A growing body of scientific evidence is linking environmental toxins to increasing rates of breast cancer and other diseases."

BCPP is particularly concerned about phthalates because recent studies have found elevated phthalate levels in girls with premature breast development.[17] "As breast cancer advocates," explained Nudelman, "the reason we care about this phenomenon is that the earlier girls experience puberty, the earlier their bodies start to be exposed to estrogen. A women's risk of breast cancer is directly linked to her lifetime exposure to natural and artificial estrogens." With this concern in mind, Janet and her colleagues girded for a fight.

The first round of the state-level phthalates debate ended badly. In January 2006 an attempt to institute a European-style ban on phthalates and bisphenol A failed in the California state legislature. Now stymied at two levels of government, advocates like Nudelman decided to take the fight to the only, if unlikely, level left: municipal government.

Despite vehement industry opposition, in June 2006 San Francisco's board of supervisors voted unanimously for a ban on phthalates and BPA in certain products. Quickly thereafter, a statewide bill flew through the legislature and landed on the desk of Governor Arnold Schwarzenegger. In October 2007 the continent's first bill restricting phthalates passed into state law. Within a few months, a dozen other states had introduced phthalate bans.

It fell to another Republican, George W. Bush, to ink a federal deal. In August 2008 the president signed one of the most significant pieces of consumer protection legislation in a generation. It permanently prohibited the sale of children's toys or childcare articles that contained more than 0.1 percent DEHP, DBP or BBP. The legislation took a precautionary approach to the other three phthalates—DINP, DIDP and DNOP—and imposed an interim ban while the science was studied further.

Nearly a decade after toxic kids' toys were banned in Europe, this "better safe than sorry" approach had finally come to America.

Of course, the phthalates story isn't over yet. This noxious class of chemicals still resides in many household items, especially in the bathroom (see chapter 1!). Even now, in 2019, despite the U.S. ban on toxic toys, some jurisdictions like Canada have yet to catch up. But thanks to the efforts of some great advocates and a few determined legislators, there's some good news and some progress to celebrate. Similar efforts have brought improvements in levels of chemicals as diverse as lead, DDT and dioxins.[18]

It's pretty simple, really. When certain phthalates, such as diethylhexyl phthalate (DEHP), were banned in kids' toys and other plastic products, their levels started to come down in the bodies of Americans and Europeans. By a lot—up to 50 percent in some cases.[19] When governments get their act together and ban or restrict a substance, dramatic improvements can happen. The graph in figure 1 tells the happy tale.

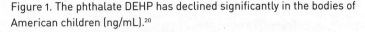

Figure 1. The phthalate DEHP has declined significantly in the bodies of American children (ng/mL).[20]

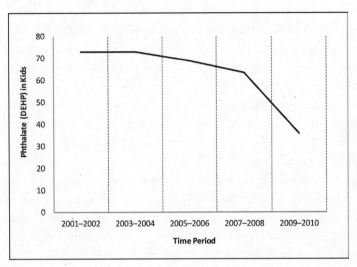

The consumer and regulatory trends we've just described illustrate one theme related to the toxic chemical issue that will recur throughout this book: *Only when people exercise their power as both citizens and consumers will there be solutions to the problems caused by damaging chemicals in the environment.* As citizens we must demand that our governments respect the health and future of all by properly restricting and managing unsafe chemicals. As consumers we need to protect ourselves and our families by making informed choices, given the lack of corporate concern for our health. It is through firing on both these cylinders that a greener future will be brought about.

Our Rubber Duck Experiments

When we set out in early 2008 to write *Slow Death*, we were full of questions. By that time, a huge number of studies had confirmed that we always carry some level of toxic chemicals in our bodies, but there was plenty we still didn't know. Where exactly do the toxins come from? What products and brands are responsible? Can they be avoided? And will changes in consumers' behaviour result in appreciable improvements in our personal pollution levels?

As we grappled with these questions an idea started forming. "Why don't we experiment on ourselves?"

What began as a joke, an offhand thought, quickly became a ten-year megaproject. What better way to demonstrate, in concrete terms, the pollution load our bodies carry than to deliberately ingest and absorb a whole bunch of these suspect substances and see whether they did, in fact, linger in our systems?

We set only one ironclad rule: our efforts had to mimic real life. We couldn't chug a bottle of mercury. We couldn't douse ourselves in Teflon. Whatever activities we undertook had to be normal things that people do every day.

In the experiments described in *Slow Death*, we explored seven chemicals that, with the exception of mercury, present a greater threat to us now than ever before. Their production is increasing. And the number of products in which they're used has exploded. At the same time the levels of these chemicals in human bodies are rising.

The goal of our experiments was to find the link between ordinary activities and a measurable increase in levels of pollution in our bodies. We (Rick and Bruce) spent one week exposing ourselves to a variety of pollutants. But while we were deliberately and voluntarily exposing ourselves to these substances, hundreds of millions of people around the world were unknowingly and involuntarily exposing themselves to the same chemicals.

In order to make changes in our toxin levels more easily detectable, we strictly limited our exposure to the pollutants in the days or weeks before the tests. Bruce avoided eating fish for a full month before the mercury test, and Rick tried to steer clear of phthalates, BPA and triclosan for forty-eight hours prior to testing for those chemicals. We measured any increases or decreases by methodically taking blood and urine samples before and after our planned exposures.

It seemed easiest to do our testing together. The bulk of our experiments took place in a rented condo over two days. We stayed in our "test room" in twelve-hour shifts, which created a pattern not unlike our regular routines. At about 3 by 3.5 metres, the room was much like any bedroom, TV room or home office in any apartment across North America. There we exposed ourselves to chemicals such as the phthalates and triclosan contained in personal-care products, the BPA that leached from baby bottles and tin cans, the mercury in tuna, and off-gassing from carpets.

Rick showered and washed dishes, drank coffee from a polycarbonate cup and ate lunch heated in a container in the microwave. Bruce ate tuna and then a little more tuna, and we had the test-room carpet treated with Stainmaster, a trademarked protective coating. There was little more to it.[21]

By the end of the week, we were freed from the confines of our little test room. Our blood and urine samples were sent to Sidney, British Columbia, to be analyzed at SGS AXYS Analytical, a laboratory that does work for governments and police forces across the continent.

Then, with our polluted bodies, we returned to our usual lives to await the results.

You can see the results of these experiments, and the conclusions we drew from them, in chapters 1 to 7 of this book.

Toxin Toxout

We followed up the experiments in *Slow Death* with some more involved, longer manipulations in our second book, *Toxin Toxout*, in which we focused on one question: Can we do anything to reduce pollutants in our bodies, and in our kids' bodies, in the short term? Answer: Yes. Lots.

We learned, again through self-experimentation and interviews with experts, that the toxins we were investigating can enter our bodies through skin absorption, eating, breathing and drinking—and we also learned a lot about how to keep them out. With the help of some friends in the beauty industry, we compared the levels of paraben and phthalate in women's bodies when green rather than conventional cosmetic products are used. Then we moved on to some groundbreaking experiments with kids to find out how organic versus conventional diets can affect their bodies' pesticide levels.

We explored the multibillion-dollar detox industry through the stories of several fascinating individuals who have devoted years of their lives to the complex, expensive and sometimes painful journey of personal detoxification. Then we took a deep dive into learning how the human body naturally removes toxic chemicals and looking at ways we can enhance those natural detox mechanisms. Getting up close and personal, we set out to try some of the better-known detox treatments to see if they actually work. Bruce travelled to California for an electromagnetic-free sleep and to Texas for an intravenous detox experience called chelation therapy. And after spending hours in an infrared sauna back in Canada collecting sweat, we discovered that detox treatments aren't necessarily for the faint of heart. Do these alternative therapies work? That was the big question, and we found the answers the hard way. Our next experiment took us to Michigan, where Rick spent an entire day in a parked SUV to check out the effects of "new car smell."

With our experiments and personal detox results in hand, we stepped back to take a look at the bigger picture, with an investigation of the burgeoning field of "green chemistry." The journey began with Bruce climbing North America's biggest toxic trash pile to see where broken toys end up and to discover ways to avoid the creation of toxic waste in the first place. We also looked at some fascinating toxin-free emerging technologies and plumbed the depths of the challenges faced by those who are trying to create a greener, less toxic world.

We detail the results of all these experiments and investigations in chapters 8 to 12 of this book.

So there you go. We've learned a lot after a decade of being human guinea pigs. The final chapter of this volume summarizes this learning within a new framework for understanding how to detox our bodies, our lives and the economy. Combining new research results with our detailed investigation of personal detox strategies and our under-standing of the potential new green economy, we created the "Slow Death by Rubber Duck Top Ten" list.

BPA Redux

In 2009, the burgeoning awareness about toxic chemicals centred on BPA in baby bottles: a fight that was actually won (check it out in chapter 7, "Mothers Know Best").

So before we jump into the chapters we've just described, let's bring the BPA story up to date, because it epitomizes much that has gone right—and wrong—with the toxic chemical debate.

First, the bad news . . .

Mary Shaw's members are exposed to more BPA every day than possibly any other humans on Earth.

Mary is a health and safety representative for the United Food and Commercial Workers (UFCW) union, one of the largest private-sector unions in the United States and Canada. She represents seventy thousand people in Ontario, and a great many of her members work in retail, including grocery stores and the hospitality industry.

In 2017, Mary was contacted by one of her members who worked part-time at a grocery store and was also a student. He was concerned about some research he'd read concerning the exposure of cashiers to BPA and a related substance, BPS (bisphenol S), through an unlikely source: the coatings on cash register receipts. Receipts are something that UFCW members handle in vast quantities every day.

"This was new information for me and the union," Mary told us on the phone from her office in Cambridge, Ontario. "It turns out that the now standard cash register receipts are coated on one side with a good quantity of BPA." When the paper runs through the register, a heat-transfer process creates the numbers on the receipt and allows for inkless printing. Prompted by her member's concern, Mary started looking at some of the recent studies showing that this BPA can come off on people's hands and be absorbed through the skin.

Mary realized the deeply worrisome nature of the situation. "As I read, I became more and more alarmed regarding worker and consumer exposure," she said. In one study that Mary came across, BPA levels in the bodies of cashiers were found to be significantly higher than in the general population because of their constant handling of BPA-coated receipts.[22]

She quickly understood that the BPA might be carried around on the hands throughout the day. "Anytime we handle thermal receipt paper, the powder comes off on your hand and you transfer that powder to your food and then you ingest it. This should be a huge concern for restaurants," she said.[23] Though some of the stores where her members work claimed to use "BPA-free" receipts, her research made clear that the main alternative to BPA is the closely related chemical BPS, and "the damaging properties of BPS are very similar to BPA."[24]

Mary started doing some calculations. "In one mid-sized grocery store in my area, they had 13,400 customers in one week. Of those, 7,300 customers went through the 'normal' lanes and 6,100 went through the express lanes. In the express lanes, the transactions will be very small. The average transaction is between about 45 and 50 seconds per customer and the average shift for a worker on the express lane is 4 or 5 hours in length." Mary concluded, "If my math is right, a worker on a 5-hour shift would handle 400 transactions—and therefore at least 400 receipts—in that time."

There's another wrinkle that Mary began to worry about. "Wet hands apparently dramatically increase the absorption rate of the BPA. And cashiers often have wet hands, because they're constantly either using hand sanitizer or handling produce."[25]

Mary is troubled about BPA and BPS on receipts not just for union members but also for consumers. "As a consumer, I'm asked every time I go into a store if I want a receipt. I usually say yes. There's really no option. This issue of toxic chemicals on thermal receipts is an enormous problem, not just for my members but for everybody. Every day. This thermal paper is being used not just for cash register receipts but for an increasing number of other things like movie tickets, transit tickets and parking tickets. It's everywhere."

Dr. Fred vom Saal is probably the first person we spoke to about the science of BPA over a decade ago. Fred is a professor at the University of Missouri and was the pioneering researcher in the 1990s who first started ringing the alarm bell about BPA's damaging effects on human health. After twenty years of studying the chemical and over seventy research papers, he's more apprehensive about BPA than ever. And he agrees with Mary Shaw that cash register receipts are one of our most significant everyday sources of BPA exposure.

"The link between BPA exposure and human disease is much stronger now than it was ten years ago, when *Slow Death* was first published. Literally every week now another new study on BPA crosses my desk," he told us from his lab in St. Louis (our phone call actually interrupted the writing of his latest BPA paper). "We now have solid evidence for BPA exposure driving things like obesity, diabetes, heart disease and neurobehavioural problems," he said. "In one recent study, we have evidence of BPA in people causing the deaths of fetuses during in vitro fertilization. The higher a woman's level of BPA during the in vitro fertilization, the lower the probability of her producing a live baby. BPA exposure results in the ovary producing less estrogen."

Vom Saal is tracking not only the ongoing prevalence and effects of BPA itself, but also the growing problem of "regrettable substitutions." Incredibly, in Canada, in the U.S., and in many countries around the world, when one toxic chemical is banned or phased out, there's no legal requirement that the replacement be any better. "This is what's happened with BPA and BPS, with the phthalates DEHP and DINP and many other toxic chemicals," Vom Saal told us. (See chapter 1, "Wellness Revolution" for more on phthalates.)

Perhaps the most egregious example he pointed to was fire retardants, the "replacement of PCBs, beginning in the 1970s, with PBDEs." (See chapter 3, "The New PCBs.") "The illogical thinking at the time was that substituting a chlorine chemical (PCBs) with a bromine chemical (PBDEs) would solve the health issues. Instead, PBDEs turned out to be very problematic and tied to many human health concerns. Now PBDEs are being phased out and replaced by toxic phosphate/PBDE mixtures, such as Firemaster 550." So, as Vom Saal points out, over the past four decades we have made the same mistake twice over, with PCBs and PBDEs—in both cases replacing one poison with a different poison.

Looking for evidence that humanity's escape from BPA exposure is on the horizon, Vom Saal keeps track of one other important metric: global levels of BPA production. Here again, it's good news/bad news. A recent report said that government regulations spurred by health concerns are the "key challenge" to further expansion of the BPA market in Canada, the U.S. and Europe, but that other applications for BPA use—including in thermal paper—are growing.[26]

So let's delve into that specific BPA issue in our typical full-frontal, up-close-and-personal, *Slow Death* way.

Poisonous Paper

Ten years ago, one of our very first experiments resulted in a 7.5 times increase in BPA in Rick's body (see chapter 7, "Mothers Know Best") from eating and drinking out of BPA-treated plastic containers and baby bottles, as well as tin cans (which are still, to this day, largely lined with BPA-containing epoxy resin). After talking to Mary Shaw, it was clear to us that the obvious—and most important—source of BPA exposure today is cash register receipts, so we decided to conduct another experiment with the chemical.

We turned to our friends and colleagues at Environmental Defence Canada—the nation's premier pollution fighters—to give us a hand. The organization's smart young toxic-chemical campaigners Muhannad Malas and Sarah Jamal volunteered to join our experiment.

After examining a few recent scientific studies on BPA and BPS in cash register receipts, we concluded that a necessary first step would be to "detox" from BPA as best we could. In order to show a potential increase in BPA in our bodies, we wanted our levels of BPA to be as low as possible to begin with. To achieve this, we would have to avoid canned food and any handling of cash register receipts for at least forty-eight hours in advance of testing day—which, we all agreed, would be extremely difficult to do. For starters, all four of us travel for work and quite often collect cash register receipts in our wallets so that we can claim expenses when the trip is over. We attempted various ways of taking receipts from cashiers without touching them and without seeming crazy. We considered wearing gloves or pulling our sleeves down over our hands. Rick finally settled on carrying a little envelope that he pushed across the counter and invited the cashier to place the receipt inside.

The cash register receipts that some retailers use are coated with BPA, while many more use paper coated with BPS or yet other substances. Because of this variation we decided to collect receipts from as many different retailers as possible. Rick contributed some that he had been collecting to document his travel expenses. Sarah, Bruce and Muhannad scrupulously saved their shopping receipts from a week of personal purchases.

With preparations made, we woke on a blustery February morning and prepared to gather at Rick's house. Before leaving home, each of us collected a urine sample from our first pee of the day and brought it with us. Then we sat down at Rick's dining room table to perform possibly the least dramatic toxic experiment in our ten-year history of crazy experiments: passing a bunch of cash register receipts around the table so that the four of us continually handled them for a fifteen-minute period.

Because there is some evidence that wet fingers increase BPA/BPS absorption through the skin, Bruce ate greasy French fries and Rick used hand sanitizer prior to the experiment. When fifteen minutes had passed, we used our BPA-coated fingers to eat some cheap sushi we had bought at a store down the street.

We waited eight hours to let the BPA and BPS be absorbed by our bodies, and then each of us took a second urine sample. We shipped all the samples to SGS AXYS Analytical, the same lab that we had used ten years before for the original *Slow Death*, and awaited the results.

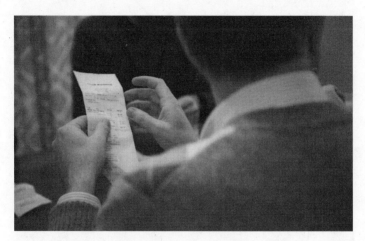

A snapshot from our BPA/BPS experiment with cash register receipts.

115 Times

The results of our experiment were stunning (see figure 2). In all cases the scale of the BPA increase surpassed the levels we were able to achieve with our baby bottle experiment in *Slow Death*. All four of us had similar levels of BPA and BPS in our bodies at the outset. All four of us after handling the receipts experienced huge increases in the levels of these chemicals in our bodies. At the high end, Rick's BPA level was 42 times higher than his starting level. Sarah's was 4 times as high. For BPS, Rick's level increased an incredible 115 times, while Sarah's was the lowest at 8 times. We think that Rick's impressive increase was due to his use of hand sanitizer before the experiment—a fact that reinforces Mary Shaw's concern for the health of her UFCW members.

Figure 2. Levels of urine BPA and BPS in Rick, Bruce, Sarah and
Muhannad after handling cash register receipts for 15 minutes (ng/mL).

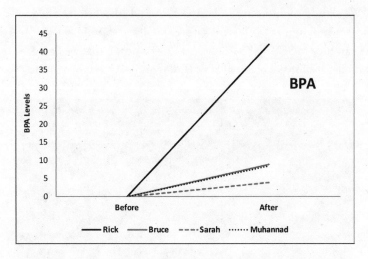

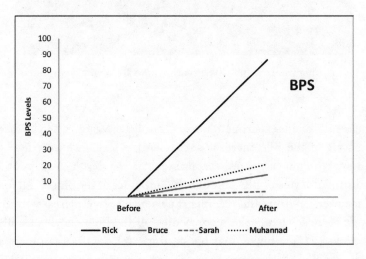

Rick caught up with Ken Cook, president and co-founder of the
Environmental Working Group, at a conference on cancer prevention
in Montreal, and showed him the stunning graphs above. Ken wasn't
surprised. EWG is the U.S. non-profit organization that first popular-
ized the notion of testing human bodies for pollution in the early
2000s. Still hard at work more than twenty-five years after EWG's

creation, Ken compared the toxic chemical issue to the legendary arcade game "Whac-A-Mole." "We were able to get BPA out of baby bottles and children's products," he recalled, and then explained the downside of that victory. "But it's now popped up in places we never could have anticipated, like cash register receipts. We were able to stigmatize BPA to a certain extent, so companies moved to what is likely another toxic chemical in BPS," Ken said.

Despite the ongoing public exposure to BPA, Ken believes that great strides have been made to keep consumers safer from toxic chemicals. "Companies have learned that once the public gets the notion that a chemical is unsafe, they have no choice—they must respond to get that chemical out. We don't have to boycott anymore. It's not 'boycotts,' it's 'buy cuts.' We know how to move consumer preferences. We can get the attention of any big company in any big market. Now it's just a matter of velocity. We need to accelerate the positive change."

As you make your personal positive changes, we hope you enjoy this updated book. It remains the definitive guide to toxic chemicals in the human body and how to get them out. We poisoned ourselves for over a decade so that you don't have to. Let the detox begin!

ONE: WELLNESS REVOLUTION

[RICK LATHERS UP]

A woman who doesn't wear perfume has no future.

—COCO CHANEL

AS THE SONG SAYS ABOUT NEW YORK CITY, if you can make it there, you'll make it anywhere. So I think it's auspicious that the Sustainable Cosmetics Summit is now an annual event in the Big Apple. After arriving at the midtown Manhattan hotel where the event was being held (in May 2012) and squeezing by Jude Law's largish camera crew (he was filming a scene in the hotel lobby), I found myself in a fluorescent-lit room with a couple of hundred people. Despite the beckoning sunshine outside, they were—as evidenced by the large coffee mugs in hand—digging in for two days of back-to-back seminars.

"Eclectic" would be an apt word to describe the crowd. Over the next few days, I met representatives of wild shea nut harvesters from sub-Saharan Africa, jojoba farmers and producers of obscure natural scents and oils. Button-down corporate types from companies like Colgate-Palmolive mingled with former (or current) patchouli-redolent hippies and über-trendy black-clad celebrity hairdressers.

What brought this diverse group together? The sweet smell, literally, of success.

Amarjit Sahota is the summit organizer and head of London-based Ecovia Intelligence, a research and consulting company specializing in the organic sector. According to Sahota, the growth of the natural and organic personal-care market is outpacing all other segments of the cosmetics industry. And we're talking here about an industry that's way more than makeup. From shampoo to shaving cream, from fragrance to facial cleanser, these people are responsible for pretty much every skin, hair and body product in your bathroom. Though still comprising less than 10 percent of industry sales in Europe and North America, natural and organic cosmetics were nonetheless worth US$9.1 billion in 2011. As of 2018, the U.S. market alone was estimated at over $13.2 billion and expected to continue to grow at roughly 7 percent a year.[1] I asked Sahota what was behind this phenomenon.

"It's really a manifestation of a broader trend," he told me. "What we are seeing globally is a general rise in ethical consumerism. People have become more discerning about the products that they buy. They're asking more questions: Where is it made? Does it have synthetic chemicals? Is it being produced in an ecological way? This is happening with food, cosmetics, household cleaning products, clothing, toys—and the list goes on."

Linda Gilbert, a Florida-based pollster who since 1990 has been tracking public attitudes related to sustainability and who presented her findings to the summit, agreed with Sahota. "The consumer interest in sustainability, and in particular limiting their exposure to pollution and toxic chemicals in their everyday lives, is a tidal wave. It's transformational," she told me. "It is impacting virtually every industry that you look at. The home-building industry, with the drive to low-VOC building materials. The food industry, with increased scrutiny of packaging. The transportation industry. The garden product industry. Consumers are becoming more and more aware of ways they can avoid chemicals in their lifestyles."

Her blunt conclusion? "If companies don't retool and reinvent themselves, they're not going to be in business." Gilbert used the example of bisphenol A in baby bottles to illustrate her point. Over the past decade, the growing consumer backlash against the hormone-disrupting chemical has ensured that non-BPA bottles came to dominate the market.

Gilbert calls this consumer awakening a *wellness revolution*. "Consumers in the United States have this growing sense that there's a personal environment that they can and should control," she explained. "They can't control the global environment, but they can control what goes in their home, what goes on their lawn, what they're breathing in because of fragrances and body lotion." She maintains that for health reasons, and often with no particular reference to environmental concerns, consumers are looking to reduce exposure to synthetic chemicals in their daily life. Though Gilbert admits that about 15 percent of the population (what she calls the "Drill, baby, drill" demographic) will never be interested in these issues, her findings indicate that among the other 85 percent the appetite for sustainable cosmetics is growing: "They are ready to make changes for a more eco-friendly lifestyle, and—significantly—willing to change brands to accomplish this."[2]

One of the great advances since *Slow Death* is that mobile "apps" abound, making it easier for wellness-savvy consumers to choose cleaner personal-care products. Take the Canadian start-up PurPicks, for example, which now has thousands of monthly users gaining access to over 1,500 clean, non-toxic products from over 250 artisanal skincare brands. They claim to be not only the world's largest directory of certified organic/nontoxic beauty and personal-care products but also the platform with the most user-generated healthy product reviews. Every product is independently certified to the highest standards and then reviewed by cosmetics users who can tell you whether that super-clean mascara is going to run or not. It is the veritable TripAdvisor of cosmetics.

In the Beginning . . .

If there's one company in the beauty industry that made natural ingredients the very core of its brand, it's Aveda (its slogan is "The Art and Science of Pure Flower and Plant Essences"). Founded by the late Austrian celebrity hairdresser Horst Rechelbacher in 1978, Aveda was subsequently sold to Estée Lauder in 1997 and has since grown into a global presence. Like the computer and electronics manufacturer Apple, which has tried to define itself with a certain green grooviness, Aveda took some flak for not paying adequate attention to its environmental standards. But it made up for lost time, now banning phthalates, parabens, sodium lauryl sulphate (SLS) and a variety of other nasties from its formulations. (See table 1 for a short primer on these and some other common chemicals found in cosmetics.) Aveda also boasts that it is the first beauty company to run its manufacturing on 100 percent wind power, and it uses all post-consumer materials in its packaging.

Table 1. A few problem chemicals.

The Chemical	What It "Does"	The Problem
Triclosan	Synthetic antibacterial agent used as a preservative in things like shaving creams, hair conditioners, deodorants, liquid soaps, hand soaps, facial cleansers and disinfectants. Also used in some products that don't make antibacterial claims.	Animal research studies have shown triclosan to be an endocrine disruptor at low levels of exposure. There's been some progress, with the U.S. FDA announcing in September 2016 a ban on the sale of "consumer antiseptic washes" containing triclosan and 18 other antimicrobials.[3]
DEP (diethyl phthalate) and DnBP (di-n-butyl phthalate)	DEP and DnBP are the most common phthalates in personal-care products—used for their ability to hold colour, denature alcohol, act as a lubricant and fix fragrance. Found in heavily fragranced products like shampoos, lotions and perfumes.	Known endocrine disruptors. Adverse health effects from exposure include asthma and increased allergenicity, reproductive and metabolic disorders, and developmental and behavioural problems.
Methyl paraben	Most commonly used preservative in cosmetics and personal-care products. Methyl paraben is most often found in deodorants, shampoos, lotions and creams.	Found to mimic estrogen, which can lead to increased risk of breast cancer and affect male reproductive functions. The FDA continues to permit use of methyl paraben in makeup, moisturizers and other self-care products.[4]
SLS (sodium lauryl sulphate)	Petroleum-based chemical added to personal-care products as surfactants and foaming agents. Commonly found in shampoos, shower gels, cleansers and toothpaste.	Links to skin and eye irritation, organ toxicity, developmental and reproductive toxicity, and endocrine disruption. The manufacturing process contaminates SLS with 1,4-dioxane, a probable human carcinogen. Both Health Canada and the FDA permit sale of SLS as a repellent and pesticide.[5]

In Canada, Ray Civello has long been Mr. Aveda. He was the first to bring the line to Canada (starting by offering it in his salon over a muffin shop in Toronto's east end), and he still has exclusive rights. In the mid-1980s, Aveda's burgeoning delivery system was a bit quirky; the product would regularly arrive frozen from its Minnesota distribution centre. Civello persevered, building double-digit sales growth, year over year, for more than two decades. A thoughtful environmentalist, opinionated about toxic chemicals and the need for more natural products, Civello has long put his money where his mouth is by supporting various charities such as Environmental Defence Canada. Civello told me that his connection to Aveda and its social mission arose out of a difficult period in his life.

"I contracted mono, lost a lot of weight and was burned out on the whole rock 'n' roll hairdresser lifestyle," he said. "It was because I got sick that I started reading about sustainability and wellness." The beauty industry wasn't much concerned with sustainability and wellness at the time, but he saw that begin to change. "Consumers are concerned. Yes, people want to look younger, but there's a line in the sand now between doing it naturally and getting it immediately." Rather than getting a quick fix like cosmetic surgery, more people are now asking questions like "Can I do this in a more gentle way? Can I be more preventative?" Civello sees this new attitude in Aveda salons every day.

Aveda's growth has been directly related to its ability to tap into the sustainability impulses of its customers. In fact, if ever there was a godfather of greenness in the cosmetics world, it was surely the stylishly goateed founder of the company, Horst Rechelbacher. If you research Rechelbacher, you'll find quite a few images that show him drinking and eating Aveda products: nothing like chugging your hairspray and noshing on your lipstick to make a point.

I was lucky to spend some time with Rechelbacher the evening before his keynote speech to the Sustainable Cosmetics Summit in New York City, a couple of years before he passed away in 2014. His full-floor Lower Fifth Avenue penthouse (part of which used to be owned by the photographer Robert Mapplethorpe) boasted a distracting, nearly 360-degree view of the city. That night it felt a bit more crowded than it might otherwise be: products from Rechelbacher's new company, Intelligent Nutrients (IN), were piled up in the living room, ready for a launch the next day. "One of the first full lines to be certified USDA Organic," he proudly told me. (Any product with this label meets the strict organic certification requirements for food set down by the U.S. Department of Agriculture.) "Cosmetics are food," Rechelbacher continued. "What we put on our body ends up in our body." After selling Aveda to Estée Lauder for a tidy sum (US$300 million), the organic cosmetics giant decided he wanted to start again.

"Activism to me is show and tell, rather than just tell," he declared, "because if you don't do it yourself, people will ask why." Rechelbacher designed IN to be a showcase of what is possible. "The Holy Grail in cosmetics is supposed to be organic, but this is only as good as the person who makes it," he said. "Even if you give a chef organic ingredients, she can still make shitty food.

"You know when people say they put lead in lipstick?" Rechelbacher added, leaning forward for emphasis. "They don't put lead in lipstick; chemists are not *that* insane. But lead shows up during chemical processing of heavy metals. It also shows up in processing carbon, which is coal. Hair dyes are based on carbon technology. You need primary colours to do all colours. So blue comes from cobalt, yellow comes from sulphite. Those are the primary colours that are used in all colourings—from cosmetics to cars. I said to myself, 'This is toxic. Why do we use this shit? What are the alternatives?'" He jabbed the air with his finger. "Food! You know there's blue corn, there's cranberries, and the list goes on. I'm the first to make a food supplement that's a lipstick, a lip colour. There are no toxins, just nutritional benefits."

The average woman allegedly eats about four pounds of lipstick during her lifetime. If she were using IN's lip products, it would probably do her body good, given the nourishing ingredients detailed in the company's promotional materials: nutrient-dense oils of açai, rosehip and black cumin and soothing, antioxidant-rich waxes and butters. Rechelbacher took more than an hour for what was scheduled to be a ten-minute keynote speech at the summit the next morning, and nobody seemed to mind. As he exhorted those assembled in the room to be "bold" and urged them to connect with their raw ingredients because "restoration starts from the ground up—with seeds," I couldn't help thinking how far cosmetics had come. What could be more refined, more urban and more . . . well . . . *antiseptic* than the beauty industry? And yet there they were, a couple of hundred industry leaders nodding along as Rechelbacher urged them to get mud on their boots and dirt under their fingernails.

Coco Chanel, that diva of haute couture, must have been turning in her grave.

Leaving the VW Vans Behind

Cosmetics companies love their creation myths. Though the industry has become huge, with recent estimates of global annual sales in excess of US$250 billion,[6] many of makeup's most recognized brands are rooted in the humble beginnings of their charismatic founders.

Of the major cosmetics firms, the largest is L'Oréal, which was started by Eugène Schueller in 1909 when he started mixing his own "safe hair dyes" and flogging them directly to Parisian hairdressers. The industry was developed in the United States shortly thereafter by hard-driving individuals whose names became synonymous with their products: Elizabeth Arden, Helena Rubinstein and Max Factor. Revlon was launched in 1932, when Charles Revson, his brother and a chemist named Charles Lachman pooled their meagre resources to create a new manufacturing process for nail enamel. Of its creator, the Estée Lauder company says that "Estée Lauder founded this company in 1946 armed with four products and an unshakeable belief: that every woman can be beautiful."[7] And famously, Coco Chanel overcame a brutally impoverished childhood and parlayed an early interest in hat design into one of the most enduring fashion houses and perfume brands in the world.

The same kind of entrepreneurial moxie was alive and well at the summit in New York City, with many representatives of the sustainable cosmetics companies I met feeling the wind at their backs and looking forward to taking on the industry's big players. Typical of this granola-to-riches tale is Tampa-based Aubrey Organics.

Curt Valva, Aubrey Organics' CEO in 2012, confirmed with a laugh that his company's founders "were a bunch of hippies selling products out of the back of their cars." He proudly rhymed off a few of the firm's long series of firsts in the cosmetics industry: first to list all of its ingredients (1967); first to formulate products with jojoba oil (1970); first to be certified as an organic processor (1984). The world is changing, Valva says. "Sustainable cosmetics are going mainstream, and that's one of the biggest challenges for us as a company." And he's not alone in trying to reconcile company growth with an ongoing commitment to making the world a better place.

Live (Toxin-) Free or Die

From his office in the woods of New Hampshire, Bill Whyte, the founder of W. S. Badger Company, told me the story of how his business went from obscurity to having the top-selling natural sunscreen in the United States and Canada. After getting out of the army and kicking around for a bit, Whyte finally settled down and started a family in the Granite State. He built his own house, gardened organically and was happily working as a carpenter.

"And then one winter," Whyte said, in what I got the feeling was an oft-recounted tale, "I had really cracked fingers from working outside. It was *awful*. They would split and bleed, so I needed to do something. I was lying in bed one night with my hands in olive-oil-soaked socks covered in plastic bags. And Katie [Whyte's wife] turned to me and said, 'You know, that's really pathetic. You can do better than that.'" The next morning, Bill went to the kitchen and started concocting various mixtures. He made a balm out of beeswax, olive oil and other ingredients, and it healed his fingers nicely. "So a light bulb went on in my head," he said. "I can sell this to carpenters and other people who work with their hands." And thus was birthed Badger, with the sum total of the company being Whyte filling tins late into the night, listening to rock 'n' roll, and delivering on weekends.

For a while after the launch of his Badger Balm, Whyte told me, he resisted the siren call of product diversification. But opportunity presented itself. "At the time, there weren't any mineral sunscreens," he told me. "Even the natural sunscreens were using chemicals as the active ingredient." Always up for a challenge, and experimenting with mixtures in his kitchen, Whyte wondered whether he could make a sunscreen that would be healthful. While researching, he learned that non-toxic zinc oxide was used for the old lifeguard sunscreens.

Whyte's timing was perfect. Little did he know that the Environmental Working Group (EWG), well known for evaluating toxic chemical levels in consumer products and in the bodies of Americans, was about to launch its first-ever "report card" on sunscreens, ranking them for effectiveness and safety.

Of all the consumer products that EWG could have focused on, there was a reason they put sunscreen in their crosshairs, according to Ken Cook, EWG's perennially energetic president. "The federal government had not done anything to require significant efficacy or safety testing or anything for sunscreens. They had some guidelines that had been pending for, like, thirty years. It was ridiculous," Cook grumbled in an interview on this issue in 2012. "We're not talking about mascara here or shampoo—something that's designed to make you look nice or make you clean; we're talking about [products that can prevent] skin cancers. And . . . companies were producing products that didn't work and advertising them falsely as staying on all day and being waterproof. Then on top of all that, you get to the chemical issues." As a result of their years of research, Cook and EWG had developed significant concerns about the chemicals in sunscreens leading to allergic reactions and immune system issues and—ironically—posing an increased risk of cancer. Fed up with government inertia, they decided to publish their own ranking of sunscreens according to rigorous safety criteria.

The public and media attention was huge. And Badger was ranked at the top of the list of safe sunscreens.

When the EWG analysis was featured on *Good Morning America*, Badger's sales exploded overnight. The company's inventory, which Whyte figured would last for a year, was gone in less than a week. And sales have been going through the roof ever since.

I've noticed over the years that the sunscreens used by parents and kids at the daycares and summer camps where I drop my kids have changed a lot over the decade. As a measure of the growing popularity of mineral sunscreens, tubes of Badger and other great brands like Canada's own Green Beaver and Attitude now have pride of place alongside smelly coconut-scented conventional products. And they're gradually taking over.

Though I'll grant you that it's not the most scientific measurement in the world, mineral sunscreens are on a roll.

Label Decoding

As I learned at the summit, some of the largest companies offering green beauty products are based in Europe. "Our company has been walking the walk since the 1920s," said the baby-faced Jasper van

Brakel, at the time the North American CEO of Swiss-based Weleda. "Using biodynamic ingredients, using organic ingredients. Never using chemicals. We manufacture holistic medicines as well as skin-care, body-care and baby-care products. The world has caught up to what this company is doing."

Now with roughly US$496 million in global sales, Weleda was founded nearly one hundred years ago as a herbal medicine laboratory by that most prototypical of hipsters, Rudolf Steiner.[8] Around this same time, the Austrian philosopher and social reformer was pioneering his Waldorf education system and a new spiritual movement known as "anthroposophy": an attempt to meld science and mysticism. Van Brakel told me that Weleda is still privately held by two foundations that exist to further Steiner's worldview. "They've owned the company forever; they're never going to sell it. And they allow us to continue to work out of a principle, rather than out of the primary objective to make money."

I asked him if he felt territorial, heading the North American operations of a company that, it could be argued, invented the whole concept of plant-based personal-care products but now had to watch some of the larger industry players crowding into the same space. "It's a huge issue for us," he replied. "There are many companies out there, some of them marketing themselves as organic and natural, that have ingredients in their products that are not great at all. . . . There are many different shades of green." Increasingly, Weleda is advising large retailers that carry its products to set up a special natural and organic section for products "that meet a certain standard."

What that standard is and how to encapsulate it in a digestible way for consumers is, van Brakel admitted, the $64,000 question.

Some things are easy to label. "Sugar-free" is pretty self-explanatory. As are the "peanut-free" or "gluten-free" tags sought by allergy sufferers. What do you do, however, when you have a beauty product and you want to advertise it as more natural or organic? How do you distinguish its complicated, unpronounceable ingredients as being healthier and safer than the equally Byzantine ingredient lists on conventional beauty products? Not an easy task, especially considering the illogical and highly variable laws that exist in different countries. As just one example, some jurisdictions do not require chemicals like phthalates to be disclosed on ingredient lists, while others, like parabens or sul-phates, must be shown.

Amarjit Sahota identified this kind of perplexity in his market-update report at the summit in New York. "There's no question that consumer confusion is the biggest challenge," he said, and went on to point out that the rise of what he called "pseudonaturals" (products whose claims of "greenness" or "naturalness" are dubious at best) was contributing to the problem. Ironically, the attempted fix for this phe-nomenon—the creation of labelling schemes to validate the benefits of truly green products—was now itself adding to the murk in the minds of consumers.

"Let me give you an example from the U.K.," Sahota explained. "Let's say you're in an organic shop and you're looking at personal-care products. You've got some products labelled 'organic' from the U.K., but then there are also a couple of different products from France. They've got two labels: one for 'organic' and one for 'natural.' Another brand from Germany has similar products, but they have different logos, and then you have two from the U.S. with two different logos again. So in this shop there are perhaps twenty brands with upwards of eight different 'organic' and 'natural' labels." The obvious effect, Sahota pointed out, is the creation of profound confusion.

Slowly, though, the outline of a more comprehensive labelling system has begun to emerge. In Europe as of 2017, rigorous green stan-dards for cosmetics are now harmonized and certified by the new COSMOS system (created as an international nonprofit association in 2010).[9] The U.S. Department of Agriculture now certifies body-care products made from agricultural ingredients so long as they fall within the standards of the American National Organic Program.[10] And the Environmental Working Group has started working directly with man-ufacturers to popularize a new "EWG Verified" family of personal-care and consumer products that are "free from EWG's chemicals of con-cern" and meet "our strictest standards for your health."

Brazilian Blowout Blow-Up

Yes, labels are good. They help consumers make more informed choices. But what happens when companies are prepared to, shall we say, economize on the truth?

In 2011, a small advocacy group based in Oakland, California, called the Center for Environmental Health (CEH) became suspicious that many manufacturers were being less than honest regarding the levels of organic ingredients in their products. California law is very clear on this score: in order to use the word "organic," you need to ensure that your product contains at least 70 percent organic ingredients. The CEH launched a time-consuming but simple exercise: it collected dozens of allegedly "organic" products—shampoos and conditioners, lotions, deodorants, toothpastes, you name it—and examined the detailed ingredient lists on the labels. Many of the lists showed few or no organic ingredients. And since ingredients are listed in order of predominance, from major to minor, the CEH calculated that each of the products contained far less than 70 percent organics. Frustrated with what they considered a clear flouting of the law, the CEH sued. The goal was to bring the companies into compliance with California law—either by compelling them to remove their improper organic claims or by ensuring that they increased the proportion of organic ingredients in their products.

"We want to encourage organics, plain and simple," said Michael Green, CEO of CEH. "You can't successfully encourage organics if people don't believe that things are what they say they are on the label. Because who is going to go out of their way to buy this stuff unless there's some truth in advertising?" The lawsuit had a quick effect, Green said proudly. "The vast majority of the companies have changed what they were doing. Most of them took the word 'organic' off the label of the products that we challenged them on, and some of them then created another line of products that they *could* put that label on." For now, CEH's lawsuit has helped reinforce the fact that the word "organic" has value and a legal meaning and can't simply be used to hoodwink consumers. Unfortunately, another recent, high-profile example of labelling gone amok hasn't ended on nearly as positive a note.

In September 2010, Jennifer Arce, an experienced hairdresser based near San Diego, decided to try a new hair-straightening product manufactured by GIB LLC, commonly known as Brazilian Blowout. "I specifically chose Brazilian Blowout because it was advertised as the only hair-straightening treatment that improved the health of the hair, caused no damage, had no harsh chemicals and, most importantly, was formaldehyde free." To get the hang of the product so that she could eventually use it on her clients, Arce arranged for her sister, also a co-worker, to do a Brazilian Blowout on her.

Arce remembers the exact day, the exact moment, because her life hasn't been the same since.

"Within minutes of her applying it to my hair, my eyes were burning, my throat was burning, my lungs were burning, and I was having a hard time breathing. My symptoms were escalating, and my sister was having all the same issues." Arce told me that even when the two women moved outside to complete the procedure in the fresh air, they continued to feel sick. That night when she went home, she was lethargic and could barely swallow, and she developed a terrible migraine. Her puzzled doctor attributed her ongoing problems to possible chemical poisoning. "In the days following the treatment, I was having a hard time doing little, simple, everyday tasks," she said. "I couldn't turn on a stove or an oven because the gas fumes coming out would make me sick. I couldn't use any cleaning products. I couldn't pump gas. I couldn't use hairspray on myself or on my clients—just being at work around all these chemicals was a struggle."

The penny finally dropped for Arce when she realized that some of her co-workers were getting sick too. "Many of them had been on and off antibiotics for months after exposure to the Brazilian Blowout chemicals, and we all had the same symptoms." She and her sister started researching and discovered that an increasing number of people were recording similar complaints online. Moved to action, the U.S. Occupational Safety and Health Administration (OSHA) began testing the product—including in Arce's salon—and discovered that, far from being formaldehyde-free, Brazilian Blowout contained up to 10 percent of this volatile cancer-causing agent.[11]

With GIB, the maker of the products, protesting all the while that they were safe, the State of California sued. Arce was one of the hairdressers involved in the action. While the public debate raged and the lawyers were on the case, she was back at work trying to make a living, having been forced to move salons when her previous boss refused to ban Brazilian Blowout in the shop. The allure of the product was too much. "Oh, yeah," Arce said when I asked if the thing worked. "My hair never looked so good after using it. It was beautiful, shiny—you barely had to dry it. Some of the clients who do know it contains the chemical don't care, because it's making their hair so beautiful. And some of them will say, 'Beauty costs!'"

After appearing on the *Today* show and other media, telling the story of her harrowing experience, Arce now gets letters from hairdressers across the country with similar heartbreaking tales. One of the things they commiserate about is the incredible ending to the story. GIB LLC was forced to pay a settlement of $600,000 to the State of California and "cease deceptive advertising that describes two of its popular products as formaldehyde-free and safe."[12] While GIB is now obliged to identify formaldehyde in its labelling and instructions, the U.S. government lacks the power to force a product off the shelf if an obstreperous company is unwilling to do so voluntarily. Though it's now banned in some countries,[13] in the U.S. Brazilian Blowout has prevailed over its detractors and is still being used today in salons from coast to coast.

If you wanted a stark example of the abject failure of the U.S. regulatory system to ensure the safety of personal-care products, Brazilian Blowout would surely be it. But the Brazilian Blowout case is not an isolated one, and this is perhaps not surprising, since the U.S. law allegedly protecting Americans from being poisoned by their bathroom products dates back to 1938—well before the creation of many modern synthetic chemicals.

When I caught up with Lisa Archer, co-founder of the Campaign for Safe Cosmetics, I asked her how bad the current situation actually was. Fifteen minutes later, she'd rattled off a list of worrisome stories and statistics as long as my arm. "There are carcinogens in baby shampoo as well as phthalates and other problematic chemicals. Another example is mercury in skin-lightening creams, and there have actually been some cases of mercury poisoning from the use of these products."

In addition to lacking the legal authority to require recalls of damaging products, current U.S. (and Canadian) law allows companies to put dozens of secret ingredients in their products without disclosing them on the label. In a recent Canadian study, Environmental Defence tested personal-care products and discovered, on average, fourteen secret ingredients per product that were—quite legally—not disclosed on the ingredient lists.[14] Archer points out the other reason that cosmetics safety is a concern in the U.S.: "In a nutshell, FDA [the U.S. Food and Drug Administration] is pathetically understaffed and underfunded. We're talking about a budget of about $10–12 million per year and roughly ten full-time staff to govern a $60 billion cosmetics industry. There's no way, given their current capacity and their current powers, that they could actually protect the public and ensure that cosmetics are safe." Though there have been some victories at the state level (such as the California *Safe Cosmetics Act* that led to the prosecution of Brazilian Blowout), in the estimation of Ken Cook from the EWG, prospects of significant further statutory gains in the United States are "very grim, unfortunately."

Despite this, Archer and Cook were surprisingly upbeat regarding the pace of change in the United States. "There's a sort of a 'girlcott' going on, versus boycott," she told me. "Instead of *opposing* certain products, women are *supporting* companies who are more honest and transparent and using safer ingredients. And it's not just with cosmetics—you see it with BPA in baby bottles, you see organic food becoming more main-stream and things like that. And that's what I think is exciting. Even if the policy change is going to take a long time to happen, people are waking up to this issue. That market shift is going to continue to happen, driven by those conscious moms, in particular, who are changing their habits."[15]

Of Mennonites and Nail Salon Workers

It's an indicator of how far these initiatives have come that phthalates, surely the most unpronounceable word ever, became such a poster child for consumer concern. Though there are many toxic chemicals that informed consumers are now on the lookout for on the labels of their beauty products—including sodium lauryl sulphate, siloxanes and quaternium-15—phthalates are top of the list.

If you want to talk phthalates, the go-to expert is, without a doubt, Dr. Shanna Swan from Mount Sinai School of Medicine in New York City. As we sat amongst the dog-walkers and pigeons on a sunny day in Madison Square Park, the first question I asked was how the scientific literature had developed on phthalates over the past few years. What had we learned?

"You know, it really depends on which phthalate you're talking about," she said. "Phthalates are a family of chemicals, and each one has a different toxicity, a different use, a different route of exposure."

She proceeded to run down some of her analyses, and the first study she mentioned involved some unique test subjects. "We did some

testing recently of phthalates in the urine of Old Order Mennonites—
ten pregnant women," she told me. "They had much lower levels of
phthalates, BPA and triclosan in their bodies than the average
American. One of the main reasons for this, we think, is that they don't
use cosmetics. One woman had used hairspray, and she was the only
one who had detectable levels of MEP [the breakdown product of DEP,
a type of phthalate common in personal-care products]."[16] Another
factor that Swan and her co-authors suspect accounted for the low
levels in the volunteers was their general avoidance of cars and trucks.
Phthalate levels in the interior air of cars can be elevated because of
off-gassing from the upholstery, and this is particularly pronounced
on warm days.[17] "Usually Mennonites get around in horse-drawn bug-
gies, but some of the women reported recently riding in a car or truck.
We saw more MEHP [the breakdown product of the phthalate DEHP]
in their urine." The third factor that Swan identified was the Mennonite
habit of eating unprocessed foods, which they'd often grown themselves. Recent studies have shown markedly lower levels of BPA and
some phthalates when unprocessed food is consumed.[18]

"It's always DEHP that predominates in food. So why is that? Well,
now I'm talking speculatively, but if you take a baby in the intensive
care unit and feed it through a tube, you will measure DEHP in its
urine. No question. A lot of it. Because the warm liquid pulls the
DEHP out of the plastic in the feeding tube. I think this is probably
what's happening with milk. Milking machines use a lot of plastic
tubing. The DEHP from the plastic ends up in milk and cheese. It's
fat-soluble, so it accumulates in fatty foods. And so when people say,
'What can I do?' I say eat organic, unprocessed, fresh food. Your levels
of DEHP will come down." In fact, a study published as we were writing this updated book confirmed Swan's suspicion: people who ate
fast food were found to have levels of some phthalates in their bodies
up to 35 percent higher than people who didn't.[19]

Another study that Swan mentioned—really the flip side of the
Mennonite coin—is a startling look at phthalate levels in nail salon
workers.[20] The levels of MBP (the breakdown product of the phthalate
DBP) were significantly higher in manicurists after their work shifts.
The use of gloves alleviated this problem, a fact that points to the nail
products as the source of MBP. "Nail polish is bad, but perfume is the

worst," said Swan, referring to recent studies that demonstrated more uptake of phthalates from perfume than from any other personal-care product.[21] In the study, women who used perfume had three times as much MEP in their urine as women who didn't wear perfume.

Given that phthalates surround us every day, virtually every human being on the planet has the stuff coursing through their veins.[22] And to further compound the creepiness, elevated phthalate levels have been found in breast milk and umbilical cord blood, meaning that moms aren't just polluting themselves; they're passing their phthalate pollution on to their fetuses and nursing babies.

This is a problem because phthalates are hormone-disrupting chemicals. Once in our bodies, they are mistaken for estrogen and can create all the changes that estrogen achieves. Shanna Swan has long researched this phenomenon, including early publications about the possible role of phthalates in creating genital malformations in little boys.[23] A more recent study hints at neurobehavioural change resulting from exposure to phthalates.[24] Another showed that elevated phthalate levels in expectant fathers can result in mutations in their sperm.[25]

Hormones are like the traffic cops of our bodies. They tell everything—all critical processes—"Stop," "Go" or "Slow down." No wonder hormone mimickers like phthalates have such dramatic effects.

And when it comes to beauty products, phthalates are only the tip of a diverse and complicated toxic iceberg.

Dangers of Deodorants (and Antiperspirants)

From the mountain of evidence linking phthalates to human health concerns, I turned next to another chemical that many alert consumers are now trying to avoid: parabens. Hormonally active chemicals that, like phthalates, mimic estrogen in the human body, parabens are added to countless consumer products—foods, pharmaceuticals and beauty products, including antiperspirants and deodorants—as a preservative. Given their widespread use, it's not surprising that they're now found in the bodies of most people, including 95 percent of the American population.[26] Though parabens have not been scientifically scrutinized nearly as much as phthalates have, the examination of this preservative and its effects inside the human body is beginning to intensify.

If there is one researcher in the world who can claim to have brought parabens into the public eye, it's Dr. Philippa Darbre of the University of Reading in England. In a widely cited 2004 study, Dr. Darbre and her colleagues found parabens in human breast tissue.[27] "There was a bit of a furor," Darbre told me over the phone from her laboratory. "Up to that point, it had been assumed that parabens, once they entered the human body, would be broken down by the liver. But something different altogether happens when they're applied directly to the skin: the parabens bypass the liver and remain intact."[28]

Darbre told me she was struck by the way that breast cancers often develop. "Between 50 and 60 percent of breast cancers start in the upper outer quadrant of the breast, near the armpit." To explain why this is completely disproportionate and striking, she gave me a crash course in breast anatomy. "The breast is divided into seven regions: four quadrants, a central region, a nipple area and an axillary (or armpit) region. So if breast cancer started equally across all areas of the breast, we would expect to see less than 20 percent of cancers originating in each of those regions. But we don't, and 50 to 60 percent are up there in the upper outer quadrant. Why? Is it because of all the chemicals being applied to that region?" This question has driven her to research the possible link between underarm products and breast cancer for over fifteen years.

To further her 2004 study, Darbre continued to look for parabens in sample breast tissue from radical mastectomies. This time she used an even larger sample, and her suspicions were confirmed.[29] "Not only did we repeat our 2004 results, but we actually found even fourfold higher paraben levels in these samples." More interesting (and worrisome) in its implications for human health was the significant difference in levels of one paraben chemical in different parts of the breast. "Propyl paraben did seem to have a gradient, with more found in the axilla region than in the inner regions, which you might expect is coming from the underarm."

Do parabens cause breast cancer? As any cautious scientist would do, Darbre is quick to put her experimental results in context. "The fact that they're in the breast doesn't mean that there's necessarily a relationship with breast cancer. It's the first question. If they're not getting into the breast, then they can't have any effect on breast cancer."

But even if they don't cause cancer, there may be other effects. Although cancer is the main concern, it actually represents only about 5 percent of clinical abnormalities of the human breast, with benign conditions such as breast cysts being the most common.

In response to the many women writing to her and complaining about painful breast cysts, Darbre started looking into aluminum levels in breasts.[30] Here again she found strong evidence linking antiperspirant use with disease. Aluminum is a common component of antiperspirants because it helps keep sweat off the wearer's skin by blocking sweat ducts. Breast cysts also occur when sweat ducts don't drain properly. Darbre has found strong evidence that, like parabens, aluminum levels are highest in the part of the breast near the armpit—also where a disproportionate amount of breast cysts are found—and that aluminum levels are higher in the fluid of breast cysts than in other parts of the body. Pretty convincing stuff.

What's the response of the chemical industry to Darbre's work? Although the presence of parabens and aluminum in breast tissue (specifically, in the part of the breast most likely to manifest disease) is now undeniable, the U.S. Food and Drug Administration continues to state on its website that "At this time, [the agency does] not have information showing that parabens as they are used in cosmetics have an effect on human health."[31] Still, Darbre has tried to respond directly with further experimentation. Though manufacturers defend their *particular* parabens, the problem is not that there is one particular type of paraben in breast tissue, Darbre maintains; it's the fact that there are many. Parabens are a family of chemicals, and it's the effect of this potent and potentially toxic mixture that's the worry. In a 2012 study, she took various parabens at the same concentrations she has measured in the human body and demonstrated that in combination they have an effect.[32] "To my knowledge," she told me, "this is the first science suggesting that parabens have the capability of turning a normal breast cell into a transformed breast cell."[33] Transformed cells cannot be controlled by the body's normal processes and may be indicative of progression to a cancerous state. Scientists are producing a body of data that lead to some valid concerns about parabens. But on the flip side, where are the data supporting claims that parabens are safe? As Darbre put it, "Where are the data showing that if you put parabens into all these things that get into people at all levels . . . that there are no effects? There aren't any such data. And my interpretation is that the current data imbalance is making companies nervous. Unfortunately, we are exposed to many chemicals each day that mimic estrogen and that have complementary action."[34]

In her own life, Darbre uses as few of these products as possible. And as Bruce illustrates in chapter 10, there is growing evidence that sweating is actually an important mechanism of the body's detox system: the more you sweat, the more toxic chemicals you get rid of. Our over-air-conditioned, sweat-averse society's antiperspirant habit reduces our body's ability to clean itself while slathering on nasty pollutants. A toxic double whammy.

"A Whole New Ballgame"

I will confess that, in university, when my hipster friends were avoiding deodorant and rubbing crystals under their arms, I . . . was not. I value personal hygiene and a relative lack of stench from my fellow humans. Until I started writing this chapter, I still clung to my not infrequent use of Mitchum antiperspirant. Why? It works. As my grandmother always used to say, "Horses sweat, men perspire and women glow." I was going one further by trying not to perspire at all. With Toronto being 40 degrees Celsius for an increasing number of summer days, it's hard to be taken seriously if you're perspiring through your shirt.

But there are now better ways to deal with the problem. Quite simply, sustainable cosmetics are more popular because products have become much better.

Just how much better was sketched out for me by Judi Beerling, technical research manager for Ecovia Intelligence. After working for over thirty years in the conventional cosmetics industry, Judi decided that the formulation of conventional cosmetics had become "a bit stagnant, with everybody doing the same sorts of things over and over." She was enticed to begin concocting formulations for sustainable cosmetics companies because of the intellectual challenge.

When it comes to sustainable cosmetics, she told me during a coffee break at the New York Sustainable Cosmetics Summit, "it's a whole new ballgame." She estimated that "85 to 90 percent of the ingredients and techniques [needed] to make sustainable cosmetics are now available, and this is increasing literally on a weekly basis. Now the challenge is to figure out how to combine them to get the best effect and to make the best cosmetics we can."

Hands down, the number one remaining challenge for formulating sustainable cosmetics, according to a number of people I interviewed at the summit, is the creation of effective preservatives to replace parabens. Curt Valva explained the problem succinctly: "Many of our products are water based. Things with high water content have to be preserved because as soon as you introduce water into something, bacterial growth starts immediately. You need something to either keep the bacteria from growing at their normal level, like we would have in drinking water, or kill them completely. The problem is those things that kill bacteria are also really not good for the human body. They're designed to kill cells—that's what they do." It's particularly important, Valva told me, to keep products like mascara, which are applied near the eye, clean and totally free from mould, fungus and bacteria.

Such is the interest in non-toxic preservatives that Judi Beerling led a summit workshop on Saturday morning dedicated entirely to this topic. It's not just the question of whether new technologies are available, but also whether they are cost-effective. "You're often looking at double the cost. Sometimes triple. If you've got really high buying power—say you're a large multinational—you'd likely be able to get that down. It also depends on what you're trying to make. Some things are easier than others."

At Beerling's workshop, I learned that natural and organic products have traditionally contained ingredients like grapefruit seed extract (rather than parabens) to act as preservatives, though new materials and technologies are gaining acceptance. She outlined these "hurdle" technologies, which create barriers to block the growth of micro-organisms by putting successive impediments in their path—each hurdle diminishing the population of microorganisms until none remain. An intelligent combination of different preservation factors can create a hostile environment for bacteria right in the product itself. Some formulations include materials that make the product ever so slightly more acidic, or add emollients with properties that can disrupt the membranes of bacterial cells. Other natural cosmetics boost their preservative systems through the use of antioxidants or tiny amounts of spice extracts or alcohol. It turns out that one of the best—and simplest—ways to reduce the need for high levels of preservatives is to improve packaging. Smaller packaging helps to reduce or remove contamination issues. Airless dispensers or pumps can dramatically cut bacterial growth—unlike the huge, goopy Oil of Olay wide-neck skin-cream jar that sat on my grandmother's bathroom counter throughout my childhood.

Not that long ago, the cosmetic industry's knee-jerk solution to the problems of preserving your lipstick, shampoo and shaving gel was always the same: "Add more parabens!" Now, through the leadership of innovative chemists like Judi Beerling, manufacturers have a larger number of less toxic options. Just how many options became obvious to me when, as a way of concluding her Saturday workshop, Judi started flashing up ingredient labels from real-life natural cosmetics and invited the crowd to start playing the game "Spot That Preservative" by yelling out the answer.

As I left the workshop to catch my plane, the cries of "honeysuckle extract," "tocopherol" and "thyme oil" followed me down the hall.

Smelling Purty
The first experiment involving phthalates that I conducted on myself was part of the original *Slow Death* "toxic condo" experience described in the introduction. The setup was simple. I identified personal-care products that likely contained phthalates through consulting the Environmental Working Group's Skin Deep database (https://www.ewg.org/skindeep). We purchased all the products at local retailers.[35] None of the containers listed phthalates as an ingredient, though all listed "fragrance" or "parfum," which are code for the presence of phthalates. And fragrant they certainly were. We stored all our purchases in a cardboard box in a corner of Bruce's condo. The combined smell of the various bottles was quite something—a sickly sweet mixture of roses and pine needles.

The experiment itself was straightforward. From Friday night through Sunday morning, I limited my phthalate exposure in every way I could think of. I ate fresh food. I didn't shower. I avoided anything with heavy scents, including all personal-care products.

From Sunday morning through Monday morning, I continued this regime. By Monday at 2 p.m. I had collected twenty-four hours' worth of urine, and from Monday at 2 p.m. to Tuesday at 3 p.m., I collected the second twenty-four hours' worth. During this period I showered, shaved and used toiletries and cleaning products in the same way I normally would, using the products listed at the back of this book.[36] We packed up the litres of urine (very, very carefully) and sundry blood samples and sent them to AXYS, and then we waited. It was over a month before the results arrived.

Of the six phthalates for which we tested, five were present at detectable levels both before and after I had slathered myself in all the smelly products (see figure 3). Levels of monoethyl phthalate (MEP)—the metabolite of DEP (diethyl phthalate)—were a lot higher in the "before" measurement than any other phthalate. This just makes sense, given how dominant DEP is in personal-care products.

The really dramatic result was that, as a result of my product use, my MEP levels—MEP is one of the chemicals that Shanna Swan connected with male reproductive problems—went through the roof, from 64 to 1,410 nanograms per millilitre (ng/mL). My MEOHP and MEHHP levels (metabolites of DEHP) declined ever so slightly (from 19 to 10 ng/mL and from 26 to 12 ng/mL, respectively).

Figure 3. Levels of different phthalate metabolites in Rick's urine before and after exposure to phthalate-containing personal-care products (ng/mL). DEP is the most common phthalate in these products, and it converts to the MEP metabolite in our bodies.

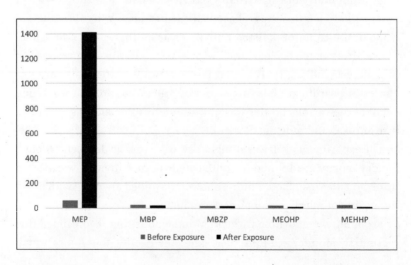

Even after that initial "detox" period in which I tried to eliminate all phthalates, five of the six phthalates still showed up in measurable levels. Where did they come from? Well, the food I ate—wholesome as it was—likely contained some phthalates. I also wondered about a couple of odoriferous air fresheners I had run into on Saturday.[37] One was in a corridor at the St. Lawrence Market; the other was in a public washroom (my son Zack had to make an emergency pit stop). All I had managed was to reduce my phthalate levels, not actually eliminate the chemicals from my body. I also showed how easy it is to crank up levels of MEP dramatically after a simple change in toiletries for only two days. Every time I used similarly smelly products on my kids, I was achieving a similar result in their bodies.

Toxic vs. Green Products

The phthalate experimentation on myself just whetted Bruce's and my appetite to go further. After doing a ton of research into the alleged merits of green personal-care products, we decided to investigate the impact of using greener products on levels of both phthalates and parabens. And we had some intrepid volunteers who were equal to the task.

Ray Civello of Aveda and Jessa Blades, one of *Glamour* magazine's seventy eco-heroes and the TreeHugger website's Best Green Makeup Artist for 2011, were up for the challenge. The idea was pretty simple. We wanted to look at the day-to-day differences in our participants' phthalate and paraben levels as they switched from using conventional, chemical-laden personal-care products to products that claimed to be greener and notionally safer.[38] The hitch with Ray and Jessa was that they'd made that switch long ago: both were already big believers that the first step in detoxing is to *avoid* harmful toxins. For the purpose of our experiment, we asked them to go back—just for a day.

Based on consultation with experts like Dr. Shanna Swan, we designed our protocol as follows.

On day 1, our participants had to undergo a twenty-four-hour "washout" phase, which meant avoiding cosmetics or personal-care products as much as possible. The logic behind the washout is that chemicals like phthalates and parabens are excreted in the urine, usually within six to twelve hours of application/ingestion/inhalation.

After twenty-four hours of cosmetics-free living, our participants gave their first urine samples on day 2, at eight a.m. That sample was used to establish their baseline body levels for the phthalates and parabens we were examining. Immediately following the first urine collection, Civello and Blades each did a one-time application of the conventional products we had sent them.[39] With the help of a study on chemicals in consumer products from the Silent Spring Institute[40] and the EWG's Skin Deep database,[41] we selected products that we were pretty sure contained phthalates and parabens aplenty.

Another urine collection was done at both the four-hour (noon) and six-hour (two p.m.) post-application marks, for a total of three urine samples from each for the first phase of the experiment. Following the two p.m. collection, we asked our volunteers to refrain from using any more cosmetics for the duration of the second washout, which would end at eight a.m. on day 4. The second phase of the experiment played out the same as the first, with urine collections at eight a.m., noon and two p.m. The only difference was that in this phase, Ray and Jessa would be applying the natural products (listed in the notes for this chapter) after their eight a.m. sample.

So there you have it. After a total of eight days, twelve urine samples and over fifty cosmetic products, the urine was packed up and sent off to our friends at SGS AXYS labs in British Columbia.[42]

Our participants were good sports about the whole thing. When I spoke to Civello as he was doing the first washout, he told me he was interested to see if his colleagues would notice. "I've smelled the same way for twenty-five years. I have a distinctive aroma that people know me by. People usually say to me, 'Man, you smell good!'" The day he walked down his office hallway stinking of Axe body spray rather than Aveda's distinctive rosemary mint, he did indeed turn some heads.

"We're really confused as to what clean smells like," Blades quipped over the phone. She doesn't normally wear strong perfumes, as she's wary of their undisclosed ingredients. But as a professional makeup artist, she concedes that there's no question that long-wear conventional products work. "If you put plastic into a product, it'll stay on. Put some of this lipstick on the back of my hand and it stays there. But women don't have to wear waterproof mascara every day. They have to wear mascara that doesn't burn their eyes and that doesn't make their eyelashes fall out."

The results of our experiment were very convincing (check out figure 4 for the story in a nutshell).

Figure 4. Graphs of Jessa's and Ray's MEP and methyl paraben levels (in ng/mL) over the course of the four-day experiment. Note the peak in the levels of both chemicals after application of conventional products.

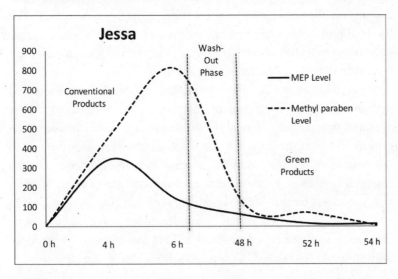

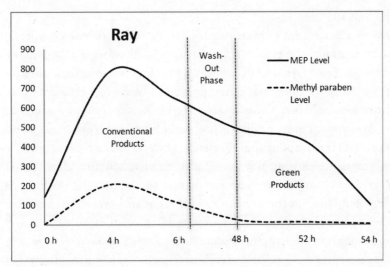

Blades's initial level of monoethyl phthalate (MEP) went from a low of 6.09 ng/mL to a high of 346 ng/mL, then back down to 12.6 ng/mL. Her methyl paraben levels started at 5.17 ng/mL, went all the way up to 805 ng/mL and then dropped to 7.69 ng/mL. Civello's levels followed the same pattern. His base MEP level was 143 ng/mL; it peaked at 786 ng/mL and fell to 99.3 ng/mL. His methyl paraben went from a low of 2.45 ng/mL to 206 ng/mL and then dropped back to 4.29 ng/mL. The levels of phthalates and parabens we found in our study match other data in scientific literature that looks at levels of these chemicals after topical application of cosmetics.[43]

While both Jessa's and Ray's phthalate and paraben levels spiked dramatically after their use of the conventional cosmetics, they declined dramatically during the subsequent washout phase of the experiment. Significantly, phthalate and paraben levels continued to fall even after application of the green personal-care products. The results from this experiment certainly support Blades's point. Women and men don't have to wear this stuff every day. Nor do they have to wear sackcloth and go without cosmetics entirely to avoid synthetic chemicals. The green products used by Blades and Civello are wonderfully effective. And they don't leave a toxic residue in the body.

Harvest Time

Here's a bonus: not only are organic and natural personal-care products better for you personally (as our experiment convincingly demonstrates), it also turns out that they're better for the earth. Back when all cosmetics companies made their products with petrochemical derivatives, you could just phone up your ingredient suppliers and get them to cook you up some new toxic goo in their lab. Easy, predictable and fast. With the rise of natural cosmetics, however, an increasing number of companies are on the hunt for previously obscure plant-based ingredients. And a new and fascinating symbiotic relationship has emerged between the producers of these plants and the companies they serve. The scramble to source reliable supplies of plant-based ingredients is intensifying; a number of people I spoke with were very concerned. One, Curt Valva of Aubrey Organics, told me that there had recently been a shortage of blue chamomile oil. "It comes from Morocco," he said. "The crop was just devastated; we got very little, and we use a lot of that particular ingredient. Our price doubled. And when a raw ingredient that is a mainstay of your product line shoots up in price like that, it becomes very, very difficult, let me tell you!"

Many natural cosmetics companies prominently mention their partnerships with traditional communities as tangible indicators of their authenticity and commitment to fair trade and sustainability. Aveda has created a whole sub-brand, "Soil to Bottle," around its tracing of raw ingredients back to their farm or harvesting co-op of origin. According to the Aveda website, the company's purchasing has resulted in improved standards of living for subsistence Indian farmers (turmeric), Australian Aborigines (wild sandalwood oil) and the Yawanawá people of Brazil (urukum seeds).

One of the ingredients most important to Bill Whyte at Badger is organic olive oil. They use hundreds of litres of the stuff every year, which they buy from a single little company—Soler Romero—in Andalusia's Jaén province in southern Spain. I spent some time chatting on the phone with Mónica Marín, the export manager for Soler Romero, from her office in the middle of the farm's six-hundred-hectare organic orchard. In the same family since the 1850s, Soler Romero had always sold its olive oil in bulk to the local co-op. Much of it was exported to Italy, where it was resold as Italian product. "Then ten years ago," Marín explained, with her hundred-year-old trees crowding outside her window, "the family decided to change the business. We received organic certification and built our own olive mill." The newly rebranded organic product soon came to the attention of Bill Whyte back in New Hampshire.

As Badger's business has grown, so have its orders of Soler Romero's olive oil. Though the bulk of her oil is still sold for human consumption, the component taken by Badger for cosmetics is increasingly important. From the point of view of Soler Romero's owners (the seventh generation of their family to try to make a go of it in the highly competitive international olive oil business), every litre of product they are able to sell to Badger is a litre they don't have to offload, at substantially lower prices, to the bulk Italian market at the end of the season.

Another businesswoman I spoke to who is grateful for the growth of the natural cosmetics market is Eugenia Akuete, then president of the Global Shea Alliance. On the phone from Accra, Ghana, where she owns a shea butter–producing company, Akuete was bullish on the

growth of her industry. "Shea nuts are harvested from across twenty-
one sub-Saharan African countries," she told me. "We're a big, a growing industry." Indeed, the Food and Agriculture Organization of the
United Nations (FAO) estimates that the shea butter industry now
employs roughly three million women in Africa, generating between
$90 and $200 million a year.[44]

Shea nuts are one of those perfect natural creations that have the
power to make even the most hardened non-believer consider the
possibility of a divine plan. If you boil them up, you can make a highly
nutritious butter that has been an important food source for centuries.
Rubbed on the skin, the vitamin E–rich oil is a useful natural moisturizer. Best of all, the nuts are produced by slow-growing, hardy trees
throughout the arid plains of mid-Africa, in an area where agriculture
is tough slogging at the best of times. The size of a large plum, the fruit
ripens at an opportune season of the year when other food supplies are
at their lowest ebb. The thin pulp is tart but edible, and the large nut
inside contains a veritable cornucopia of nutritious oils and fats. Much
of the annual harvest is consumed by millions of households locally,
but it's now also a valuable export commodity: as an ingredient in foods
such as chocolate (where it is often used as a substitute for cocoa
butter) and, increasingly, as a base for natural cosmetics.

In 1994, 50,000 tons of shea nuts were exported from West Africa. By
2012, that number had increased fivefold. From a standing start in the
mid-1990s, about 24,000 tons of shea nuts are now exported for cosmetics each year, a number that continues to increase rapidly.[45] As of 2013,
the *Africa Dispatch* reported that West Africa exported roughly 350,000
metric tons of shea butter a year.[46] I asked Eugenia Akuete whether, given
that it's a semiwild crop and supplies are presumably limited, there is
further room to grow the shea harvest. "Yes!" she replied. "Every year, an
estimated one million tons of shea nuts are harvested. And we think
there's an additional one million tons that are not used and left to rot."

Akuete told me a funny story about trying to get her company's ship-
ment of shea butter through the American border in the 1990s. She
was trying to answer a border agent's questions when another border
agent overheard the conversation. "You don't know what shea is?!" the
second agent asked incredulously, before taking it upon herself to educate her colleague about the miracle butter's many virtues.

With fans like that, it's clear this grassroots industry is only getting started.

The New Normal

When I started at the University of Guelph in 1987, the "Royal City," as it's known, had long been an island of latter-day hippies adrift in suburban southern Ontario. Parties would often end with "Rise Up," the gay rights anthem by Toronto's Parachute Club, or Midnight Oil's "Beds Are Burning." We rocked out at U2's Joshua Tree tour with socially conscious songs like "Bullet the Blue Sky." I got arrested at peace and environmental demonstrations, grew my hair and sideburns really long and determined that I should buy more organic food and products. At the time, the only place in town to purchase the requisite organic granola was the food co-op. This was a dank subterranean room—think Rome, Christians and catacombs—for which you needed to pick up a special key at the business upstairs. But in the space of a short (I mean, 1987 wasn't that long ago, right?) period of time, all things organic and natural—cosmetics, food, cleaning products—have become much more available. My neighbours and I can now get many of the goods we need from the substantial organic and natural section of our local Loblaws— one of the 2,300 supermarkets run by Canada's largest food retailer.[47] And back in 1987, though it wasn't the Summer of Love by any means, there was still a tight correlation between how you looked (long hair and tie-dye), how you cooked (did anybody really like the brown rice in that damn Enchanted Broccoli Forest?), what you thought (Nicaragua's Sandinistas were the cat's meow) and even how you smelled (patchouli still turns me on). Today? Not so much.

"The appeal of green cosmetics is super-broad," says Adria Vasil, who for years wrote a column called "Ecoholic" in Toronto's *NOW* magazine. "I get questions from yummy mummies made up after yoga, from businesswomen, from guys in suits—it's definitely changed.... If you want that vixen red lip and that smoky eye, no problem." Sustainable cosmetics are well on their way to becoming the new normal. Are people changing everything overnight? Of course not. Florida-based pollster Linda Gilbert's research has shown that people usually change up their brands in a gradual way. "In our discussions with consumers, we find that, perhaps counterintuitively, conventional products and green products will co-exist in the bathroom cabinet," she told me. "It's the same phenomenon that we observed twenty years ago, when we realized that just because someone buys organic cereal doesn't mean they'll buy organic milk. People really do pick and choose, and it's always this balancing act between brand trust, performance and considerations related to health and environment. So they may use Tom's of Maine toothpaste but also gargle with Listerine."

Bottom line? Gilbert has identified "three things that consumers tell us are getting in the way of buying more organic and natural products." The first is availability. The second is price. And the third is effectiveness or practicality.

As I hope has been obvious from reading this chapter, all three of these obstacles are well on the way to being removed. You no longer need to be an Old Order Mennonite to avoid phthalates and parabens.

TWO: THE WORLD'S SLIPPERIEST SUBSTANCE
[BRUCE TRAVELS TO TEFLON TOWN]

[Open on suburban kitchen, Wife and Husband arguing]

WIFE: *New Shimmer is a floor wax!*
HUSBAND: *No, new Shimmer is a dessert topping!*
WIFE: *It's a floor wax!*
HUSBAND: *It's a dessert topping!*
WIFE: *It's a floor wax, I'm telling you!*
HUSBAND: *It's a dessert topping, you cow!*
SPOKESMAN: *Hey, hey, hey, calm down, you two. New Shimmer is both a floor wax and a dessert topping! Here, I'll spray some on your mop . . . and some on your butterscotch pudding.*
—"SHIMMER," *Saturday Night Live*, 1975

IT'S WELL KNOWN THAT TEFLON—and its chemical relatives (called PFCs, or perfluorinated compounds)—are used to coat non-stick frying pans. Less well known is the fact that they're used to line pizza boxes and that they are a component of windshield wipers, bullets and computer mice. They're also a key ingredient in cosmetics and clothing.

"It's Everywhere," says DuPont's tagline for Teflon. And that is precisely the problem. It's not supposed to be everywhere. Not in the flesh of ringed seals in the Arctic.[1] Not in the blood of 98 percent of Americans[2] and certainly not—as we shall see—in the drinking water of the residents of Parkersburg, West Virginia.

PFCs are so prevalent and persistent and their uses are so varied that they've made one of my favourite *Saturday Night Live* skits, which aired over forty years ago, seem downright prescient. In the skit Dan Aykroyd is spraying creamy foam into his bowl while Gilda Radner is using the same product to clean the kitchen floor. The first time I saw it, I thought it was hilarious. Now it isn't quite so funny, because something very similar is happening with PFCs in real life.

The Chemical That Lasts (Almost) Forever

Teflon has the honour of being declared the world's slipperiest substance by the *Guinness Book of World Records*. Like the other well-known non-stick coatings Silverstone and Capstone, it is a DuPont brand, a type of perfluorinated compound. In addition to their prevalence in our kitchens, PFCs are also common in our bedroom closets: Gore-Tex is a brand name for PFC water-repellent fabric, as are Scotchgard and Stainmaster. The PFC group of chemicals have long been plagued with controversy. For example, in 2000, 3M, the maker of Scotchgard, voluntarily removed the PFC perfluorooctane sulphonate (PFOS) from its products when it discovered how persistent the chemical had become in the environment. In a notice to Environment Canada, the U.S. Environmental Protection Agency advised Canadians of the voluntary phase-out, stating that PFOS "appears to combine persistence, bioaccumulation and toxicity properties to an extraordinary degree."[3] Unfortunately, PFOS remains widespread in the environment.[4]

Like its chemical cousin PFOS, perfluorooctanoic acid (PFOA)—or C8 as it's also known, because of the eight carbon atoms in its molecular structure—has a lot of problems. It is considered by many scientists to be toxic and to cause birth defects, developmental problems, hormone disruption and high cholesterol.[5] The EPA has labelled it a "likely carcinogen,"[6] and it's now found in every corner of the globe.[7] Yes, it is amazingly durable, it resists other chemicals, it is fireproof and nothing sticks to it. But the very properties that make PFOA commercially desirable—durability, slipperiness and resistance to breakdown—create a major problem. Nothing gets rid of it. Not sunlight. Not our stomach acids. Once PFOA is created it may persist in the environment for centuries. Every molecule of the compound that has ever been created is still around and will be around for the foreseeable future.

DuPont is the sole U.S. manufacturer of PFOA, which the company uses to make Teflon and many other products in a West Virginia town called Parkersburg. Over the years, quantities of the chemical have escaped into the local air and water, and PFOA-linked health concerns have become an issue there.

In addition to being directly emitted into the environment, PFOA is indirectly created as a breakdown product of a specific kind of PFC called fluorotelomers, which are sprayed onto fabric or fabric-covered furniture by manufacturers or consumers. Danish researchers recently found that levels of PFOA and other perfluorinated compounds in polar bears have increased by 20 percent or more since 2000.[8] More recent research has uncovered PFOA in the body fat of polar bears migrating from East Greenland to Iceland.[9] Scott Mabury, a chemist at the University of Toronto and one of the world's leading researchers in this area, has found the chemical in many species and ecosystems.[10] I spoke with some of his research team, and their conclusion is that this ongoing and increasing pollution can be explained only by the fact that the fluorotelomers found in various products degrade into PFOA.

Mabury described the process in a 2006 interview with the Canadian Broadcasting Corporation:

> What we've discovered is that we can measure in the atmosphere fluorotelomers (also known as fluorinated alcohols) that we think are escaping from a variety of consumer products: carpet, coatings for water and stain repellency. . . . We can measure it all across North America. . . . We know it will last in the atmosphere about twenty days, sufficient time to be transported to really remote areas, like the Arctic. We know that Mother Nature, in trying to rid itself of chemical pollutants, transforms that fluorinated alcohol into much more persistent and bio-accumulative materials called perfluorinated carboxylic acids, things like PFOA.

Manufacturers dispute this theory. They believe the chemicals in the coatings are stable and not getting into the environment the way Mabury describes.

Parkersburg, West Virginia, then, is at the centre of the PFOA story—in which one small town is responsible for contaminating not just itself but the entire world and almost every living thing in it. In order to tell this story, I had to see it for myself.

The Tennants of Teflon Town

As I left Wood County Airport in my little red rental car and entered town, the temperature on a sign at one of the local banks read an even 100 degrees Fahrenheit. It was so hot I couldn't help thinking of the pro-verbial egg frying on the sidewalk. Because, of course, in Parkersburg you wouldn't have to worry about it sticking.

The quaint little town where DuPont has long manufactured Teflon sits at the confluence of the Little Kanawha and Ohio Rivers. The area's combination of forests, arable land, coal and the rivers made it a natural location to support early industrial development. In 1860 it was the site of the first producing oil well in the state, and by the late nineteenth century Parkersburg was a bustling merchant town with tanneries and ship-building facilities. Over one hundred years later, Parkersburg became ground zero for the global fallout of PFOA and the centre of an Erin Brockovich–like legal battle.

A mile or so downriver from downtown Parkersburg is DuPont's Washington Works chemical plant. It is located on what are called the "bottomlands"—the floodplain adjacent to the Ohio River.

Directly across the river from the DuPont chemical factory is the drinking-water well field for the town of Little Hocking, Ohio. As I stood in the well field, the DuPont facility dominated the view across the river. I could see pipes going in every direction, including under the river and emerging on the Ohio side, where I was standing. I could also see a newly constructed water filtration system, installed in 2006 to remove contaminants from the Little Hocking water supply, as part of a legal settlement with DuPont.

The Tennant farm, located a short distance from the Washington Works, was a typical family farm—until the cattle began to waste away and die. Jim and Della Tennant farmed for many years on their beauti-ful acreage, raising their extended family and their cattle, until things started to go awry in the early 1980s, shortly after they sold a portion of their farmland to DuPont.[11] According to Callie Lyons, a local jour-nalist and the author of *Stain-Resistant, Nonstick, Waterproof and Lethal,* a book that chronicles the story of the C8 contamination in the Parkersburg area, the Tennants started to notice strange things on their property: local wildlife were dying and minnows had disap-peared from their stream—the same stream their cattle drank from.

They watched helplessly as their animals died and others were born with serious abnormalities.

By the late 1990s the Tennants' herd was decimated. In an interview for National Public Radio, Della Tennant described the scene of a dying cow: "It had the most terrifying bawl, and every time it would open its mouth and bawl, blood would gush from its mouth. And there was nothing you could do. It was suffering, and there was nothing you could do. And whenever you think about feeding all those animals to your children, all the time they were growing up, it's something that puts a lump in your throat you can't take away."[12] Sure enough, family members were by then suffering from respiratory ailments and various cancers.

The Tennants discovered that the piece of land they'd sold to DuPont was being used as a dump for hazardous waste from the Washington Works plant, and they would later find out that it was heavily contaminated with PFOA. Working with Rob Bilott, a Cincinnati lawyer with roots in Parkersburg, they sued DuPont for damages. DuPont settled privately with the Tennants in 2001. The details of the settlement are not known. It certainly helped keep PFOA contamination—temporarily—out of the public eye, but it didn't keep it out of the water or out of Parkersburg's other citizens.

Joe

The real story of Parkersburg is not about a single contaminated farm; it's about widespread chemical contamination in the local watershed. It all started when Joe Kiger and the other residents received a letter from the Lubeck Public Service District (LPSD), advising them that a substance called PFOA had been found in their drinking water.

I met with Joe in the oak-panelled library of the historic Blennerhassett Hotel in downtown Parkersburg. He had just come from coaching the high school football team, and it was obvious that his breathing was laboured. He suffered from asthma, he told me; he also had a liver condition, had had eight prostate biopsies, and had five stents in his heart.

Joe was a big guy but fit. He looked very much the part of a high school football coach, sporting a full head of grey hair cropped short in a flat-topped brush cut. He never worked for DuPont, but he was born and raised in Parkersburg and had more than a passing interest in PFOA. He was the lead plaintiff in a class action lawsuit against DuPont.

Filing the lawsuit was something "I just had to do," Joe said. "What good are you if you can't stand up for yourself?"

Joe told me how he first got involved in one of the largest environmental class action suits in U.S. history. The letter from the Lubeck water utility contained an assurance that, according to DuPont, the PFOA levels in the drinking water were safe. Why, Joe wondered, was DuPont telling the water utility that the water was safe? Shouldn't it be the other way around? Joe held on to the letter. Over the next several months, many of his friends also started suffering from health problems, and stories about unsafe chemical use at the DuPont plant were popping up in the news. Word of the Tennant farm lawsuit was spreading around town, too. It dawned on Joe that something was up. "I said to the wife, 'Where's that letter?'"

Joe called the Lubeck water utility, which he said was evasive at best. Then he got in touch with the West Virginia Department of Natural Resources and the Department of Environment. According to Kiger, everyone he phoned treated the issue "like the plague." DuPont, he said, was of little help. "It was like a wall went up."

After getting no help locally, Joe called the U.S. EPA regional office in Philadelphia. They asked him to fax a copy of the letter he'd received from the Lubeck Public Service District. The letter noted that "the DuPont Company has established its own drinking water guideline" and "DuPont has advised the District that it is confident these levels [of PFOA found in Lubeck drinking water] are safe." Seeing the letter, an EPA employee said to him, "What the hell is PFOA doing in your water?" This employee sent Joe the name of a lawyer: Rob Bilott, the one who'd taken on the Tennant farm case. On August 30, 2001, with Kiger as the lead plaintiff, Bilott filed a class action suit against DuPont. The lawsuit alleged, among other things, that the actions of DuPont, together with those of the Lubeck Public Service District, "were conducted with such intentional, malicious, wanton, willful, and reckless indifference to the Plaintiffs . . . and flagrant disregard for the safety and property of Plaintiffs"[13] that they were liable for punitive damages.

The lawyers didn't mince their words, although the plaintiffs in the class action suit were well aware of the important economic role DuPont played in the community. They made it clear from the outset that their goal was not to shut down the DuPont plant but merely to get answers to their questions, and fair compensation. The plaintiffs wanted to know whether the PFOA in their water was a health problem or not.

DuPont provides nearly two thousand direct high-paying jobs in the community and at least as many indirect jobs. As Joe said, "It was like eatin' possum: the more you chew, the bigger it gets." He endured various forms of abuse from members of his community, which was quietly divided between those who were loyal to DuPont because they worked there or had family members working at the plant (known locally as DuPonters) and those who wanted to know more about perfluorinated compounds (PFCs) and their health. Some of the DuPonters were vocal and intimidating. Objects were thrown at Joe's house and harassment was always in the back of his mind. When a neighbour's house accidentally caught fire and burned to the ground, a friend of his quipped, "They must have gotten the wrong address."

Health issues in Parkersburg and at the Washington Works plant were a well-kept secret prior to the class action suit. A little too well, in the opinion of the EPA, leading the agency (in yet another legal action against the company) to sue DuPont for failing to disclose the fact that it had found PFOA in the blood of its workers at the Washington Works plant as early as 1981. The lawsuit was settled in December 2005 and DuPont was fined $16.5 million, the largest administrative penalty the EPA has ever obtained under U.S. law.[14]

A Discovery at the Plant

It turns out that DuPont knew of health risks associated with PFOA as far back as 1961, when company researchers discovered that rat livers were enlarged when exposed to very low doses. An internal DuPont memo on PFOA and related chemicals advised that "all of these materials . . . be handled with extreme care. Contact with the skin should be strictly avoided."[15]

3M is another major corporation that manufactured and used PFOA and conducted health studies on its workers (but has since phased out the production of PFOA, PFOS and PFOS-related products). One study found that 3M workers directly exposed to PFOA were three times more likely to die of prostate cancer than the least exposed workers.[16] 3M discounted the results because the death rates were still within the average range for unexposed men, and in fact they used the study to claim that PFOA was safe despite the cancer deaths.[17] The health effects are complex, the doses are very low and the human studies involve small numbers of people, so no single study on its own provides conclusive evidence of harm to humans. But putting all the information together, the weight of the evidence suggests that PFOA is a big problem. It is this assessment that led the EPA to deem PFOA a "likely carcinogen." Yet DuPont remains confident that PFOA is safe, stating: "DuPont believes the weight of evidence indicates that PFOA exposure does not pose a health risk to the general public."[18]

I headed off to Charleston, West Virginia, to meet with Harry Deitzler, the lead litigator in the class action suit against DuPont. Like Joe Kiger, he was born and raised in Parkersburg. He described the situation of the local citizens with a conviction and eloquence that helped explain his success as the country's leading PFOA prosecutor.

Harry told me about the DuPont study in 1981 in which the company was looking to see if there were birth defects among the children of workers who'd been exposed to PFOA. Studies of rats showed very specific facial birth defects: cleft palates, nostril deformities and, according to Harry, an unmistakable tear duct deformity that seemed unique to PFOA.[19] DuPont chose eight women who worked with the chemical. If one birth defect was found among the eight women, Harry claimed, DuPont was planning to chalk it up as "coincidence," even though one birth defect in a sample size of eight would be highly unusual. If two or more birth defects were found, DuPont would know they had a problem on their hands. It turned out that two of the eight women did have children born with birth defects—the same kind of eye and facial problems found in the studies of rats exposed to PFOA. DuPont's response? Transfer the women to another part of the factory, cancel the ongoing health studies and keep the results a secret. Harry's distaste for this episode was visible as he spoke to me. Perhaps those were the acts of "reckless indifference" and "flagrant disregard" he had in mind when he used that language in the class action lawsuit.

In early 2003 the Lubeck Public Service District settled privately, leaving DuPont as the sole defendant in the lawsuit. Following the judge's order to seek mediation, DuPont settled in February 2005. Over the course of the three-year civil action, Harry Deitzler estimated that they reviewed more than 1.5 million pages of documents, and the legal team racked up fees and related costs of over $22 million, all of which were paid by DuPont.

The legal settlement included a $71 million health and education project, the installation of a $15 million state-of-the-art water treatment facility to allow the six local water districts to remove PFOA from the water supply to the "lowest practicable levels," and the creation of a $20 million science panel to determine whether there is a probable link between PFOA exposure and adverse medical effects.[20] In the original settlement DuPont agreed to pay up to $235 million to cover medical costs for plaintiffs who could demonstrate direct personal harm.[21] In 2017, DuPont and spin-off company Chemours, operator of the Washington Works plant in Parkersburg, agreed to pay $670.7 million in compensation to the affected residents and claims to have discontinued use of PFOA in 2015.[22]

This is one of the largest environmental class action settlements won to date. To put this amount in context, however, it is roughly equivalent to only one-tenth of one year's after-tax profit for DuPont, based on over $3 billion in profits and revenue of $30 billion in 2007 alone.[23]

Out of the Frying Pan . . .

The non-stick frying pan is surely the icon of the world of perfluorinated chemicals like those produced at the Washington Works plant. In centuries past, canaries were lowered into coalmines, and if they died, miners knew that the air below ground could be toxic to them as well. Perhaps we should heed the modern-day equivalent: non-stick coatings literally kill canaries in kitchens.

It seems that the delicate respiratory systems of birds cannot tolerate the fumes from non-stick pans when they are heated to high temperatures. Their little aviator lungs hemorrhage, becoming filled with fluid and causing the birds to drown.[24] This rapid and deadly syndrome has been known for thirty-five years and even has a name: Teflon toxicosis. Non-stick frying pans, toaster ovens, cookie sheets and pizza pans have all been implicated in pet bird deaths. And the bird killings are not restricted to cooking devices. Irons, space heaters, carpet glues and new sofas have also destroyed the sensitive lungs of pet birds, causing them to suffocate. More than one incident of mass bird deaths has been reported in the vicinity of non-stick coating factories in Canada and Great Britain. And there are also reports of birds dying from self-cleaning ovens, heat lamps and oven interiors with non-stick coatings.

As you might imagine, this is a touchy subject. No manufacturer likes to be called a pet-killer. And having one of your prized brands followed by the word "toxicosis" is not exactly a marketing dream come true. DuPont gives this advice: "Sadly, bird fatalities can result when both birds and cooking pots or pans are left unattended in the kitchen—even for just a few minutes. Cooking fumes from any type of unattended or overheated cookware, not just non-stick, can damage a bird's lungs with alarming speed. This is why you should always move your birds out of the kitchen before cooking."[25] The advice from DuPont does not mention Teflon. The question remains: Do non-stick cooking utensils pose a greater and substantial risk of possibly causing health problems for the humans who use those utensils? The jury is still out on this, but there's some convincing evidence to suggest that non-stick coatings can heat up quickly to levels where numerous toxic gases (some carcinogenic to humans) can be released. According to both manufacturers of non-stick coatings and independent studies, the coatings start to break down between 400°F (200°C) and 550°F (260°C), and highly toxic fumes, including known human carcinogens, are emitted when the pans are heated above 680°F (360°C).[26] The manufacturers claim that these temperatures are rarely reached under normal cooking conditions. This is where the disagreement, and contrary evidence, emerges. Independent studies commissioned by the Environmental Working Group (EWG) show that pans with non-stick coatings can reach over 700°F (370°C) in five minutes or less when preheated on "high" on a conventional electric stove.[27] That means "normal cooking conditions" can result in temperatures high enough for non-stick coatings to break down and toxic fumes to be released.

There are now an increasing number of non-stick products (including broiling pans and oven interiors) that are used in such a way that they guarantee that higher than "normal" cooking conditions will be reached. This is because broiling is a much higher-temperature method of cooking, and when an oven interior is heated, the surface temperatures inside the oven become much hotter than what's cooking in it. The EWG report notes that non-stick stovetop drip pans (the trays that fit under the elements on electric stoves) can reach temperatures as high as 1,000°F (540°C).[28] At temperatures this high the nonstick coatings break down further and the noxious gases that are released include perfluoroisobutylene (PFIB), a relative of the World War I nerve gas phosgene. That ought to do Polly in if the toxins released at "lower" temperatures don't.

Although birds appear to be the most sensitive species, they are not the only ones affected by heated non-stick coatings. In more than one experiment, non-stick pans heated to 800°F killed a group of rats within four to eight hours.[29] In several cases of bird deaths after exposure to fumes from Teflon, the bird owners were also hospitalized with what is known as "polymer fume fever," which causes flu-like symptoms, including difficulty breathing, accelerated heart rate, chills and body aches.[30]

In another strange twist, smoking in the presence of Teflon is exceptionally toxic. Minuscule Teflon particles can decompose in a burning cigarette, causing polymer fume fever in smokers who work in non-stick coating factories. It's not known to what extent problems are caused by smoking at home while heating non-stick pans, but since both practices are fairly risky on their own, it might be wise to avoid that butt while sautéing your mushrooms in a non-stick pan.

I happen to think I'm pretty handy with a frying pan, so here are a few very specific pieces of advice from my own cooking experience on how to kick non-stick.

First, your frying pan doesn't need to be a high-end gourmet item, but it must have a reasonably solid base, so it can heat quickly and evenly and retain heat at a constant temperature. Even if you spend a bit more per pan, it will actually save you more money than if you buy less expensive non-stick pans every few years after the coating has been scraped off and consumed with your scrambled eggs.

There are three basic categories of pots and pans to consider (and many variations on these): cast iron, stainless steel and enamel-coated cast iron. My favourite, and the all-American classic, is the basic black cast-iron skillet. The beauty of cast iron is that if it is treated properly and cared for, it outperforms non-stick. The only things that you should not cook in cast iron are high-acid vegetables such as tomatoes, because they concentrate too much iron if they are cooked for a long time.

There are three main reasons food sticks to a pan. First is that the pan is not hot enough. (And a pan must reach the correct temperature *before* any food is placed in it.) The second reason is not having a nice coating of oil in the pan. And the third is using a plastic spatula instead of a metal one. (Plastic spatulas tend to act more like shovels than spatulas.)

So follow this simple advice: make sure the pan is hot enough and that it has a nice coating of oil—and use a metal spatula—*et voilà!* You can relegate your non-stick pans to the dusty back of your cupboard.

A Sticky, Stain-Ridden Future

Working as an environmentalist for the past thirty years, I have often been frustrated to see government and industry ignoring intelligent environmental analysis. In the early 1970s environmental health experts developed the concept of assessing chemicals as persistent, bioaccumulative or toxic (PBT); these categories were proposed as a gauge for targeting substances to be phased out. The rationale for using PBT analysis is fundamentally sound from scientific, ecological and ultimately even economic perspectives. When substances that are found to exhibit all three of these properties are in widespread use for decades, one can be almost certain that human health and/or ecological problems will surface, often resulting in costly legal settlements.

I was sitting in my little red rental car before departing from the historic but slightly dog-eared town of Harmar, Ohio, just up the river from Parkersburg. It was late in the day and several merchants were chatting on the sidewalk after closing up their antique shops. I was not paying much attention to their conversation, but oddly enough I overheard one of them say, "You're soaking in it," and then another made reference to Madge's whereabouts. Madge, of course, was the fictional manicurist from the old Palmolive commercials who, for a twenty-five-year period, would tell her customers not to worry about the fact that they were soaking their hands in dish detergent. Her famous line "You're soaking in it!" is apropos for Parkersburg residents and PFOA. It also correctly describes the prevalence of many other toxic chemicals—PBT: persistent, bioaccumulative and toxic—in all of our lives.

Dish detergent is a mild (in fact, "more than just mild," as the TV commercial proclaimed) proxy for many of the chemical exposures we face today. We are eating, drinking and soaking in tens of thousands of potentially toxic substances, most of which we know little about. When all these chemicals are combined in our drinking water, we know virtually nothing about how they interact with each other or our bodies, and even less about how they affect developing brains and fetuses. Medical experts have no idea whether twenty different carcinogenic chemicals in the water are twenty times more likely to cause cancer or a hundred times, or whether their effect is likely to be no different from that of just one chemical. In fact, this area of study, called "cumulative risk assessment," is still in its infancy, and studies of the health effects of multiple chemical exposures are rarely undertaken, because of the complexity and lack of scientific understanding of chemical interactions in humans. It is hard enough to understand the effects of one chemical, because it often takes fifty to one hundred years of use and study to figure that out.

Today we are told by real people who work for chemical companies (not fictional manicurists) not to worry, even though we are essentially soaking ourselves, our furniture, our clothes, our food, our packaging and most other things in our lives in a toxic brew, with unknown consequences.

Tap water, sadly, is where the legacy of toxic chemical manufacturing emerges in its most nefarious form. PFOA is no different. The storylines of small American towns contaminated by industrial pollution are remarkably similar in the best-known cases. They start when citizens notice unusual health effects in the community and raise concerns with local officials. It is an all-too-familiar tale, and I often wonder how many of these stories are happening every day around the world, in places where citizens either have no legal recourse or there simply isn't a strong enough leader to fight the battle.

Off-Gassing and Us

We're often asked whether our self-experimentation made us feel ill. Did our bodies respond to the chemicals we were subjecting them to? Mostly the answer is no, with one big exception. The only experiment that hit us both really hard was the one involving perfluorinated chemicals. Ironically, it was also the one that—in the unique way we were defining success—flopped.

The experiment was simple. We wanted to see whether we could increase the level of PFOA in our blood. After speaking to a few experts, we decided to try measuring the effects of inhaling the off-gassing from a "normal" stain-repellent treatment. We needed a dedicated space, and I had an unused room in my condo that fit the bill.

The test room was 3 metres by 3.7 metres, with a large walk-in closet and a small hallway. It was 2.4 metres in height. We furnished it with the local thrift shop's finest: a wall-to-wall beige carpet remnant, a pink loveseat, a brocade easy chair and gold curtains. Man, it was ugly. The loveseat looked as though it could have used a good thick coating of stain repellent twenty years sooner.

Once we had the room ready, we booked an appointment with a carpet professional we found online (there were many companies to choose from). The guy arrived at the condo with a canister on his back, full of what he claimed was Teflon Advanced fabric protector. With no breathing equipment of any kind (I hate to think what his PFOA levels are), he sprayed the carpet, chairs and curtains just as he would for any client. The whole procedure cost sixty dollars.

We asked him how long we should air out the room before starting to use it again. "About twenty minutes should do it," he replied.

Not a chance. The stain-repellent stench after twenty minutes was completely over the top. The intense chemical odour—not unlike a reeking dry cleaning shop—caught in our throats and made our eyes water like crazy. It was more than two hours before we could spend any time in the room, and even then Rick and I took turns in the early part of the experiment poking our heads out the door to gulp some fresh air.

For two days we sat in the room with the windows and doors closed and the air vent plugged. We ate, we watched movies and lots of CNN (since it was the U.S. presidential primary season and all), we played *Guitar Hero* and we tried our best to get a bit of work done while breathing the fumes in our stain-free environment. The taste and smell lasted in my mouth for days after the experiment—because of the persistent quality of PFCs, no doubt. At one point when I stepped outside the room (we left for only a few minutes at a time during the two days to get food from the kitchen, which we brought back into the room to eat on the sofa), I nearly fell flat on my face. The PFC coating on the bottom of my shoes had made them so slippery I could hardly stand. At one point Rick's wife, Jennifer, came to visit and told us we both looked pale, completely red-eyed and zoned out as we lounged with our feet up on the coffee table.

Before the test began Rick and I had levels of four perfluorinated compounds in our blood that were similar to those measured in male Americans by the National Health and Nutrition Examination Survey

(NHANES)(see table 2). My PFOA level was 2.8 nanograms per millilitre (ng/mL), and Rick's was 3.5 ng/mL, compared to the NHANES mean value of 4.5 ng/mL.

Table 2. Bruce's and Rick's perfluorinated chemical blood levels compared to a sample of over 1,000 U.S. males as measured by the National Health and Nutrition Examination Survey (NHANES)[31]

PFC Type	Bruce's Results (ng/mL)	Rick's Results (ng/mL)	NHANES Geometric Mean (ng/mL)
PFOA	2.8	3.5	4.5
PFOS	31.1	27.1	23.3
PFNA	1.2	1.1	1.1
PFHxS	1.9	2.7	2.2

As we sat in our room, we were convinced that if any test could guarantee dramatically skyrocketing personal pollution levels, it was this one. With bisphenol A and the other things we were experimenting with, the actions we were undertaking were subtle. The chemicals were invisible, tasteless and (with the exception of the phthalates and personal-care products) odourless. The PFC experiment, by contrast, was dramatic. You could cut the off-gassing with a knife. We were sure we'd find hugely high levels of these chemicals in our bodies.

But it was not to be. As our blood tests showed, for the four chemicals of interest, including PFOA, there was no measurable increase in us over the two-day period. What had happened? We went back to Dr. Scott Mabury for some answers, along with his colleague at the time Craig Butt.

"There could be two explanations for the lack of increase," said Butt. First, the high background exposure of PFCs and the relatively long half-life (about three to five years) of these compounds in our bodies likely make it difficult to raise levels above the existing baseline. In addition, Butt pointed out, in experimental parlance we hadn't "controlled" for the product used by the carpet applicator. Although the guy told us he was using Teflon Advanced, which Mabury's lab has tested and confirmed that it contains the precursors to PFOA,[32] we never did see the original product container. This is in contrast to our other experiments, in which we purchased the sources of pollution (such as tuna steaks, BPA baby bottles and antibacterial products) ourselves.

"I'm not surprised the experiment didn't work," concluded Butt. "Over the span of a few days it will not be possible to raise your blood levels above the background levels. Air exposure is probably an important exposure route, but it would probably take several weeks or, more likely, months of exposure to raise the levels above background."

Based on our experimental protocol, Butt did an approximate back-of-the-envelope calculation for Rick to illustrate his point.[33] His conclusion? Even if we had assumed unrealistic uptake and conversion rates, it would have been highly unlikely for Rick and me to see an increase in blood levels of PFOA over the two days of the experiment. Could a few weeks or months of exposure to the multiple sources commonly found in our homes and offices crank our levels? Yes. And it clearly does, judging from the levels of PFOA in all of us. But a few unpleasant days of trying to raise them deliberately did not work.

Too bad we hadn't figured this out before we spent two days sitting in that stinky room.

THREE: THE NEW PCBS

[RICK FANS THE FLAME-RETARDANT FIRE]

> *Well it's been so long*
> *And I've been putting out fire with gasoline . . .*
> —DAVID BOWIE, "CAT PEOPLE (PUTTING OUT FIRE)," 1982

THIS PART OF THE STORY started with some snuggly pyjamas. Really nice ones, covered with friendly penguins and dinosaurs, that my sister had brought back for our two young boys after some cross-border shopping at Carter's (a well-known chain of children's stores) in Buffalo, New York.

One day in late autumn, as one of the coldest winters in living memory started to settle in, it was bedtime and I had our squirmy one-year-old, Owain, on his back. I started to put on the new one-piece pyjamas and stopped midway, the zipper halfway zipped, the upper part of the pyjamas bunched around his fat little baby belly.

"Sweetie!" I yelled down the stairs to my wife, Jennifer. "Have you seen this honkin' washing label on Owain's pyjamas?"

"What do you mean? No!" she yelled back. Owain tried to make a break for it. I grabbed him and pulled him back.

"Well, it's huge and talks about the material in these things being flame resistant."

Jennifer was coming up the stairs. She knew where I was headed. "Does that mean you're not going to put them on now?" she asked in a tone of voice typically reserved by harried parents for the supper/bath/bedtime dash.

"Ummm . . . right. But I'll make you a deal: I'll phone the company and find out what flame retardants they put in these, and if it's not harmful I'll put them back on."

"Sure you will," she said, her face conveying her cumulative annoyance with my chemical skepticism, the non-stick pans relegated to basement storage, every plastic container upended and the symbols on the bottom scrutinized, every fine-print ingredient list on our shampoos examined.

But more on those pyjamas later.

Quest for Fire (Retardants)

In the climactic scene of the 1981 classic caveman flick *Quest for Fire,* our Neanderthal hero Naoh is taught by the Cro-Magnon Ivaka tribe how to make fire by rubbing sticks together. The fact that you can start a fire from scratch is a bit of a revelation for Naoh. Once lit, though, a fire can do a lot of damage. How much do you want to bet that the very next thing our prehistoric ancestors learned how to do after starting a fire was how to quench an accidentally out-of-control blaze?

We humans have been trying to master the chemistry of fire prevention for quite a while. In ancient Egypt and China, vinegar and alum were painted on wood to increase their fire resistance.[1] During the siege of Piraeus by Sulla in 86 BCE, alum-soaked wood survived the fires of battle. In seventeenth-century Paris, flame-retardant treatments were pioneered for canvas, and in 1820 French king Louis XVIII commissioned the chemist Joseph-Louis Gay-Lussac to find better ways of protecting fabrics used in the theatre. Gay-Lussac is generally credited with being the first person to figure out the scientific basis of fire retardancy with his concoction of ammonium salts of sulphuric, hydrochloric and phosphoric acids. At about the same time, bromine was discovered in a French saltwater marsh, and our species' fire-fighting was transformed forever.

Bromine is an element related to chlorine, fluorine and iodine (together called the "halogen" elements); it's a smelly brownish liquid obtained from saltwater brine deposits. It turns out that bromine is pretty good at quenching fire. Usually when something burns, the fragments interact with oxygen to keep the fire going. With the right kind of brominated mixture, the bromine atoms capture the burning fragments and prevent the combination with oxygen from happening. As a result the fire smoulders rather than spreading. Of the approximately 175 flame-retardant chemicals used at present, some of the most common—and most controversial—are "brominated."[2]

Because of this specific key ingredient, one of the unusual aspects of this family of chemicals is that its production is controlled by a very small number of companies with reliable access to bromine wells. The largest bromine reserve in the United States is located in Columbia and Union Counties in Arkansas. China's bromine reserves are located in Shandong province, and Israel's bromine reserves are contained in the waters of the Dead Sea. That's pretty much it for the world's current sources of bromine.

I caught up with Stockholm University's Dr. Åke Bergman, one of the world's foremost authorities on brominated fire retardants (BFRs), at a conference in Victoria, B.C., dedicated to the bromine chemicals. He explained that BFRs were products in perpetual search of a new use and that their application as flame retardants emerged with the demise of leaded gasoline. In the 1920s tetraethyl lead was invented as a gasoline additive, but it also left a corrosive byproduct in the engine. The solution hit upon at that time was to add a chemical called ethylene dibromide (EDB) to the mix. At the time, gasoline additives accounted for about three-quarters of the bromine consumption in the United States.[3]

When leaded gasoline began to be phased out in the U.S. in the 1960s, bromine companies needed to dream up new applications for their product, and fast. The Great Lakes Chemical Corporation—then the largest supplier of bromine products—decided to use EDB domestically as a pesticide. This plan ran aground, however, when in 1983 the U.S. Environmental Protection Agency issued an "emergency suspension" of all agricultural uses of EDB—the most restrictive measure the EPA can take under the law—because of evidence that EDB was a carcinogen and a mutagen and was contaminating groundwater supplies in a number of states.

But another use for bromine grew in the twilight of leaded gasoline: it began to be produced and marketed as a flame retardant. Great Lakes Chemical built several new flame-retardant plants in the early 1970s, and production of BFRs has been increasing ever since. As the use of BFRs mushroomed, so did the controversy.

Mutagenic Pyjamas

The story of tris-BP (2,3-dibromopropyl phosphate), the first type of flame retardant to gain public notoriety, highlights the tight relationship between the rise of BFRs and increasingly stringent flammability regulations that governments began to adopt in the 1970s. In the U.S., the *Flammable Fabrics Act* was first passed in the 1950s to regulate the manufacture of cool (and combustible) *Grease*-style clothing such as furry pink brushed rayon sweaters. The legislation was amended in the late 1960s to allow standards to be set for many additional consumer products.

In 1973, for the first time, the U.S. Department of Commerce set mandatory fire-resistance standards for children's nighties and pyjamas. Up to that point kids' PJs had mostly been made of soft cotton. Tris-BP quickly became the favoured chemical treatment and, because it was difficult to use with cotton, sparked the transition to polyester, the fabric most often used in kids' pyjamas to this day. Dollops of tris-BP totalling about 5 percent of fabric weight were layered onto the pyjamas of about 50 million U.S. children between 1973 and 1977. As the *New York Times* pointed out at the time, "the complicated tale of Tris . . . is a classic tale of good intentions—and of the sad truth of the axiom that, too often, the road to Hell is paved with just such generous or compassionate impulses, at least for the Federal Government."[4]

Though there was some early evidence that the new fire safety standards somewhat reduced the number of infants killed by their pyjamas igniting, evidence started to quickly mount that tris-BP was a mutagen and a carcinogen. As a result, in early 1976 the Environmental Defense Fund (EDF) made big headlines when it petitioned the Consumer Product Safety Commission (CPSC) for action. Because the evidence linking tris-BP to cancer was still somewhat equivocal, the EDF petition simply asked for tris-BP garments to be labelled with a tag that said "Contains the flame retardant Tris. Should be washed at least three times prior to wearing."

The companies that manufactured tris-BP pooh-poohed the petition, one of their spokespersons saying at the time that potential hazards from the chemical were minimal.[5] The target of the petition, Richard Simpson, chairman of the CPSC, said in an address to the American Apparel Manufacturers Association that "based on what I've examined . . . I would doubt that there is a problem. There is a great leap from the tests [cited in the petition] to a conclusion that the chemical is a carcinogen. And I am skeptical when a petition which raises the spectre of cancer suggests the remedy of a label asking people to wash the clothes three times before wearing. If there is a real problem, there should be a ban, not a label."[6]

Simpson had spoken too soon. In February 1977 the EDF obtained yet more evidence from National Cancer Institute testing that it claimed showed tris-BP was a "potent" cause of cancer (one hundred times more powerful than the carcinogens in cigarette smoke) and that the chemical could be absorbed by children through the skin or by "mouthing" tris-BP–treated clothing. The fund filed yet another petition—this time for a complete ban—with the CPSC.

Under pressure, the industry caved. Sander Allen, a spokesman for the major manufacturer of tris-BP, the Velsicol Chemical Corporation of Chicago, said in response to the fund's petition that the company did not agree that tris-BP caused cancer but had discontinued making it for garments, because the safety testing necessary to assuage growing public concern was too costly.[7] And public concern there certainly was. In fact, the public debate sparked by the Environmental Defense Fund's first labelling petition had caused demand for tris-BP–treated garments to collapse. Between 1976 and 1977 tris-BP sleepwear went from about 60 to 70 percent of the U.S. market to only 20 percent.

With the heavy lifting completed by the EDF and the way cleared for its decision, in April 1977, exactly a year after Richard Simpson's dismissive comment, the CPSC acted on the National Cancer Institute's testing and banned the treatment of garments with tris-BP. Not a moment too soon: a study published shortly afterwards in the journal *Science* actually found the chemical in the urine of children who were wearing or who had worn tris-BP–treated sleepwear.[8]

Almost overnight an estimated 20 million garments in retail inventories were pulled from the shelves. Because of tris-BP's toxic properties, the government prohibited disposal of these pyjamas; they could only be buried or burned or used as industrial wiping cloths. What to do with this cancer-causing mountain of material? The answer quickly became evident as advertisements started popping up in the classified pages of publications like *Women's Wear Daily*: "TRIS-TRIS-TRIS . . . We will buy any fabric containing Tris-BP."[9] By some estimates, millions of tris-BP–treated pyjamas were shipped quietly out of the U.S. to Europe and other parts unknown to be sold between the time tris-BP was banned in 1977 and June 1978, when the CPSC also stopped tris-BP exports.[10]

Propelled by the memory of the tris-BP controversy, public demand for comfortable pyjamas made of natural fabric grew throughout the next few decades, and in 1999 the CPSC finally relaxed its regulations on the flame retardants that needed to be added to PJs. At present less than 1 percent of children's sleepwear is treated with flame retardants, although, as we will see later in this chapter, the word "treated" as used by government and industry has a narrower definition than would be assumed by the average person.

As the tris-BP fiasco was playing itself out over the U.S. airwaves, another geographically specific—though no less horrifying—BFR scandal was set to explode: the contamination of much of Michigan by polybrominated biphenyls (PBBs).

Cattlegate

One of the worst chemical disasters in U.S. history started on a farm.

Rick Halbert knew there was something wrong with his dairy cows. His four hundred animals in southwestern Michigan were becoming increasingly unhealthy; they had decreased appetites and milk production and they were developing really weird symptoms: hematomas and abscesses, abnormal hoof growth, hair matting and loss, and severe reproductive abnormalities. In the autumn of 1973, after his veterinarian was unable to diagnose any disease, Halbert suspected problems with his recent order of high-protein feed pellets, supplied by Michigan Farm Bureau Services, the state's largest feed distributor. Luckily for the people of Michigan, Halbert was no ordinary farmer. Before returning to the family business, he had completed a master's degree in chemical engineering and had worked three years for the Dow Chemical Company. After repeated lack of response from Farm Bureau Services and the Michigan Department of Agriculture, Halbert spent five thousand dollars to conduct his own testing of the feed.

Though chemical contamination can have major effects, it often results from minuscule amounts of product. Sensitive equipment is needed to detect organic compounds such as those Halbert suspected were present. The more common chemical contaminants that were first considered—such as dieldrin, DDT (both of which pesticides were then in use) and polychlorinated biphenyls, or PCBs (of which PBBs are a very close cousin)—show up as early-emerging peaks on the read-out produced by a scientific instrument called a gas chromatograph. Because of its extreme stability, PBB shows up as a late-emerging peak. Nothing was evident in the analyses of Halbert's feed until one day in January 1974, when the researchers running the chromatograph forgot to turn the machine off during their lunch break. When they returned, a remarkable and unfamiliar reading had appeared.[11]

Halbert passed this result to a scientist at the U.S. Department of Agriculture who, by coincidence, recognized it as a compound that he had been working with: PBB, a flame retardant produced by the Michigan Chemical Corporation for use in moulded plastic parts such as the cases of televisions, typewriters and business machines. The company also sold magnesium oxide to Farm Bureau Services, which then added this supplement to dairy feed to increase cows' milk production. There had been a mix-up at the company's plant.

When first informed of the situation in April 1974, Michigan Chemical rejected the idea that Firemaster, its PBB product, could have been substituted for Nutrimaster, its magnesium oxide product.[12] It was quickly proven wrong. As the state and federal governments moved in to investigate, it became clear that the mistake had happened when the company ran out of preprinted bags and employees hand-lettered the two similar trade names on identical plain brown bags. After a bit of rough handling and smudging of labels, between 225 and 450 kilograms of PBB were accidentally shipped to the Farm Bureau Services mill and incorporated into animal feed.

About nine months after the chemical first entered the Michigan food chain and Rick Halbert's cattle, the source was finally identified. It would be another year and a half before all the contaminated livestock and poultry were tracked down. By this point the contamination was widespread: several thousand farm families and their neighbours had consumed poisoned meat, eggs and milk, and the general public in Michigan had been exposed to a wide array of PBB-contaminated products. The Michigan Long-Term PBB Study has tracked the health of Michigan residents since the incident, and its results point to a potential link between high PBB exposure and an increased risk of cancers of the breast and the digestive system, lymphoma, elevated rates of spontaneous abortion and menstrual complications.[13]

By the end of 1975, about 28,000 cattle, 5,920 pigs and 1.5 million chickens had been destroyed. About 785 tonnes of contaminated animal feed, 8,137 kilograms of cheese, 1,192 kilograms of butter, 15,422 kilograms of milk products and nearly 5 million eggs were buried in huge pits throughout Michigan. Estimates of the total cost for statewide decontamination reached the hundreds of millions of U.S. dollars. And perhaps most shockingly, five years after the incident, about 97 percent of state residents still had measurable levels of the chemical in their bodies.[14] No surprise that one of the most popular Michigan bumper stickers at the time read "PBB—Cattlegate Bigger Than Watergate." Many investigations and much finger-pointing ensued, and in 1982 the U.S. government, the State of Michigan and Velsicol Chemical announced a consent judgment of $38.5 million to settle clean-up costs associated with PBB and other contamination from the Michigan Chemical Corporation.

As the 1970s drew to a close, a number of commentators expressed the hope that the newly adopted U.S. *Toxic Substances Control Act* (1976) would prevent tris-BP and PBB-type disasters in the future.[15] But it was not to be. As Sonya Lunder, a scientist at the Environmental Working Group, so eloquently put it, "When we look at the history of fire retardants, we can assume that public health protection arrives late if at all."[16]

Yushō

PCBs, mentioned a few times already in this book, are familiar to many people, and with good reason. Short for "polychlorinated biphenyls," PCBs, along with the pesticide DDT, are perhaps the most infamous of environmental contaminants. Manufactured for industrial applications that include plasticizers, fluids in electric capacitors and hydraulic oils, PCBs were first detected in the environment in 1996—in the bodies of white-tailed sea eagles. Soon scientists were measuring PCB levels in unlikely places all over the world, and this family of chemicals very quickly began to exhibit, in the words of the understated Dr. Åke Bergman, "very obvious toxic effects." Years earlier, in the summer of 1968, a terrible disaster had occurred in the western part of Japan that dramatically illustrated the dangers of PCBs. PCBs leaked from the heat exchanger at a company that manufactured rice-bran cooking oil and contaminated some cans of oil that were then purchased by consumers. About 1,800 people were affected by what became known as *yushō* (oil disease). Many fell gravely ill, babies were stillborn and about three hundred people died in the ensuing years from the poisoning. A whole host of very graphic symptoms were developed by sufferers, including angry sores on their faces and bodies (called "chloracne"); dark skin discoloration (even on newborn babies born to afflicted mothers); enlargement of and hyper-secretion from glands around the eyes; and respiratory and neurological problems.[17]

A very similar incident (causing an illness known in Chinese as *yu-cheng*) occurred in Taiwan in 1979. The combination of the growing evidence of widespread environmental contamination by PCBs and the horrible illnesses and fatalities stemming from *yushō* and *yu-cheng* moved governments the world over to act in unprecedented ways. Within the next few years, many nations had banned the production, and most uses, of PCBs. PCBs remain the only chemical specifically banned by a vote of the U.S. Congress (in an amendment to the U.S. *Toxic Substances Control Act*). And the international Stockholm Convention on Persistent Organic Pollutants brought a complete end to PCBs in 2001.

The banning of PCBs is one of the greatest environmental and human health success stories. Yes, the global environment remains contaminated with them three decades after they were banned, and most humans tested throughout the world have detectable levels in their bodies. But PCB levels are going down. I know this personally. As part of Environmental Defence's ongoing Toxic Nation campaign, I've been tested for these chemicals (see figure 5). I have nine kinds of PCBs at detectable levels in my body. A major drag, but I represent a point on an improving curve: the number of PCB compounds in my body, and the levels at which these substances were measured, are somewhat lower than in the study participants who are older than I am, and much higher than in children who were tested.

Figure 5. The number of PCBs detected in Rick and the median number detected among Canadians tested in the Toxic Nation studies.

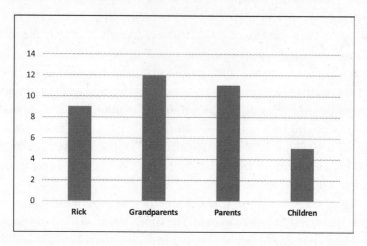

Another chemistry lesson is necessary at this point in our story. PCBs are a member of a family of chemicals called polyhalogenated POPs. Translation: they are persistent organic pollutants (POPs) that contain many halogen (chlorine, bromine, fluorine or iodine) atoms. These chemicals have long half-lives in the environment and in the bodies of animals—about two to ten years. Other members of this chemical family include various chlorinated and brominated compounds such as PBBs (of Michigan cattle fame, now phased out around the world) and polybrominated diphenyl ethers (PBDEs)—currently among the most common flame retardants. The PCBs and PBDEs and others—let's call them subfamilies—each make up a group of individual chemicals called "congeners." Each congener shares the subfamily's chemical backbone but has different numbers and positions of halogen atoms attached.

Persistent organic pollutants have three chemical characteristics that make them intrinsically hazardous: they are stable (persistent), they are stored in fat tissue for long periods (that is, they are "lipophilic"), and they have the potential to act as endocrine (hormone) disruptors. The stability and lipophilic nature of POPs causes them to "biomagnify" up the food chain. This means that the higher-level predators store all the POPs from the lower-level animals and plants that they eat—in their fat tissues. And top-level predators—like us—concentrate and store the most. Once POPs are released into the environment, they find their way into pregnant or nursing mothers, where they pass through the placenta to the developing fetus or concentrate in the fat of the breast milk and are ingested by the nursing infant.[18]

Some POPs—like PBDEs—can bind to our cell receptors and create effects similar to those caused by hormones. Several carry out estrogen-like activities, whereas others have antiestrogenic effects. Health effects as diverse as shortened duration of lactation in mothers, neurodevelopmental cognitive and motor deficits, intellectual impairment in children and greater risk of cancer have been attributed to polyhalogenated POPs.[19]

In short, PBDEs and PCBs are so similar that some scientists are increasingly referring to the former as "the new PCBs." But as we shall see, unlike the case with PCBs, the challenge of global contamination with PBDEs and other toxic flame retardants is a long, long way from being solved.[20]

Mother's Milk

As Dr. Deborah Rice tells it, it was the similarity of PBDEs to PCBs that first caught the interest of the scientific community. Rice, a scientist at the Maine Center for Disease Control and Prevention and a well-known expert on brominated flame retardants, spoke with me on the phone from her office in Augusta. "Analytical chemists looked at the structure of PBDEs and they said, 'Wow! This looks a lot like PCBs and some of the other chemicals that are out there that we know are persistent, that we know are bioaccumulative, and gee, I wonder if that's what PBDEs are doing out there in the environment.'

"We came to recognize that, just like PCBs, these chemicals are indeed persistent," she said. "They bioaccumulate through food chains all over the world, and of course we're terminal predators [at the top of the food chain] so we get a concentrated dose. When you take PBDEs into the laboratory and look at them for endocrine disruption, for disruption of thyroid hormones and for developmental neurotoxicity, they have the same effects, the effects you'd expect them to have based on their similarity to PCBs."

"We never seem to learn!" Rice exclaimed. "To me it's really a very sad tale that as we were banning PCBs in the late 1970s, we were putting PBDEs and other flame retardants into the environment."

In a prominent 1977 *Science* article about the tris-BP controversy, Arlene Blum and Bruce Ames actually warned of the possibility of more widespread global pollution by flame retardants. This last sentence of their article encapsulates both their impatience and the growing challenge in dealing with an avalanche of synthetic chemicals: "While waiting for the effects of the large-scale human exposure to the halogenated carcinogens—polychlorinated biphenyls (PCBs), vinyl chloride, Strobane-toxaphene, aldrin-dieldrin, DDT, trichloroethylene, dibromochloropropane, chloroform, ethylene dibromide, Kepone-mirex, heptachlor-chlordane, pentachloronitrobenzene, and so forth—we might think about the avoidance of a similar situation with flame retardants."[21]

But in much the same way that the world began to wake up to the dangers of PCBs only in the late 1960s, after they started to be found in wildlife, Tom Webster, a senior researcher at the Boston University School of Public Health, dates the first awareness of the dangers of PBDEs to a very specific moment: "With PBDEs they were pretty much under the radar until about 1998," he told me at the Victoria BFR conference, "and that's when this group in Sweden did [a] . . . retrospective study of breast milk. What they found is that the levels of PCBs and dioxins had started coming down from about 1970 to 1998 and levels of PBDEs were going up. That totally got everyone's attention. Because PBDE levels are going up exponentially and they're basically cousins of PCBs."

The Swedish results were a bombshell. Humans are at the top of the food chain for sure, but nursing babies are at the very top (though it's important to point out that the health benefits of nursing still outweigh the downsides). Using banked breast milk sampled from thousands of Swedish women between 1972 and 1997, the researchers were able to show diametrically different results for PCBs and some other contaminants and PBDEs. The level of PCBs in the milk banked in 1997 was 30 percent of the level found in milk from 1972. In stark contrast, the concentration of PBDEs in the milk increased exponentially between 1972 and 1997, doubling every five years.

These results were widely publicized, and with each passing year the massive dimensions of the problem have become clearer. Listening to the presentations at the Victoria conference was overwhelming. The titles of the studies by the assembled international scientists tell the tale: "Association Between PBDE Exposure and Preterm Birth"; "PBDEs in the St. Lawrence: New Contaminants to Be Monitored"; "PBDEs in Harbor Seals from British Columbia, Canada, and Washington State, U.S.A.: An Emerging Threat"; "Levels and Patterns of PBDEs Measured in Human Tissues from Four Continents and in Food and Environmental Samples from Selected Countries."

You get the picture. They're everywhere.

Dust to Dust

One of the basic questions that PBDE researchers continue to wrestle with is how PBDEs get into people. They seem to be quite different from other persistent, bioaccumulative toxins that enter the human body, mostly through food. In fact, for a number of years, the levels of PBDEs being measured in Americans didn't make any sense to scientists at all. In some people the levels were low, while in others they were hugely elevated—from 100 to 500 percent above the national average. With food-borne pollution, levels across populations are similar, because everyone eats food. There was obviously some other, unidentified source of PBDEs in everyday life that could cause marked differences between individuals and households. But what was it? Heather Stapleton, an academic at Duke University, was one of the first to solve this riddle.

She recalls that shortly after PBDEs were noticed by the scientific community, everyone started measuring levels in water, soils and sediments. And yet PBDEs are used in objects like sofas, rugs and television sets. "I remember thinking to myself that we were measuring for these things in external environments when they're actually found in internal environments." So Stapleton took a sample of house dust that she had been testing for pesticides and lead, and analyzed it for PBDEs instead. She was shocked at the results. Levels of flame retardants were much higher than she had expected.

Next she measured dust samples from sixteen homes in the Washington, D.C., area. Again she found very high levels of PBDEs. It turns out that PBDEs leach out of the products they are put into: the squishy foam in a sofa, the padding in a mattress, the back of a TV set. They waft into the air in our houses and offices and cars and sailboats and settle to the ground as dust.

PBDEs and Rug Rats

Stapleton's research points to the extreme risk PBDE pollution poses to children. Because they're closer to the floor, because they play in places where dust lurks (such as under the bed), children are uniquely vulnerable to this sort of indoor pollution. Further, PBDEs were not around when my grandparents were born. They spent much of their life unexposed to these toxins. In my childhood PBDEs existed, but they were not as common as they are now. My two young boys are wallowing in the stuff every day and will bump up against this pollution for the rest of their lives. Younger people have higher levels of PBDEs than older people do. In contrast to our PCB success, PBDEs—and some other newer pollutants—are a legacy we are leaving our children.

Heather Stapleton has continued her research. She presented a study at the Victoria meeting on two new kinds of BFRs that she had recently found in household dust: 2 (ethylhexyl) 2,3,4,5-tetrabromobenzoate (TBB) and bis (2-ethylhexyl) tetrabromophthalate (TBPH). These chemicals are the basis of the new flame-retardant mixture Firemaster 550, manufactured by the Chemtura Corporation (a new company formed by amalgamation of Great Lakes Chemical and the Crompton Corporation in 2005). Stapleton was told by chemical and furniture manufacturing companies that "they would be very surprised" if she found the new BFRs in household dust. Well, she did. Three to four years after Firemaster 550 first appeared on the market as the preferred flame retardant for the polyurethane foam used in many North American sofas, its chemical ingredients were present at detectable levels in household dust.

Who knew that dust bunnies could be such dangerous beasts?

With all this evidence of contamination and harm, with all these similarities to PCBs and the discovery that PBDEs are now polluting the most private recesses of our homes, the million-dollar question is obviously "Why haven't PBDEs been completely banned?"

Deborah Rice, of the Maine Center for Disease Control and Prevention, thinks it's because there's been no *yushō*-style catastrophic accident with PBDEs so far. Whatever pollution is happening is slow. It's quieter and more insidious than PCBs. Nobody has died from a huge dose of the stuff, so there's been no graphic illustration of the damage it can do. If there had been, people would be able to extrapolate and realize the harm being done to them over time by much smaller doses. To be crass about it, the bromine industry has not been held to account because no one has yet been able to produce a dead body linked to PBDE poisoning.

"You're Human!"

I went to the Victoria meeting armed with my PBDE blood-test results. Unlike with other chemicals to which I'd subjected myself for our books, I didn't try to manipulate the levels of PBDEs in my own body. I just offered up ten vials of blood for a one-time test and called it a day.

I decided on this approach because, according to the experts I spoke to, PBDEs are so prevalent and have such long half-lives (measured in years) that it would be impossible for me to significantly affect levels in my blood in just a few days. Actually, that's not entirely correct. I probably could have jacked up my levels of PBDEs very quickly, but in order to do so I would have had to stray into outlandish activities, and thereby violate the one immutable law that Bruce and I agreed would define our experiments—that we would stick with "everyday" activities.

Short of jumping up and down on a decaying old couch for hours on end, filling a room with PBDE-laden dust and aspirating it with vacuum-like zeal, or eating dust bunnies for breakfast, I could not alter my PBDE levels in anything less than weeks or months, not days. (Interestingly, however, in Victoria, Åke Bergman presented the results of a brand-new study in which eight Swedish travellers showed significantly increased PBDE levels after taking long-haul flights overseas and returning home a number of days later. Aircraft, with all their upholstery and foam insulation and closed air systems, are extremely high in PBDE contamination, so perhaps under other specific conditions like that, PBDE levels can be affected relatively quickly.)

In my own body it turns out I have eight detectable PBDEs (see Table 3). "You're human!" joked Coreen Hamilton, then director of research at SGS AXYS Analytical Services, the lab that evaluated many of our blood and urine samples. "Everyone's got similar levels. These look pretty typical."

Table 3. Rick's PBDE results are shown in comparison to the National
Health and Nutrition Examination Survey (NHANES) results. The
NHANES data are based on blood samples collected from U.S. citizens
and analyzed for PBDE levels.

BDE Type	My Results (ng/g lipid)	NHANES Geometric Mean (ng/g lipid)	NHANES Median Mean (ng/g lipid)	NHANES 25th Percentile (ng/g lipid)
BDE 15	0.1	NA	NA	NA
BDE 28	0.4	1.2	1.1	<LOD
BDE 47	8.1	20.5	19.2	9.3
BDE 49	0.1	NA	NA	NA
BDE 99	1.3	5.0	<LOD	<LOD
BDE 100	1.2	3.9	3.6	1.6
BDE 153	4.1	5.7	4.8	2.4
BDE 154	0.1	*	NA	NA

* Not reported; 75th percentile is 0.8.
"NA" means not measured by NHANES.
"LOD" means result less than level of detection of analysis.

I dug a bit deeper with Tom Webster of Boston University, asking
him how my results compared to the findings of the huge National
Health and Nutrition Examination Survey (NHANES) study—a regular
survey of levels of environmental contaminants in the U.S. population
by the Centers for Disease Control.[22]

Webster contrasted my results with the geometric mean, the 50th
percentile and the 25th percentile of the 2,062 NHANES study participants. "As you can see, for all reported congeners, your values are less
than the geometric mean and 50th percentile. For BDE 47 and BDE
100, you're also less than the 25th percentile. For BDE 153 you're
between the 25th and 50th percentiles. So overall, I'd say that your
PBDE[23] concentrations are less than the typical U.S. resident. There
have been some suggestions that Canadians have lower levels than
Americans, on average, but until we have a representative sample of
Canadians, we won't know for sure."

I couldn't stop thinking about Coreen's offhand comment: "You're
human." How strange and disturbing that the defining characteristics
of most humans on Earth now include, along with two eyebrows and
ten toes, measurable levels of brominated diphenyl ether #153.

If they want to, future archaeologists will be able to define toxic eras in human history by analyzing the telltale levels of these potent, globally distributed chemicals in our race's desiccated remains. The classifications might go something like this: Era PCB (1950 to 2030); Epoch PBDE (1980 to 2075); Age of Firemaster 550 (2005 to ?)—like the rings of a tree or the layers in sedimentary rock.

The Global Bromine Oligopoly

Deborah Rice thinks there's a second big difference that explains the relatively quick ban on PCBs as opposed to the excruciatingly slow progress on PBDEs. Quite simply, the bromine industry is organized.

As *Chemical Marketing Reporter* put it, "the global bromine industry is essentially an oligopoly controlled by Albemarle, Great Lakes [now LANXESS Corporation], and the Dead Sea Bromine Group [now ICL Israel Chemicals]."[24] In 1997 these companies banded together with the Tosoh Corporation to form the Bromine Science and Environmental Forum (BSEF), an association that lobbies for their common interests. Together, BSEF members control over 80 percent of the global production of brominated flame retardants, a sort of OPEC of BFR.

They have been very successful advocates for their product. Market demand for flame retardants increased from 372 million kilograms in 1996 to 450 million kilograms in 2006. By 2015, global flame-retardant consumption totalled $6.29 billion. and this figure is currently expected to grow to $11.96 billion by 2025.[25] PBDEs are now found in a huge number of common consumer items, with the majority being used in the ever-increasing panoply of electronic devices, gizmos and gewgaws that fill our lives.[26]

Unlike other industrial groups I've dealt with over the years, the bromine barons push their products through lobbying, in many cases for *more* government regulation. Industries usually avoid regulation like the plague, engaging in huge lobbying offensives to derail it entirely or to make sure it's so toothless that they can safely ignore it. And, of course, as we'll see in a moment, BSEF members do their fair share of this. Bromine companies work relentlessly to persuade governments to leave their affairs as unregulated as possible, and at the same time they push for tighter and tighter regulations on the business of others, for instance by promoting increasingly stringent flammability standards on manufactured goods. As we've seen, going all the way back to the use of tris-BP in pyjamas, fire-prevention standards mean darn good business for bromine companies. The higher the standards, the better. Not surprisingly, the BSEF is represented on key committees in major jurisdictions that actually make the decisions on new flammability standards.

I met Joel Tenney, then the North American advocacy director for Israel Chemicals, and the BSEF's Canadian lobbyist, Chris Benedetti, at the Victoria meeting on brominated flame retardants. Listening to them, you'd think that BSEF members are really in the business of public service, just doing their part to save lives and property and combat accidental fires (and, of course, they can quote chapter and verse on the number of accidental fires specifically avoided due to the wonders of BFRs).[27] The seeming reasonableness of the industry's message and its spokespeople is belied by the ruthless way they have dealt with their critics over the years, seeking to stall any progress on bromine regulation.

The PCB Playbook

When PCBs were banned, industry's attempts to forestall the inevitable lasted only a few years. The evidence of global contamination and human health problems linked to PCBs, along with numerous PCB spills throughout Europe and the United States, quickly made it clear that the jig was up. An insight into the industry's thinking can be gleaned from a fascinating 1969 internal discussion paper from Monsanto—the only PCB manufacturer in the U.S. at the time. Titled "PCB Environmental Pollution Abatement Plan," the document acknowledges that "PCBs are a worldwide ecological problem" and sets out three possible courses of action, noting the pros and cons of each.

Here are some excerpts from the Monsanto "playbook." Under "Courses of Action," they list:

A: Do Nothing. We would most likely be forced out of this business. Other product areas would be adversely affected. We would project an image as an irresponsible member of the business world . . .

B: Discontinue Manufacture of All PCBs. Although we all realize this could be an eventually [sic] unfortunately the solution is not this simple. . . . Other product areas would be affected. . . . Competition would take advantage on all fronts. We would be admitting guilt by our actions. . . .

C: Respond responsibly, admitting that there is growing evidence of environmental contamination by the higher chlorinated biphenyls and take action as new data is generated to correct the problem. . . . We could maximize the corporate image by publicizing this act. . . . Additionally we could gain precious time needed to develop new products and investigate further the lower chlorinated materials.[28]

Monsanto chose option C (seem reasonable on the surface but do everything possible to delay) over option A (refuse to take action; be patently unreasonable) or option B (do the right thing). Similar approaches are taken by bromine companies today.

In 1970 Monsanto announced that it would no longer sell PCBs for use as water-resistant plasticizers or as hydraulic fluid but that it would continue to manufacture the chemical for use as a coolant in electrical transformers.[29] In spite of the unstoppable momentum behind a PCB ban, the company kept producing PCBs for almost six more years. It wasn't until early 1976 that Monsanto announced it was planning to phase out the manufacture of PCBs completely. Even then the company spokesman said he couldn't give an exact timetable for the phase-out.[30]

Fast-forward to Europe in the late 1990s in the wake of the Swedish breast milk study. While protesting all the while that their products were safe, BSEF members started to soften their public line defending penta-BDE (referred to as "penta"), one of the three commonly used PBDEs, but they retrenched around defending the other two PBDEs, "octa" and "deca." When the European Union and California proceeded to ban penta and octa in 2003, Great Lakes Chemical announced it would voluntarily phase out those two chemicals by 2005 but ramped up its defence of deca and newer products like Firemaster 550. "Deca-BDE is the most widely used of the three and has been tested extensively by the National Academy of Sciences, the World Health Organization, and the EPA [the U.S. Environmental Protection Agency]," the BSEF said at the time. "All have given deca-BDE a clean bill of health."

Since we published *Toxin Toxout* in 2012, progress to finally get rid of deca has accelerated. In 2017, the E.U. decided to ban the use of deca in consumer items in quantities greater than 0.1 percent. The ban takes effect in March 2019. Unfortunately, items placed on the market prior to that are exempt, as is the ongoing use of deca in aircraft and certain other applications. As a result of negotiations with the EPA, the manufacturers of deca voluntarily agreed to phase out its use in the U.S. by 2013. A voluntary phase-out happened in Canada around the same time. Deca continues to be used in many other places in the world.

Tris-BP and PBBs in the 1970s. Ethylene dibromide in the 1980s. Penta and octa in the 1990s. Deca and Firemaster 550 today. The bromine industry's use of the "PCB playbook" has succeeded for almost forty years.

Putting Out Fire with Gasoline

For a few years, I will confess, my wife and I were addicted to the TV series *Mad Men*. The reality depicted in the show would be the kind of world the flame retardant industry would really enjoy. *Mad Men* follows the lives of a handful of hard-drinking, philandering advertising executives in New York City in the early 1960s. Everyone in the show smokes—at work, in boardrooms, offices, bathrooms, beds, cars. Such a world, with so much potential for house fires caused by lit cigarettes, is a flame retardant industry executive's dream. The more fires there are, the more loss of life, the more property damage, the more support there would surely be for infusing every household item with flame retardants.

One of the greatest challenges to the industry's ongoing attempts to convince companies to flame-retard so many products has come from an unlikely source: the international movement to legislate self-extinguishing or "reduced ignition propensity" (RIP—an unfortunate acronym) cigarettes. Canada became the first country to require, in 2005, that cigarettes be made from special paper that has bands, or "speed bumps," to slow the burn. Europe now has a similar continent-wide standard. In the U.S., all fifty states have mandated RIP guidelines for cigarettes since 2011.[31] To the extent that smouldering cigarettes are the leading cause of fire deaths—and that this new kind of cigarette will, by some estimates, eliminate three-quarters of these fatalities—the flame retardant industry may have finally met a flammability standard from which it derives no benefit. Less risk of fire equals less traction for its arguments in favour of chemical flame retardants.

Nonetheless, the industry's intransigence is incredible. In a fascinating development it turns out that many of the top lobbyists for the flame-retardant industry formerly worked in the tobacco industry. In a blockbuster series of articles in 2012, the Chicago *Tribune* explored this tight connection and exposed other shady practices that the flame-retardant industry has used to push their products.[32] Lobbyists for the flame-retardant industry spearheaded efforts to oppose the spread of self-extinguishing cigarettes and founded an organization of fire marshals to advocate for the use of flame retardants. The fire marshals then petitioned the Consumer Product Safety Commission to require manufacturers to make upholstered furniture that would resist ignition by an open flame, a severe standard that would best be met with pounds of flame retardants in a couch. Dangerous cigarettes and toxic flame retardants: a match made in heaven (or perhaps hell).

After years of the industry getting its way, I'm delighted to report that, since *Slow Death* was first published, the tide has . . . just maybe . . . started to turn in the flame-retardant debate.

There is no more stalwart opponent of damaging flame retardants than Arlene Blum. In the late 1970s it was Blum's research that exposed the problem of toxic tris-BP flame retardants in babies' sleepwear, and she's been one of the global leaders in the fight for rational regulation of flame retardants ever since. Though she wouldn't use the word "optimistic" in reference to the current state of the debate when she spoke with me over the phone from California, she certainly sounded more positive than she did when last we spoke ten years ago.

"With flame retardants, the debate revolves around standards," Blum says. "In the U.S. and internationally we've been very successful. The California furniture standard was changed in 2014 so flame retardants are no longer needed in furniture or baby products across the U.S. and Canada. That's pounds less toxics in every home. And despite industry opposition we've prevented new standards that would have resulted in unnecessary flame retardants in items as varied as pillows and computers. Nonetheless, large amounts of unwarranted flame retardants continue to be used in TV cases and building insulation."

The results of the efforts of Arlene and her allies have started to pay off in major ways: levels of PBDEs in the breast milk of California women significantly decreased between 2003 and 2012.[33]

Arlene's goal is to move away from the flawed approach whereby governments evaluate the toxicity of chemicals one by one. "To reduce the use of unneeded and harmful chemicals and protect our health and environment, we need to think about whole classes of chemicals of concern and ask if they are necessary given the potential for harm," she told me. To this end, she's delighted by the September 2017 vote by the CPSC to move towards a ban of all halogenated flame retardants in a range of consumer products. "This is a historic ruling. It has the potential to prevent the common practice of banning a harmful chemical only to replace it with a similar chemical that causes similar health problems. I think it will set a precedent of regulating chemicals by class and can prevent harm from exposure to the entire chemical class." She went on: "The CPSC recommendation should send a signal to manufacturers to limit use of all flame retardants in products where they do not provide a fire safety benefit. After all: there is already data suggesting that alternative flame retardants may pose similar health problems."

With any luck, Arlene Blum's forty-year quest to detox us from flame retardants may be coming to a successful end.

Owain's Pyjamas

Jennifer was right, of course. I never did get around to phoning about the penguin pyjamas in time to use them that winter of 2008. Our kids continued to wear their somewhat ratty hand-me-downs to bed. And it was just as well. After the PJs had sat on my desk for eight months, I finally got tired of looking at them and phoned Carter's to ask some questions.

"There are no flame retardants in our 100 percent polyester pyjamas," I was assured by the nice woman at the other end of the customer service line. "They're all natural. The polyester is naturally fire resistant." Not aware that polyester is "all-natural" anything, I asked if she could send me something in writing to confirm this. Within minutes (leading me to believe that perhaps they'd heard this question before), I received a short document by email, emphasizing that Carter's products "are made of polyester which complies 100% with CPSC guidelines."

After doing a bit of research on what those CPSC guidelines were at the time, I discovered that most polyester in sleepwear was infused with a few different kinds of flame retardant. They aren't painted on the surface of the garments as tris-BP was (the CPSC calls this "treated") but rather bonded right into the fabric.[34] Chemicals used in this way included halogenated hydrocarbons (chlorine and bromine), inorganic flame retardants (antimony oxides) and phosphate-based compounds. I e-mailed Carter's, asking exactly what flame retardant was being mixed into their polyester, and a week later I received this message from the "Quality Department": "We rely on the natural flame resistant properties of polyester. When manufactured in a clean environment we meet all applicable state and federal regulations." That didn't really answer my question. And the penguin pyjamas were forever consigned to a dusty box in the corner of our basement.

Ten years on, most children's sleepwear isn't being made with halogenated chemicals. And that's a great thing. But we still have some way to go to make sure that kids—and all of us—aren't being haunted by toxic flame retardants when we go to sleep at night.

FOUR: QUICKSILVER, SLOW DEATH

[BRUCE EATS MUCH TUNA]

I was eating tuna four times a week. I had crying spells, low-grade depression, loss of memory, and brain fog, which is where I would be talking to you and I would get disoriented.[1]

— DAPHNE ZUNIGA, ACTRESS

ALL SHE WAS DOING WAS EATING "your average Hollywood stay-in-shape diet, a ton of fish and low carbs," actress Daphne Zuniga told *ABC News* in 2005. Perhaps best known for her starring role in the 1990s TV series *Melrose Place*, Zuniga recollected that she "would go out for sushi and think, 'Oh, great, at least we're not going for Italian, with all the oil and carbs.'"[2] Over time, however, she noticed unusual symptoms, including an itchy rash all over her body that landed her in the emergency room. She saw plenty of doctors, but nobody seemed to have a clue. It was only after reading a commonly quoted statistic from a U.S. Environmental Protection Agency study to the effect that one in six women of childbearing age has elevated mercury levels that she thought she should go for tests. Sure enough, her blood mercury levels were significantly over the safe level. She changed her diet and the symptoms largely disappeared within six months.

That mercury poisoning of TV stars made headlines was somewhat of a breakthrough for a toxin that has been quietly haunting humans for thousands of years. The mercury story is one of human tragedy, industrial malfeasance, government collusion and the shocking inability of humans to act prudently when presented with the facts. There are powerful lessons to be drawn from mercury that help shed light on some of the other substances Rick and I tested. Why, for example, does it take so long for a toxic chemical to be banned from use in products humans consume when we know it causes harm? And how is it that we continue to believe the corporations that profit from toxic pollution when, time after time, substance after substance, they are proven to be wrong and the public pays the price? By asking these questions I am hopeful that we are starting to make some progress on the solutions.

Bruce's Tuna Feast

It's Saturday and the tuna-eating experiment is about to begin. I love tuna. I love tuna sandwiches, I love tuna sushi, I love grilled tuna steaks. Because of my love of this fish and, frankly, all seafood, I tend to eat more of it than the average North American or European. It's not unusual for me to eat about eight fish meals in a week. Fish, after all, is an important source of protein and fatty acids. So, with the task of figuring out who was going to expose themselves to which toxic chemicals, I, of course, jumped at the chance to be the tuna guinea pig. How difficult could it be to eat a little tuna?

Given my high level of fish consumption, I needed first to try to bring my background mercury level down to one more like that of a typical North American. We did no pretesting at this stage, but to be safe I avoided tuna and most other sources of fish for about six weeks. Given that the half-life of mercury in our bodies can be several months, this probably had only a modest impact on my actual mercury levels.[3]

Colleagues of mine at the University of Quebec in Montreal are among the leading mercury researchers in the world. Whenever they do field research, they test their mercury levels in advance of their travels and upon their return. Invariably their mercury levels increase noticeably as a result of eating the local fish at the places they visit. From this I knew that it was theoretically possible to measurably increase the level of mercury in my blood by eating fish that presumably contained mercury. What I did not know was whether eating a few meals over the course of forty-eight hours would make a detectable difference. I was worried that, given the large amounts of fish I eat regularly, a few extra tuna meals would not have much effect.

After drawing my first blood sample to determine my pre-tuna mercury levels, I got to work making a tuna sandwich. We regularly purchased many varieties of canned tuna, but I chose my favourite: solid white tuna. Solid white also happens to have the highest levels of mercury. Flaked or chunk light tuna has lower amounts of mercury because the fish used in flaked tuna tend to be smaller. Smaller fish have lower concentrations because they are younger and eat smaller fish themselves, so the effects of biomagnification tend to be less pronounced. ("Biomagnification" is the term used to describe how levels of toxins increase with the larger and higher in the food chain a predator is— because it keeps not only its own toxins but also the accumulated toxins of the prey it eats, the prey its prey eats and so on.) The larger fish are also usually older and have had more time to bioaccumulate mercury in their diet over many years. Tuna can live for twenty years and reach weights of up to 700 kilograms (1,500 lb). These are the most prized for sushi.

Most readers will be familiar with the classic tuna sandwich or tuna salad, but we all have our favourite variations. My tuna sandwiches are usually made with a can of tuna, a tablespoon or two of real mayonnaise, a chopped celery stalk and a big squeeze of lemon. Unfortunately, on day 1 we were out of celery, so the tuna salad was a little bland. I spread the filling on commercial whole-wheat bread.

Without celery as filler, the tuna seemed to disappear easily into the bread, and before I knew it I had managed to get an entire 5-ounce (170 mg) can of tuna into my sandwich. Six minutes later I'd downed it. Rick stared at me with an evil glint in his eyes and then turned to the other tuna cans on the counter.

"Surely," he remarked, "that little tuna sandwich didn't fill you up. How about another?" As a matter of fact, I was still a little peckish, so I accepted the challenge.

It was day 2, another twenty-four hours had passed, and once again I made a tuna sandwich for lunch (to be followed by a blood sample at 5:15 p.m.). Rick and I were in the middle of breathing perfluorinated stain-resistant chemicals at the time (see chapter 2), so the chance to get out to the kitchen was a welcome break from the nasty fumes. This time I ate only one sandwich, filled with an entire 7.5-ounce can of solid white albacore tuna. I also had a cup of tea, but not in polycarbonate plastic (see chapter 7); deliberate exposure to two or three nasty chemicals at a time is enough for me. Tea, according to a recent paper by my mercury-studying colleagues in Montreal, can remobilize mercury stored in your body.[4] That means it adds old mercury, probably from your liver, to the new tuna mercury. On the other hand, tea (green and black) seems to reduce the bioaccessibility of mercury as it is ingested.[5] So who knows.

At 5:45 p.m., after a few hours of sitting and breathing PFOA, I downed a healthy trayful of tuna sushi and sashimi takeout. For non-aficionados of this delicacy, sushi is raw fish on a little bed of cold sticky rice, and sashimi is just a piece of raw fish on its own. I ate them with wasabi (Japanese horseradish) and soy sauce. This was just an appetizer. Soon, after happily gobbling down the contents of my tuna sushi tray, I was presented with another tray of (much nicer-looking, I must admit) tuna sashimi, sushi roll and nigiri sushi—for dinner. It took me a good forty minutes to polish off this batch, and I was forced to wash it down with a beer or two.

Day 3 looked remarkably like day 2, with another tuna sandwich for lunch. It was not a very memorable sandwich, to be honest, or perhaps that was the mercury kicking in, since I don't remember much of day 3; frankly, it was a hellish day. I am generally very relaxed, easygoing and almost unflappable, but by day 3 in our condo, I was miserable. It suddenly occurred to me that perhaps this feeling of intense and uncontrollable irritability was the mercury building up in my body. Was I experiencing a Daphne Zuniga "brain fog"? At this point I had no idea whether or not my mercury levels were, in fact, any higher, but I was definitely experiencing an unpleasant anxiety.

Amazingly, I was looking forward to another tuna dinner—a couple of big, thick tuna steaks from the fish market. I was more than happy to cook them. By now—after reading chapter 2—you may have guessed that they were cooked in a frying pan with a non-stick coating. This was not to keep the tuna from sticking, of course, but to make sure we were not missing any opportunities to add to the perfluorinated chemicals Rick and I were inhaling in the other room.

I rubbed the tuna steaks with a combination of white and black sesame seeds and seared them in the hot frying pan with a little olive oil. We had a small salad and a little wasabi mayonnaise and, of course, an icy beer or two. Despite this being my seventh tuna meal or snack in three days, I had no trouble consuming a hunk of tuna that weighed just over a pound (500 grams), far larger than a typical serving. At close to twenty dollars a pound, fresh tuna is so expensive that only rich people can poison themselves in this way.

There are, of course, cheaper ways of elevating your mercury blood levels, especially if you enjoy sport fishing. Most lakes in North America have advisories warning against eating certain fish, and 80 percent of fish advisories are due to mercury contamination.[6] If you can catch good-sized fish like pickerel or walleye on a regular basis, you'll have no trouble poisoning yourself. In fact, this happened to a fellow living in Minnesota, who became seriously ill to the point where he was hospitalized and unable to walk.[7] After numerous tests and medical consultations, one doctor finally asked the man's wife if she could think of anything unusual about what he was doing or eating. She thought for a moment and mentioned that he loved to fish and that he ate much of the fish he caught. In fact, she said, he ate fish virtually every day of the week. The doctor immediately tested his blood for mercury, and sure enough, he had levels high enough to qualify him as having Minamata disease, so named after a town in Japan where mercury poisoning was rampant. More on that infamous incident later in this chapter.

Although I suspected my mercury levels would have increased, only blood tests would determine whether, in fact, there was enough of the chemical in my seven meals and snacks to make a noticeable difference in the concentration of mercury in my blood. As with all our blood samples, these were taken according to standard medical research protocols and the blood was centrifuged on site. My mercury blood samples were sent to Brooks Rand Labs in Seattle and tested using EPA Method 1631 protocols.

I was familiar enough with the literature to know that it was possible to elevate mercury levels in blood, and I certainly knew my colleagues in Montreal had demonstrated this. But I was still not convinced that seven meals and snacks would do the trick. What would a substantial increase look like anyway? If I increased my mercury levels by 10 percent, or 50 percent, was that really a big deal?

After five weeks of waiting, I received the results (see figure 6). My first blood test (taken on day 1 before I ate my two large tuna sandwiches for lunch), showed that the mercury concentration in my blood was 3.53 µg/L (micrograms per litre). The North American average is less than 1 µg/L, so I had about four times the average mercury level in my blood before my tuna eating even began. And this was after not eating fish for six weeks.

After three mercury meals/snacks, the mercury in my blood shot up to 7.55 µg/L, more than doubling in less than forty-eight hours. This also sent my mercury levels above the U.S. Environmental Protection Agency reference dose level of 5.8 µg/L. The reference dose is the "safe" level set by the U.S. government, and anything above 5.8 µg/L is definitely cause for concern, primarily for women of childbearing age.[8]

In my final blood test, the morning after my tuna steak dinner on day 3, my mercury blood levels reached 8.63 µg/L. After seven meals/snacks in three days, I had managed to *more than double* the mercury levels in my blood! The experiment had worked. Not only did it reveal high levels of mercury in several sources of tuna, but it also demonstrated how easy it is to spike mercury levels by eating just a few sandwiches and a couple of tuna dinners.

Figure 6. Bruce's blood mercury levels (in µg/L) increased significantly as a result of eating fish.

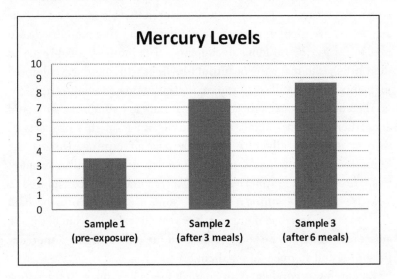

Magical Mercury Tour

Mercury is cool stuff. About twenty-five years ago I started working on issues around mercury—its uses, effects on health and sources of mercury pollution—with a Canadian environmental group called Pollution

Probe. How is it, we asked ourselves, that given all we know about mercury, we are still putting it in skinny glass tubes and sticking those tubes in people's mouths—and other places, for that matter?

Anyone who has broken a thermometer knows how strange and fascinating it is to watch the mercury inside turn into tiny silver-coloured balls that split apart and scatter. Even more bizarre is pushing the tiny balls back together, taking ten or so separate little blobs and watching them recombine into one perfect larger sphere. It's an amateur alchemist's dream, the human equivalent of crows being drawn to shiny objects.

Given these alluring attributes, it's no wonder that many cultures believed mercury had mystical properties, including the power to prolong life. In certain Latin cultures it is said to ward off evil spirits: mercury amulets can still be purchased at street markets throughout Mexico and parts of Central America. Perhaps one of the more dangerous practices was sprinkling liquid mercury in infants' beds to protect them from evil spirits and keep them healthy.[9]

Mercury has been used for many other purposes over the centuries.[10] A Danish researcher has recently discovered that six medieval monks appear to have died of mercury poisoning from using mercury-based inks to transcribe religious documents.[11] The monks probably licked their brushes to make the beautiful fine lines with mercury-laden red pigments that are still so vibrant in their illuminated manuscripts.

The ancient Romans discovered that mercury combines with gold and other precious metals and took advantage of this property to recover gold and silver in the early days of mining. During the Renaissance the physicians of the day believed in its healing properties. Throughout the American Civil War, mercury was considered to be a cure-all for everything from skin lesions to constipation. Abraham Lincoln was prescribed mercury tablets called "calomel," but being the smart fellow he was, he soon recognized the telltale signs of mercury poisoning and stopped taking them.[12]

Research was conducted on Spanish mercury miners in the 1960s that included memorable images of the miners' attempts to trace a curved line on paper.[13] The miners were unable to follow the curve at all and instead produced a jagged, squiggly line resembling a child's attempt to draw lightning. Uncontrollable trembling is one of the early signs of serious mercury poisoning.

We are all familiar with stories of Spanish galleons carrying tonnes of gold and silver looted from the Indigenous peoples of Central and South America. Much less well known is the fact that many tonnes of mercury were transported in those same ships from Spain to the "New World," to mine even more gold and silver. My colleague Luke Trip from Environment Canada visited Zacatecas, Mexico, where up to 34,000 tonnes of discarded Spanish mercury was thought to be present.[14] Luke said it's possible to scoop up a handful of dirt and squeeze liquid mercury from it. To put this in context, one tonne equals one million grams, and if the conditions are right, half a gram can contaminate the amount of water in two hundred Olympic-sized swimming pools.

The height of eighteenth-century European fashion was the beaver felt hat, or what we think of as a typical black top hat. Owing to its fungicidal properties, mercury was used in the manufacture of these hats to ensure that the fur would not "go off." Unfortunately, the hatters (manufacturers) would often go mad as a result of breathing the toxic mercury fumes—hence the phrase "mad as a hatter."

Mercury pollution these days is more complex. We now worry less about direct exposure causing disease and potential death and more about long-term exposure to tiny amounts in our food, which can cause insidious neurodevelopmental problems, especially in children.

Mercury is different from the other substances Rick and I are writing about, because it is a naturally occurring element, not a manufactured chemical. It's been around forever—literally. It occurs naturally in rocks, plants, water and most living things. So volcanoes, forest fires and oceans all release mercury into the atmosphere. This is called "natural" mercury, because the source of the release into the environment is natural. There is also "anthropogenic" mercury, which results from human activity. All mercury released by human-made sources (such as waste incinerators, coal-fired power plants, mercury thermometers and fluorescent lights) fits into this category. These various sources impact us in different ways, as we shall see.

Is Mercury Really Dangerous?

People often ask me, "I used to play with mercury as a kid whenever a thermometer broke. Was that dangerous?"

"Well, probably not really, as long as you didn't play with it for hours on end, day after day," I'd reply, knowing that lots of people (like me) had.

Then I tell the story of the dentist in British Columbia who decided to heat mercury on his stove.[15] It seems he had a great fascination with mercury and for some unknown reason decided to boil some up. Mercury vapour is highly toxic, and the vapours killed him. Not only that, his apartment building was condemned because of the mercury levels, forcing all the residents into a local motel.

Then there was the boy from Ohio who was hospitalized with a mysterious debilitating illness, later discovered to be mercury poisoning.[16] It turned out there had been an accidental mercury spill in his family's apartment, and the mercury vapours caused the fifteen-year-old to become very ill. His symptoms included a rash, sweating, cold intolerance, tremors, irritability, insomnia and anorexia. He was diagnosed with measles, sent for psychiatric treatment and even accused of having psychosomatic symptoms before mercury poisoning was identified as the cause.

In another case a nine-year-old boy was being treated for neurological and kidney problems after a blood pressure device broke, spilling mercury in his house.[17] Unfortunately the boy's mother vacuumed up the spilled mercury, thus inadvertently turning the vacuum cleaner into a mercury vapour distribution device. Each time the vacuum was operated, the warm air from it sprayed highly toxic mercury vapour throughout the apartment.

And consider the terrible tale of a chemistry professor at Dartmouth College.[18] Karen Wetterhahn was very concerned about the toxic effects of mercury on humans and the ecosystem and was working with a particularly toxic form of the metal called dimethylmercury. This rare form is used in research because it produces the effects of mercury very rapidly, allowing studies to take place over short periods of time. Special precautions are required when handling it, and Wetterhahn was wearing latex gloves and working under a fume hood to protect herself. It is believed that one or more drops of the lethal liquid spilled onto her latex gloves. The mercury leaked through the latex and reached her skin. The tiny amount was quickly absorbed by her body and led to devastatingly high mercury levels in her blood. Wetterhahn knew the effects of mercury poisoning and witnessed first-hand some of the classic symptoms: shaking, slurred speech and tunnel vision.

Less than a year after this exposure, Wetterhahn was dead. Her brief exposure to dimethylmercury represented nearly one hundred times the lethal dose. The most tragic part of the story is that if governments and industry had acted responsibly over the past fifty years and banned mercury uses when it was obvious they were causing harm, she probably would not have needed to be doing that research in 1996.

Exposure to high levels of everyday mercury (let alone dimethylmercury) can cause permanent brain damage, central nervous system disorders, memory loss, heart disease, kidney failure, liver damage, cancer, loss of vision, loss of sensation and tremors. It is also among the suspected endocrine disruptors that do damage to the reproductive and hormonal development of fetuses and infants. A growing body of research links mercury to neurological diseases such as multiple sclerosis, attention deficit disorder and Parkinson's.[19, 20]

Medical researchers at the University of Calgary have identified the exact cause of mercury damage to the brain.[21] When mercury concentrates in major organs like the brain or kidneys, it dissolves neurons. The Calgary researchers created a video (available on YouTube) that shows mercury molecules destroying brain neurons as though they were little Pac-Mans munching away on brain cells. Alzheimer's and autism are associated with the kind of brain neuron damage caused by mercury.

So in case there is any doubt, mercury is a seriously potent neurotoxin that will kill you if you breathe it, eat it or otherwise expose yourself to high enough levels. Even moderately high levels taken in over an extended period of time will cause serious physical and mental impairment.

Cool Liquid Metal

Mercury is the only metal that is a liquid at room temperature. Most other metals need to be heated to hundreds or thousands of degrees Celsius before they melt. Liquid mercury, on the other hand, can be stored safely in a plastic bottle.

As with other metals, mercury conducts electricity, and the unusual combination of its being both liquid and an electrical conductor has led to its use in electrical switches. Remember the round household thermostats that first came into use in the 1950s? Or how about the silent wall switches popular in the 1970s? Just one of either of those devices contains enough mercury to contaminate a twenty-acre lake to the point where the fish in the lake should not be eaten.

So why is there mercury in switches? It's quite simple: the little blob of liquid mercury slides back and forth each time the switch is flicked, resulting in an electrical contact forming or being cut off and the light turning on or off. Check to see if you still have a silent light switch at home. It's easy to tell because, rather than clicking on or off, they're very smooth and quiet, and they give almost no resistance to being flicked.

You might think that mercury switches are a pretty limited application, until you realize that so-called "tilt switches" are everywhere. Anyone for ice cream? When you open up the freezer lid, a little blob of mercury slides down the switch and, presto, the light comes on. How about trying to find the tire iron in the trunk of your car? Luckily, a little light goes on when you open the trunk, thanks to tilt switches and the mercury they contain.

Mercury has other uses as well. Because it's a highly volatile substance and vaporizes easily, it is used in virtually all fluorescent and neon lights. The metal vapour conducts electricity inside the glass tube, causing various gases to fluoresce when an electrical current is introduced. Mercury also has the unique property of expanding evenly with pressure and temperature, and this makes it perfect for thermometers, barometers and manometers.

Mercury can be used with other metals, creating combinations called amalgams. (The other metals dissolve in mercury like salt in water.) The best-known mercury amalgams are made with silver and are used to fill cavities in teeth. The average "silver" filling is one-half mercury by weight. Some dentists continue to use mercury, but it is largely being replaced with white composite resins.[22] Controversy and active debate surround the health effects of mercury fillings. A segment of the population appears to have hypersensitivity to mercury, and these people often have their mercury fillings replaced (although removing a large number of mercury fillings at one time is not advisable, since that can result in very high temporary mercury exposure). To this day, dental associations continue to defend the use of mercury.

Perhaps mercury's most obvious property is that it kills living things, including mould and fungus (conveniently preventing bacterial infections in the mouth when used to fill cavities). These properties were well known in the fifteenth and sixteenth centuries, and ailments ranging from constipation and ringworm fungus to syphilis were treated with mercury into the early twentieth century. This has led to speculation that some of the crazy antics of famous emperors and leaders of the past may have been caused by mercury poisoning from their syphilis treatments.

Throughout the twentieth century mercury was used widely in bathroom, kitchen and hospital paints to prevent the growth of mould and mildew, and mercury emissions from drying paint were significant. Most Western countries have now banned this practice. In countries like Canada, where the regulation of toxic substances has been virtually unknown until recently, manufacturers follow international standards. The Canadian market is relatively small— compared to markets in the U.S., Europe or Japan—so Canada rarely sets industry standards that exceed those of other nations. We have not technically banned mercury from paint, but companies operating in Canada agreed voluntarily not to sell paint containing mercury. Mercury has also been used as an agricultural fungicide, notably on potatoes. The high frequency of unusual cancers among potato farmers in Prince Edward Island may be linked to specialized potato fungicides and pesticides.[23][24]

Dancing Cats and Human Tragedy

The devastating effects of mercury poisoning burst onto the international stage in 1956 when residents of Minamata, Japan, started to become very, very ill. Strange behaviour in cats was the first sign that something was awry in this fishing town on Japan's southernmost island, Kyushu. Throughout the town, cats were literally jumping, twisting and doing back flips, which led to the term "dancing cat disease" in reference to the uncontrollable muscle spasms and tremors seen in the poisoned felines.[25] Further research on the cats led local health scientists to the conclusion that mercury contamination in fish and shellfish was the cause of this strange and lethal disease. In addition to dancing cats, seabirds were dropping from the sky, unable to fly.

Seafood was, and still is, the primary protein in Japan and the most important part of the diet of any fishing village. Along with the cats, people in Minamata started to show the telltale signs of mercury poisoning, including trembling, numbness, irritability and tunnel vision, but at the time mercury poisoning was not commonly known in the medical community.

The Minamata poisoning episode provided local medical researchers with the hard evidence that first linked mercury pollution in water to mercury contamination in fish and ultimately mercury poisoning in humans.[26] Based on studies of the deceased, no-longer-dancing cats, specialists identified the cause specifically as methylmercury. It is important to point out that methylmercury is the organic form of mercury, making it much more dangerous in food. This is because organic chemicals ("organic" used here in the sense of substances composed of carbon and hydrogen atoms, not food produced on environmentally friendly farms) can be most easily incorporated into human blood and tissue.

Once the methylmercury link was made, it was not long before the source was discovered to be a chemical plant in Minamata that manufactured polyvinyl plastic. The mercury-laced industrial waste was being dumped directly into Minamata Bay—the same bay where local fishers placed their nets and traps.

Tragically for people in Japan's fishing industry, methylmercury bioaccumulates and biomagnifies more powerfully than almost any other substance known. Even at very low rates of bioaccumulation or with relatively low concentrations of mercury in the water, top predator fish can have mercury concentrations that are hundreds or thousands of times— possibly even a million times—greater than concentrations in the water in which they swim. And this was why eating large fish out of Minamata Bay was deadly.

Eating poison fish, sadly enough, was not the greatest tragedy at Minamata. Government officials ignored the well-established evidence of the local medical researchers for more than *ten years*. Without any government action, the chemical company continued to poison the people of Minamata. Stillbirths, serious deformities and the poisoning of tens of thousands of people might have been largely avoided had the government and the chemical company not acted with such blatant disregard for human suffering.

Today, the symptoms of severe mercury poisoning are still referred to as "Minamata disease." In Japan court battles continue even now between the citizens of Minamata and the Japanese government over compensation for the poisoned families. Despite the devastation and gross negligence on the part of the government and the chemical company, the Japanese government is still fighting to minimize the official estimate of those affected, thereby limiting the compensation it will have to pay. The official government line is that roughly 3,000 people were poisoned by methylmercury. Kumamoto University researchers put the number at 35,000. Many severely debilitated survivors are still living in Minamata today, but many, many more are no longer with us.[27]

Paper, Rock, Fish

Soon after the tragic mercury poisonings in Japan, a number of serious incidents occurred in North America. In 1969 a pulp and paper mill polluted the English-Wabigoon river system in northern Ontario, contaminating the water so severely that the fish were no longer safe to eat. Not only did this destroy the primary food source for the local people, it destroyed their traditional way of life.

Mercury is used in what are called chlor-alkali plants as part of the pulp and paper manufacturing process. It was common practice for a mercury cell chlor-alkali plant to be constructed by a paper mill. It was also common practice for tonnes of mercury to be dumped into local rivers from these plants.

One such paper mill in northern Ontario was located upstream of the Grassy Narrows and Wabaseemoong First Nations, where testing has revealed people to possess high levels of mercury in their blood and hair, levels high enough to suggest symptoms of Minamata disease.[28] Federal and provincial governments claimed that the mercury levels were only modestly elevated, and that they had warned the community in time not to eat the fish. Independent studies suggested otherwise. The Grassy Narrows poisoning made international headlines again in 2017 when a new study found that over 90 percent of the community still showed signs of mercury poisoning.[29] And the *Toronto Star* reported that the Government of Ontario knew in the early 1990s about mercury poisoning upstream from the Grassy Narrows First Nation, but repeatedly failed to inform members of the local community.[30] In June 2017, the Ontario government announced $85 million in funding to clean up, finally, the fifty-year-old poisonous mess.

The negligence that led to enormous quantities of mercury being dumped into the river system, at a time when mercury poisoning in

Japan was making international headlines, is still shocking. Similar incidents occurred across North America, causing the closure of commercial fisheries and destroying the food supply for dozens of local communities.

The mercury from chlor-alkali plants is elemental mercury, meaning it is pure metallic mercury, as opposed to the much more toxic organic form, methylmercury, which was being dumped directly into the ocean at Minamata. The English-Wabigoon River fish were, however, contaminated with organic methylmercury similar to that found at Minamata. How could this be so? you may ask. The answer requires a final chemistry lesson. To make a long story short, mercury undergoes a process called "methylation," and methylation is critical to understanding how mercury ends up in fish—and cats and birds and humans, for that matter.

Methylation is the process through which mercury is converted from inorganic to organic mercury. Organic mercury contains carbon atoms, making this form of the metal much more absorbable by living things. Methylation occurs naturally and to a significant extent in lakes and rivers around the world if the conditions are right. In fact, most lakes, especially northern lakes in North America, contain methylmercury. Places like Minnesota, Ontario, Quebec and Wisconsin seem to be particularly well suited to methylmercury formation, and this has to do with a number of factors, including the type of rock, the acidity of the water and the presence of organic matter in lakes where mercury is found.

To explain the rest of the process, let's look at the reservoirs of hydroelectric dams, where elevated levels of mercury were found in fish in the late 1970s. This type of pollution still exists in dam reservoirs today and is of special to concern to Canada, where so many hydroelectric dams are in operation. Unlike the mercury from chemical plants in Japan or pulp and paper mills in North America, the mercury in hydropower reservoirs is not dumped directly into the water. It comes from the soil. Mercury levels in lakes are also affected by additional mercury that is deposited with the rain, mainly blowing across the North Pole from coal-fired electric plants in China and Eastern Europe.

Mercury is a naturally occurring element found in rock and soil, and it is affected when a river is dammed. First, the dam causes a large area of land to be flooded. Next, when dams flood large areas of forest, the trees die and decompose in the reservoir. This is a critical step, because the rotting plants produce perfect conditions for methylating micro-organisms. The mercury found in the rock underlying a hydro reservoir is released by methylation caused by the increased bacterial activity associated with the decomposition of plant life in flooded areas. And with increased methylation come elevated levels of methylmercury. Some of the world's largest hydro dams are found in northern Quebec; after their construction, the mercury level in large predatory fish in the dam reservoirs was found to be so high that it was several decades before the local Cree population was allowed to consume them.[31]

From a health risk perspective, a toxic substance is only as danger-ous as its ability to get inside your body and harm critical bodily organs and functions. Methylmercury has these characteristics in spades, including two of the most serious toxicity traits: it crosses the blood–brain barrier and it crosses the placental barrier. In fact, not only is it able to get into our brains, mercury seems to prefer hanging out in our grey matter—hence the term "neurotoxic." Mercury also binds to pro-teins. (This is different from "lipophilic" chlorinated chemicals such as pesticides or PCBs, which are stored in our fat.) So in addition to collecting in brains, mercury tends to concentrate in major organs such as the heart, liver and kidneys, and kidney failure is one of the major causes of death from mercury poisoning.

In case it is not now obvious, the mercury dumped into the English-Wabigoon river system was converted to methylmercury by the micro-organisms in the river. The fish (the ones that survived, that is) were soon too contaminated to eat, and the locals lost their food supply and a large part of their livelihood. Meanwhile, we got nice white paper.

Getting Polluted Is Easy

Even when not eating massive amounts of tuna for the purposes of experimentation, I participate directly in mercury pollution. We all do.

The Inuit people of the Canadian Arctic live in what is considered to be the most pristine and fragile ecosystem on earth. Sadly, it is also the world's toxic tailpipe. Poisonous chemicals of all kinds, including mercury, end up concentrating in the Arctic because of global weather patterns and the nasty emission sources located in the northern hemisphere. Arctic animals such as whales, polar bears and seals also happen to be large, long-lived fish-eaters, making them prime candidates for high levels of mercury. In some Arctic communities in Canada, nearly one-third of the women have mercury blood measurements higher than the levels the World Health Organization deems to be a concern.[32] This is in addition to their toxic levels of PCBs, dioxins and fluorinated chemicals. Governments largely abandoned Inuit people's right to a toxin-free traditional diet, and the alternative of eating frozen chicken dinners and other substitutes instead of local wildlife is neither appealing nor healthy.

The major sources of mercury pollution today are atmospheric, and the two largest atmospheric sources are coal burning, to produce electricity, and waste incineration. In the case of incineration, most of the mercury comes from products that are discarded, including fluorescent lights, old batteries, drywall with mercury paint, and electronics. The mercury in coal occurs naturally, and in coal-fired electrical plants it is released up smokestacks when the coal is burned. Once in the atmosphere, mercury can travel thousands of kilometres and be deposited in rain or snow far from the original source.

The atmosphere is not a great place to practise the "dilution is the solution to pollution" motto (which was popular in the 1980s). It's that kind of thinking that has led to the pollution problems we face today. Mercury in the atmosphere can circle the globe, but areas downwind of major pollution sources are usually the hardest hit. In Canada, mercury levels increase from west to east across the country, blown by prevailing winds from coal-fired electrical plants and waste incinerators.[33] Similar patterns of mercury deposits can be found along the paths of prevailing winds around the world.

Medical researchers discovered that mercury poses a health risk even at very low, continuous doses at about the same time that scientists studying atmospheric mercury shifted focus from direct local emissions to pervasive global pollution. Teams of medical researchers studied children who live in the Faroe Islands (in the North Sea) and the Seychelles Islands (in the Indian Ocean).[34] They chose these places because they're far away from any direct sources of mercury and because fish is a major part of the local diet in both locales. After years of study they determined that there is no safe level of mercury. The old way of thinking (that there is a "safe threshold" and that we can pollute up to that level with no effect) was dismissed. Studies, the most famous of which were carried out by Dr. Philippe Grandjean and his team of researchers in the Faroe Islands, found "cognitive deficit" and "impaired motor skills" in children with very low levels of mercury in their blood.[35] The mercury the children were consuming did not come from a local factory dumping waste into or near fishing grounds; it was simply the background mercury found in the ocean today.

These studies led to a major revamping of mercury health standards and the issuing of special bulletins around the world, warning pregnant women not to eat *any* high-mercury fish while pregnant. The studies indicated that fetuses and infants are susceptible to even the tiniest amounts of mercury in their developing brains.[36] The Catch-22 is that for many women around the world, local fish is one of the most important sources of protein and omega-3 fatty acids, so not eating fish during pregnancy may be more harmful to an unborn baby than eating mercury-contaminated fish. Not a great choice. And in spite of the risks, Indigenous peoples of both genders in Canada have been advised to continue eating contaminated fish because of its importance as a protein source.

So where do all these observations and edicts leave us today? There is good news and bad news. The good news is that, thanks to government regulations (mainly in Europe and the United States), mercury use in consumer products has dropped dramatically over the past three decades. Most batteries, paints and switches are now mercury free. Mercury thermometers and thermostats are being phased out.[37] Fluorescent lights still contain mercury, although less now than they did at the end of the previous century. More recently, billions of energy-efficient compact fluorescents (CFLs) have been installed in North America. If your electricity comes from coal, using these low-energy bulbs effectively lowers mercury emissions. That benefit is offset, however, when the bulbs are tossed in the garbage (or broken) and their mercury vapour escapes. Recycling programmes, usually involving a trip to your local municipal recycling depot or IKEA store, recover most of the mercury when the lights are discarded, but a better lighting solution has arrived.

CFLs have turned out to be a short-lived technology with the rapid advances and price reductions in LEDs (light-emitting diodes). LEDs have overtaken CFL sales more quickly than anyone predicted ten years ago, and global lighting giant GE has announced that it will soon be stopping CFL manufacturing altogether. LEDs are the best choice for many reasons; they also save energy and money, but they last for up to twenty years and they are totally mercury free.

As for the coal burning that generates so much of our household electricity, coal continues to be the source of about 40 percent of global electricity production, but coal burning is on the decline. In the United States, for example, coal use is dropping like a black stone, thanks to natural gas and renewable energy. In Ontario, coal-fired electricity has been phased out completely—that's not just good news, but great news! This means coal burning, the largest source of mercury emissions, has turned the corner, and we can happily assert that global emissions of mercury are on the decline for the first time since the Industrial Revolution.

All this good news about mercury in our emissions and products doesn't help when we are still shovelling it into ourselves by the mouthful. Tuna lovers, sushi eaters, pregnant women and children should seriously limit the high-mercury fish they eat. Unfortunately, governments are offering no help in this regard. In Canada, fish with mercury levels that exceed the government's own health guidelines can be purchased at any fish market. My tuna steaks were almost certainly in this category. Recently Environment Canada updated its recommendations and now categorizes tuna as a fish "to be eaten less often." The ministry counsels, specifically, that the general population limit its consumption of tuna to less than 150 grams per week.[38]

I asked Canadian government officials to explain how they could justify such a faint-hearted set of recommendations. I was told fresh tuna are considered by the Government of Canada to be an "exotic specialty fish." The Ferraris of the piscine world, I suppose. The thinking behind the exemption seems to be that fresh tuna is so expensive that average people cannot afford to eat enough to poison themselves.

I think I proved that theory wrong.

FIVE: GERMOPHOBIA

[RICK GOES ANTIBACTERIAL]

I don't like germs. That's why I don't like to shake hands. You just never know what that person did with his or her hand right before it was offered to you to shake. . . .

One final germ warning. Avoid touching the first floor button on the elevator. It is absolutely swarming with germs. I think from now on, I'm taking the stairs.

—DONALD TRUMP, 2006

THERE'S TRICLOSAN IN my garden hose.

Of all the chemicals we're writing about in this book, triclosan was the only one that I was feeling smug about. If you look hard enough, its presence as the active ingredient in many "antibacterial" products is usually labelled, and my family and I have been shunning it for years. So I was pretty sure I had completely banished it from the house.

But there I was one evening, watering our little vegetable garden and looking down at the hose. I noticed for the first time that there were words printed on it. The letters were very small and the words were repeated the entire length of the hose, so at a glance they blended together into a solid stripe. But as I wiped off the grime and stared hard, I could just make out the phrase "Microban Protection." Microban is a producer of antibacterial products that most often contain triclosan as the active ingredient.

Unbelievable! I looked up at the tomato plants that I was unknowingly dousing with germicide, courtesy of my decidedly un-green green rubber hose. As I watched the triclosan water soaking into my backyard soil, I felt a wave of exasperation. Were consumers really suffering from a plague of germy garden hoses in need of a laboratory-engineered solution?

Ciba's Baby

Dr. Stuart Levy, a professor of microbiology at Tufts University, chuckled sympathetically when I told him about my hose. He agreed that the craze for "antibacterial" products has got out of hand; triclosan has indeed crept into some ridiculous places. "We have antibacterial chopsticks here in Chinatown. . . . Toyota advertises antibacterial steering wheels and certain other features. You've got a hose. I've seen a hot tub. I mean, come on, already. If you're really going to advertise it as a product for health, then put it in something where it's going to work. Microban has succeeded in putting it in everything. You can now get a total triclosan bedroom, complete with pillows and pillowcases and slippers!"

So successful have the purveyors of triclosan been, in fact, that the list Levy quickly rattled off is just the tip of the iceberg. The Environmental Working Group has found the chemical in household items as disparate as toothpaste, underwear, towels, mattresses, sponges, shower curtains, phones, flooring, cutting boards, fabric and children's toys. One hundred and forty kinds of consumer products in all.[1] And this is by no means an exhaustive list.

In 2016, the U.S. Food and Drug Administration banned use of triclosan in hand soaps, but the chemical remains an integral part of a wide range of commercial products.[2]

In many ways the history of triclosan resembles that of the brominated flame retardants I talked about in chapter 3. They are both products in perpetual search of new (and increasingly ridiculous) applications. Microban and other manufacturerers of triclosan realized they could take a chemical that had previously been limited to hospital applications, build the term "antibacterial" into a saleable brand, water down the chemical's concentration and insert it into products as diverse as deodorant and countertops.

The slogans used to sell triclosan extol the many virtues of the germ-free life. "Spread love, not germs," said the U.S. Soap and Detergent Association (SDA) in one Valentine's Day press release. An advertisement for pet shampoo says that its "gentle yet effective antibacterial action and the crisp scent of fresh green apples destroys odor and leaves your dog's coat clean and shining." And another company tells us to "wipe-out acne bacteria and excess oil with these towelettes. Medicated with antibacterial Triclosan and Salicylic Acid to help to prevent future breakouts." The growing use of triclosan rang alarm bells for Stuart Levy. In addition to being the director of the Center for Adaptation Genetics and Drug Resistance at Tufts University, Levy founded and continues to serve as president of the Alliance for the Prudent Use of Antibiotics (APUA). As explained on its website, APUA's mission is to "strengthen society's defences against infectious disease by promoting appropriate antimicrobial[3] access and use and controlling antimicrobial resistance on a worldwide basis."[4]

This is no easy task. Infectious microbes are wily beasts. And the way they adapt to antibiotics is a constant challenge for doctors. APUA recognizes it has a major job on its hands, given that "antimicrobials are uniquely societal drugs because each individual patient use can propagate resistant organisms affecting entire health facilities, the environment and the community." As a result "wide-scale antimicrobial misuse and related drug resistance is challenging infectious disease treatment and healthcare budgets worldwide."

This was the backdrop against which Levy started wondering whether antibacterial products might also be contributing to resistant bacteria. "It was at the very beginning of this [antibacterial] phenomenon and Hasbro was impregnating triclosan into some of their toys and claiming it would protect kids from infectious disease transfer. Then [kitchen equipment retailer] Joyce Chen came out with her impregnated plastic cutting board. . . . Corporate marketers discovered that the use of the term 'antibacterial' would be a good marketing ploy; so they started advertising it. I mean, one of the funny parts was when you looked at the Reach toothbrush; the triclosan wasn't in the bristles, it was in the handle. And yet it was advertised as the antibacterial toothbrush."

Dr. Philip Tierno, the director of Clinical Microbiology and Diagnostic Immunology at New York University's Medical Center, also dates his interest in triclosan back to the Hasbro toys incident. Unlike Stuart Levy, however, Tierno is in favour of triclosan in some applications (he personally uses triclosan toothpaste and soap). However, he is withering in his criticism of others. "There are certain products that incorporate triclosan because they want to jump on the microbial band-wagon and make money rather than prevent transmission of infection from one person to another," he says. "One in particular is a pizza cutter which has a wheel—a metal wheel that you would use to slice pizza—and a plastic handle, and the plastic handle has the triclosan incorporated into it." Tierno calls this an "example of a useless product," given that you have to wash the cheese and other pizza bits off the wheel anyway and therefore wash the handle as well. Tierno adds that "many of the formulations of triclosan contain either too little triclosan to be effec-tive or contain it in a ratio that is not ideal for maintaining its germ-killing ability." He'd like to eliminate these products, he says, "because they are taxing the environment—both the human environment and the environment at large—with unnecessary extra levels of triclosan over and above that which is useful from an antibacterial standpoint."

Interestingly, even the company that invented triclosan has become queasy at some of the uses to which its chemical is being put. Klaus Nussbaum was global business head of the hygiene division at Ciba Inc., the company that first introduced triclosan for use in hospital surgical scrubs in 1972. Ciba was at that time the dominant manufacturer of the chemical worldwide. I spoke with Nussbaum at length over a crackly speakerphone (a PR rep was sitting in on the interview) from his office in Basel, Switzerland. Not surprisingly, he was quite positive about the chemical. He pointed out that it's been in use for forty years and rhymed off a number of papers that have pronounced it safe for widespread use. Near the end of the interview, however, Nussbaum made a passing refer-ence to triclosan disappearing "from some applications we're not in favour of." When I pressed him on this point and expressed surprise that there were any uses of triclosan Ciba wouldn't support, given the com-pany's oft-expressed view that the chemical is not harmful to the envi-ronment or human health, he said that it was a "positioning issue for the product." He singled out "widespread, one-use" items like triclosan-infused garbage bags as being of concern to the company.

Even Ciba, it would seem, can't justify its invention sitting in land-fill sites forever, leaching triclosan into our waterways. Even the chemical industry will acknowledge that bacteria actually belong in some places in this world.

The Germs Bite Back

The over-triclosanitization of the planet wouldn't be such a big deal if it weren't for a few niggling problems: (1) mounting evidence that, in many products, it works no better than competing products that have no triclosan; (2) increasing levels in people and the environment that have now been linked to health problems; and (3) the biggie, the emergence of a solid case that it's contributing to bacterial resistance, a.k.a. the rise of "superbugs."

Let's look at each of these in turn.

First off, are antibacterial soaps really no better than "normal" products? Well, in household settings, this would seem to be the case. Studies published by the American Medical Association, the U.S. Food and Drug Administration and the Centers for Disease Control and Prevention's journal *Emerging Infectious Diseases* come to similar conclusions: that in household settings, there is no evidence to suggest that the use of antibacterial soap is more beneficial than the use of soap and water in reducing bacteria or the rate of disease.[5] Another study, of two hundred American households, concluded that people who use antibacterial products have no reduced risk for infectious disease symptoms.[6]

Recently, another large study of American households found that soaps containing triclosan were generally no more effective (and possibly even less effective) than plain soap at preventing infectious illness symptoms and reducing bacteria on the hands.[7] Regardless of where the samples were gathered, there was little benefit associated with the use of soap containing triclosan compared to using plain, regular soap.[8]

Stuart Levy, one of the authors of this study, points out that "in household products, triclosan is probably somewhere around one-fifth or one-tenth the concentrations that are used in hospitals." Levy supports the prudent use of triclosan ("it's great in hospitals") but objects to its use in lower concentrations in a more widespread way. Enough chemical is being put in the products to tout them as "antibacterial" but not always enough to actually kill the germs on our hands.

Second, evidence of the bioaccumulative and persistent nature of triclosan is mounting. It tends to build up in animal and human fat tissues and has been detected in umbilical cord blood as well. Swedish studies have documented high levels of triclosan in breast milk.[9] In one paper published in 2002, it was found in three of five breast milk samples. The

Centers for Disease Control and Prevention found triclosan in the urine of 75 percent of the more than 2,500 Americans tested.[10]

As the use of triclosan becomes more widespread in consumer products, the likelihood of its being emitted into waterways also increases, since approximately 95 percent of products containing triclosan end up going down the drain. Triclosan was one of the most frequently detected compounds in a U.S. geological survey of American streams, likely a result of its presence in discharges of treated waste water.[11] While wastewater treatment can remove much of the triclosan and other compounds, not all of it will be removed. And triclosan risks having toxic effects on algae and aquatic ecosystems. Japanese studies of fish have demonstrated androgenic effects in fish exposed to triclosan, causing changes in fin length and sex ratios.[12] Studies on frogs have shown that low levels of the chemical can interfere with normal thyroid function, triggering rapid transformation of tadpoles into adults.[13] In Scandinavia, government officials have discouraged the use of triclosan as a result of possible endocrine disruption as well as potential bacterial resistance. Concerns have also been raised about triclosan's interference with thyroid activity. In a study of mice, it was found that triclosan affected body temperature, lowering it, and caused a depressant effect on the nervous system.[14]

And finally, the superbugs. The question of whether the prevalence of triclosan is causing bacterial resistance is the hottest debate surrounding this chemical. The American Medical Association went so far as to recommend against the use of antibacterial products in the home, citing evidence of antimicrobial resistance.[15] More recently, the U.S. Food and Drug Administration banned use of triclosan in "health care antiseptics."[16]

Not surprisingly, Brian Sansoni of the American Cleaning Institute (the lobby group for the cleaning-products industry) in the United States calls the allegations about bacterial resistance a "common suburban myth." He points out that the only evidence for bacterial resistance stemming from triclosan exposure comes from the lab and that "there is no real-world evidence linking the use of antibacterial products and their ingredients to antibiotic resistance—none." Sansoni thinks it unfortunate that "continuing to hype this hypothesis" detracts attention from the major contributor to antibiotic resistance, "which is crystal clear: it's the overprescription and the overuse of antibiotic drugs. What we've seen, unfortunately, is both of these scenarios equated in the same breath—you know, antibiotic drugs and antibacterial products. It's like comparing Mount Everest to a molehill."

As one of the primary targets of Brian Sansoni's criticisms, Stuart Levy is careful with his words. "I have said clearly that the use of triclosan is not the primary reason for the bacterial resistance that we face today. It's misuse of antibiotics in humans and animals." Levy continues, "But that doesn't mean we should complacently say that antibacterials aren't an issue. We should look at it and evaluate it and continue to evaluate, but better than that we should ask whether there is a benefit to the consumer if in fact there is the threat that it could be harmful." Levy acknowledges that the existing evidence comes from the laboratory and says, "The word I've always used is 'potential.' If we can observe this in the laboratory, it's certainly likely to happen in the outside world. If you use antimicrobials enough, you'll get resistance."

Germophobia

West Nile virus. Bird flu. Listeria. SARS. Flesh-eating disease. Methicillin-resistant *Staphylococcus aureus*. So often, it seems, there's a new microbe for people to fear.

And not without reason, notes Dr. Chuck Gerba. Gerba, known as "Dr. Germ" in his popular writings, is a professor of microbiology and environmental sciences at the University of Arizona and a noted authority on germs and how they spread. In his book *The Germ Freak's Guide to Outwitting Colds and Flu,* Gerba makes the point that a hundred years ago, infectious disease was the leading cause of death. By 1980 it had fallen to number five, but even as of 2017, infectious diseases represented three of the world's top ten global causes of death, according to the World Health Organization.[17]

Gerba feels strongly that we need to take stock of the situation and "reinvent hygiene" for this century. We need to do so for two reasons. First, he says, "the population is a lot more susceptible in terms of serious outcomes. One-third of our population falls into this group and these tend to be the elderly, babies, and compromised people—like cancer chemotherapy patients—and pregnant women. We're an aging population. Common diseases like diarrhea are just a mild inconvenience for most people, but if you're over sixty-five it can be quite life-threatening."

The second reason, Gerba says, is "the lifestyle changes we've undergone" that put us in contact with more germs than ever before: "More of our food supply is being imported from the developing world, which is exposing us to more varieties of pathogens than we've ever seen before. Eighty percent of us now work indoors in offices, whereas a hundred years ago most of us worked on a farm, in a field, and went into town once a week. Today we spend our days in office buildings, in supermalls, we have cruise ships that have gone from one hundred people to three thousand people, we have stadiums of an enormous size, and basically we're sharing more space with more people than ever before. When you do that, you are sharing more germs with more people than ever before."

Germs are tough and adaptable, and "every time we have a lifestyle change, they take advantage of it," says Gerba. He mentions the SARS virus: "It looks like it came from bats. It got into other animals largely because of the expanding human population and closer contact."[18] Another microbe, the *Legionella* bacterium, likes warm water; in the natural environment it would have been a problem only "if you sat in a hot spring." But in a world full of showers, hot tubs and fountains—ready-made artificial habitats—*Legionella* has thrived and presents a real threat to human health.

So what to do? Unlike Stuart Levy, Gerba is not convinced of the evidence linking triclosan to bacterial resistance. He is sure, however, that it's just not necessary in many cases. "I have my concerns about triclosan largely because I don't think it's been proven to be efficacious in everything it's been used in," he says. "I think people shouldn't go overboard with this. . . . You don't have to disinfect everything you come in contact with. I mean, even when you go out in public, just washing your hands is a good enough strategy."

Unfortunately, Gerba's common-sense approach is too rarely taken to heart.

The target of our modern-day cleaning obsession—the microorganism—was not even widely recognized as the cause of disease until the turn of the twentieth century. For most of human history, people thought that disease was spontaneously generated or was caused by a noxious form of bad air called "miasma." The miasmatic theory of disease became popular in the Middle Ages and was still being defended in the late nineteenth century by people as prominent as the Crimean War nurse Florence Nightingale. People didn't worry about germs. They worried about nasty smells from things like rotting meat, garbage and putrefaction. In order to combat those, they were obsessed with ensuring good ventilation. It wasn't until scientists like Joseph Lister (after whom Listerine and *Listeria* are named) conducted experiments demonstrating the dramatic benefits of antiseptic measures—such as the reduction of hospital infections by hand washing—that people actually believed germs were real.

In the late 1800s soap became cheap enough that the middle class could afford it. Until that point most people had soap for washing clothes and floors but not bodies. And with this new refinement, which included better body soap, broad-scale advertising was born. As Katherine Ashenburg, author of a great book called *The Dirt on Clean*,[19] explains, soap and advertising grew up together. "Advertising by fear"—which targeted the insecurities of the average person—quickly became a staple of the industry. Listerine advertisements in the early twentieth century claimed that "halitosis" was a nationwide epidemic and suggested that bad breath would inevitably upset the natural bond between a mother and child: "Are you unpopular with your own children?" And unmarried women were targeted with lines like "Skin that says, 'I do!'" or "Till BREATH do us part."

Ads were aimed not only at women but also at men. The Cleanliness Institute, an organization supported by the majority of soap manufacturers in North America, ran an ad in the late 1920s with the line "There's self-respect in SOAP and WATER" and a graphic of a well-dressed man with a briefcase looking down at an unshaven, dishevelled man. The recent marketing of "antibacterial" products is simply a continuation of the long and beautiful relationship between advertising and soap.

Rather than buying into the common notion that our ancestors didn't care about cleanliness because they simply didn't have access to the right technology or plumbing or water delivery systems, Ashenburg flips this argument on its head. She believes that technology follows desire. "The Romans had technology for water delivery and plumbing and heating in their imperial baths. That knowledge was not really lost, but until the nineteenth century, people weren't interested in it. The English, who were more interested in being clean in the nineteenth century than the French, were able to have plumbing in the majority of London houses by the 1830s. The French knew about this but declined to follow suit. All of this was really about mentality. The French didn't care to be clean in the 1830s and for some complicated historical and sociological reasons, the English cared more." Ashenburg's conclusion is that people could have been clean in lots of countries centuries earlier, but it was not a matter of interest to them. "Cultures that believed more in a communal sense were much less bothered by the fact that they smelled or their neighbours smelled."

The current unparalleled Western obsession with hygiene—"pretending that we're not of this earth," as Ashenburg says—reflects some very recent changes in societal desires. She concludes that our "germ craziness and all these antibacterial things" are connected to fears like "terrorism and 9/11. Germs, like terrorists, are unseen enemies, and you never know when they're going to strike. I think a lot of the current hygiene thinking is about the American wish to control things."

The irony being, of course, that the current rate of antibacterial use has unleashed a wave of triclosan on the population in an entirely uncontrolled and largely unmonitored manner.

Pesticide Toothpaste

Looking at the array of highly scented, luxuriously packaged, triclosan-infused toiletry items I had assembled for our experiment—surely the pinnacle of soap evolution—humanity's former longstanding disregard for bathing and tolerance of stinkiness seemed very remote indeed.

As opposed to the other chemicals dealt with in this book, our triclosan experiment was comparatively easy to organize. Triclosan is well labelled on products, and if "antibacterial" appeared anywhere on a container, the product wouldn't normally make it into our house. But for the purposes of our experiment, I purchased a variety of off-the-shelf products containing triclosan at local grocery stores and used them in a normal way over a two-day period (see table 4). I felt a little strange deliberately exposing myself to triclosan because, unlike phthalates and bisphenol A—which stay in the body for only a few hours—triclosan sticks around for several days.

In preparing our experiment we had looked at a few studies of triclosan to try to gauge what to expect. Researchers using laboratory preparations of the chemical in skin cream and mouth rinses had demonstrated how easy it was to increase levels in the urine through those single sources.[20] But there are now so many triclosan products on the market that people can easily be exposed to multiple triclosan sources simultaneously.

Table 4. Rick's Triclosan Shopping List.

Bathroom
Colgate Total toothpaste
Clean & Clear foaming facial cleanser
Dial Complete triclosan hand soap
Gillette shave gel
Right Guard deodorant
Dettol pine fragrance shower soap
Kitchen
Dawn Ultra Concentrated dish liquid/antibacterial hand soap
J Cloth (apple blossom scent with Microban)

I used these products for a mere two days, but the effect on my urine level of triclosan was stunning, sending it up from 2.47 nanograms per millilitre (ng/mL) to 7,180 ng/mL. The difference between these numbers is hard to depict visually: because of the huge increase, you can barely see my starting value on the graph (see figure 7). And why, given the fact that we've banished triclosan from our home for years, wasn't my starting value zero? Likely because of the levels of triclosan that are now found in water and food that we all absorb day in and day out.[21]

Figure 7. Levels of triclosan in Rick's urine in two 24-hour urine collections before and after deliberate exposure (ng/mL).

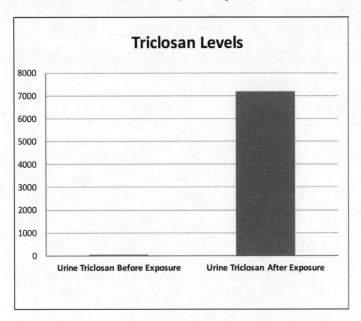

My results were very interesting when compared with recent testing by the U.S. Centers for Disease Control and Prevention (CDC). In 2003 and 2004 an analysis of triclosan levels in the urine of over two thousand Americans revealed that the geometric mean was 13 ng/mL, with a range in values from 2.3 to 3,790 ng/mL.[22]

So after two days, my self-experimentation took me from the very bottom of the heap to far above the highest value recorded to date in the U.S. population. To accomplish this, I used eight different products containing triclosan all at once, a number not likely used by many people. But judging from the hundreds of nanograms of triclosan in the urine of some of the CDC test subjects, the simultaneous use of a few triclosan products is not uncommon.

When I told Klaus Nussbaum from Ciba about the triclosan levels in my urine, he said, "It shows that your body is working very properly in removing triclosan." When I asked if 7,180 ng/mL was at all cause for concern, he answered, "It's high for the moment. Your body is working properly, but you should know that the human body usually adapts in the metabolism of triclosan." I was struck by Nussbaum's use of the word "adapt." The concept that our bodies need to adapt to synthetic chemicals is an interesting one, and biologically true. Given that triclosan is a human creation, the metabolic pathways necessary to break it down and excrete it are indeed things that our bodies need to learn how to do.

I don't know whether the future form of humans is being determined by the chemical soup we're living in, or whether the definition of our evolution as a species has now changed from "survival of the fittest" to "survival of the chemically immune." What I do know is that the ubiquity of synthetic chemicals like triclosan in our daily lives and their accumulation in our bodies are an unjustifiable imposition by the industries that manufacture the chemicals and by the government regulators who are supposed to keep such things from causing harm.

And I certainly don't want any new metabolic pathways for triclosan being activated in my body without my consent.

Nano and the Toxic Treadmill

As if triclosan weren't a big enough problem, the latest incarnation of the runaway antibacterial train presents an even more complicated challenge: nanotechnology, the creation of super-small particles that are only a few atoms or molecules in size. In recent years—with no fanfare and largely unknown to consumers—brand-new kinds of nanotechnology have become commonplace. According to the Project on Emerging Nanotechnologies, an inventory of nanotechnology-based consumer products, the number of products increased threefold between March 2006, when the inventory was released with 212 products on the market, and August 2008, when there were 609 products. As of 2016, several "online repositories" listed more than 2,000 commercially available products incorporating some element of nanotechnology.[23]

According to Dr. Andrew Maynard, director of the Risk Innovation Lab in the School for the Future of Innovation in Society at Arizona State University, average consumers will regularly encounter these nanomaterials and not even know it: "There's quite a range of nanomaterials at present," says Maynard. "People will come directly in contact with things like nano-sized silver particles that are used as antibacterial agents. They'll come in contact with nano-sized titanium dioxide and zinc oxide in cosmetics and sunscreens. They will come across some nano-encapsulates that are used in some cosmetics. They will also indirectly come in contact with things like cerium oxides being used as a fuel additive and carbon nanotubes that are usually embedded in a product. So people aren't going to be directly exposed to them, but they'll be using products that contain them."

And what's the point of nanosilver? As Maynard explains, silver has been known as an effective antimicrobial agent for centuries, but it's not that easy to use. It's very difficult to put a large lump of silver into a product. The only other available option is to use it in chemical form, such as silver ions. Over the past few years, manufacturers have discovered that if you melt silver into very small particles—about 20 or so nanometres in diameter—you can effectively incorporate those particles into a wide range of products, thereby giving them some degree of antimicrobial capability. "So now you're seeing nano-sized silver particles appearing in things like surface coatings, clothing like socks, surfaces of food containers and refrigerators. Almost any product where you can see this foreseeable market for antimicrobials," says Maynard. According to a report from Global Market Insights, antimicrobial coatings (including those using nanosilvers) created over $1 billion in U.S. revenue in 2015. The same company predicts that the American market will double in size by 2024.[24]

While nanoparticles may be new, our scientific understanding of silver is not. The EPA classifies silver as an environmental hazard because of its toxic effects on aquatic plants and animals. A study published in 2005 found that nanosilver is forty-five times more toxic than regular, standard silver.[25] Another study found that nanosilver has the potential to destroy beneficial bacteria used in wastewater treatment.[26] According to a paper published in September 2008, nearly one-third of nanosilver products on the market in September 2007 had the potential to disperse nanosilver into the environment. More recent research notes that nanosilvers generate considerable "oxidative stress" in our bodies, damaging the cellular components of DNA, activating antioxidant enzymes and degrading cell membranes.[27]

In 2006 Samsung introduced a SilverCare washer that released silver ions into the wash. These ions were then released into the waste stream with each load of laundry. Even when socks containing nanosilver are washed, nanosilver is released into the water discharged from the laundry and eventually makes its way into watercourses. The Stockholm Water

Authority claimed that households in Sweden using the nanosilver washing machine would emit two to three times more silver than would be emitted without the use of the washing machine.[28]

In another recent study, the first of its kind, researchers experimented with six different pairs of socks, all of which had been marketed as anti-odour and impregnated with nanosilver. They found that the socks released varying amounts of silver. Some released silver after the first wash, other socks gradually released the silver after multiple washes and others released no silver. More research is needed to find out just how much of the silver particles make their way from the sock into the washing water and ultimately into waste water and the broader environment, including aquatic life and humans. Meanwhile, for the average consumer standing in front of a display of nanosilver socks in a store, there is virtually no way of knowing which socks will release silver and which will not.

Given the lack of monitoring of nanosilver and what Andrew Maynard calls the "very complex" behaviour of nanosilver particles in the environment, more research in particular is needed concerning the impact of nanosilver on soils. Bacteria, after all, are what make soils work. So having soils peppered with a potent "space-age" antibacterial agent is a bit of a problem. The few studies that exist suggest that nanosilver is toxic to bacteria that consume inorganic material and thus release crucial nutrients that are essential to the formation of soil.[29] Toxicity can also affect a bacteria-driven process known as "denitrification," in which nitrates are converted to nitrogen gas in some soils, wetlands and other wet environments. This process is critical because excess nitrates reduce plant productivity. They can also result in "eutrophication in rivers, lakes and marine ecosystems, and are a drinking water pollutant."[30] Nanosilver's toxicity has also been demonstrated in studies that show its effects on mammalian liver cells, stem cells and even brain cells.[31]

While writing the original edition of *Slow Death*, I went to an evening panel discussion on nanotechnology in Toronto. It featured some experts in the field and focused on the prospects for properly regulating this new and exploding class of products. I must admit that in my darker moments that evening, listening to the extent to which nanomaterials are entirely unregulated and learning that even many manufacturers admit they do not fully understand what they're dealing with, I was struck with a feeling that we're on a sort of toxic treadmill. No sooner do we deal with one chemical that's harming our health than we see another one coming along. We can't get off the treadmill and never seem to learn from our mistakes.

I put it to Andrew Maynard that nanosilver is a classic example of this phenomenon, but he was actually more positive than I expected. "It's good that we're still at the starting stages of different types of nanotechnologies being developed and already we're having a fairly broad debate about how you would bring these technologies forward responsibly," he says. "Even though things seem to be a little bit dicey, we're doing a lot better with this technology than we have with previous ones."

The Merchants of Fear

The bottom line is that there's a little of the famous germophobe Howard Hughes in all of us, and the chemical industry preys on this big time.

The avalanche of advertising extolling the (in many cases) nonexistent virtues of triclosan and fomenting a society-wide germ panic is the prime example of this, but the use of fear to peddle chemicals is a theme you'll find in other chapters of this book as well. Fear of fire sells more flame retardants. Fear of insects sells more pesticides. Fear of the odours of daily life sells phthalates.

The irony in all this is that environmental advocates, including yours truly, are frequently accused of "fearmongering" by the chemical industry. "Our products are safe. Don't listen to the scare tactics suggesting otherwise" goes their refrain. An industry representative once called me a "chemophobe," which I thought was a cool word, even though I disagreed with the guy's premise.

So let me put it on the table: I love chemicals. Most of the chemicals in my daily life, including caffeine and alcohol and even the low-VOC paint on the walls of my home, are just dandy.

In my third year of university, I tried my hand at a summer of tree planting in the wilds of British Columbia. One day the bugs were so bad I thought I was going to lose my mind or scratch my eyes out or both. I pulled my long-sleeved shirt over my head so my face was framed by the neck hole and I doused myself—including my head—with a full bottle of the strongest DEET-ridden insect repellent imaginable. DEET is a chemical so strong it actually melts plastic, and you can't even buy bug dope now in the concentrations I was using twenty years ago. But there was no other option on the cut block that day.

So here's a message to the chemical industry: I'm no chemophobe. I'm downright chemophilic in some circumstances. What I object to are the chemicals, like triclosan, that aren't necessary, are possibly dangerous and are foisted on us every day without our knowledge or consent.

A lawn is nature under totalitarian rule.

—MICHAEL POLLAN

HEALTHY GREEN LAWNS ARE lovely to look at and great to lie on. It's no wonder they're the object of envy in the famous saying "The grass is always greener on the other side." I have vivid memories of mowing, watering, fertilizing and chemically treating my family's lawn as a teenager. There was great satisfaction in seeing a freshly cut weedless green lawn with clean diagonal mower tracks. And maybe even some pride in having people think that the grass truly was greener on our side of the fence.

Green lawns require work. But are they worth the risk of children suffering from respiratory disease? Or lawn-care workers getting non-Hodgkin's lymphoma? Or future generations of kids suffering from learning disabilities?

The truth of the matter is that lawns are pesticide guzzlers. They consume ninety million pounds of pesticides and herbicides each year in the United States.[1] Insecticides kill bugs and herbicides kill weeds. Lawn and garden fertilizers that control weeds, known as "weed and feed" products, contain the chemical 2,4-D, the most widely used herbicide in the world.[2] And 2,4-D is a major problem.

DDT Is Good for Me-e-e!"

Most sayings have deep roots, but "The grass is always greener on the other side" is strangely contemporary. Its first recorded use in print was in 1957, only two years before the peak use of DDT in North America, which came in 1959.[3]

Extensive pesticide use had begun after World War II. With mosquito-borne diseases, mainly malaria and typhus, wreaking havoc on the troops in southern Europe, North Africa and Asia, the war had brought large-scale chemical pesticide manufacturing to the United States. Before the war, synthetic pesticides were not in wide use, or even well understood, for that matter, and DDT did not even exist. But between 1943 and 1944, military demand for the potent chemical pesticide had shot up from 4.5 metric tonnes a month to 770 tonnes a month.[4] Desperate for DDT, the U.S. government provided 100 percent tax write-offs on the construction of DDT-manufacturing plants and forced Geigy, the patent owner, to give DuPont a licence to produce DDT, even permitting sales after the conclusion of the war.[5]

After the war, American companies were left with huge DDT production capabilities but no market. Manufacturers were well aware of the economic potential for DDT, and in some ways they viewed the demand for the chemical during the war as simply a means for them to develop government-subsidized production capacity. Despite concerns raised by scientists, DDT became an overnight sensation, and American farming rapidly shifted to the chemical-input model of today. DDT was also used to eradicate garden pests and houseflies, and its huge success led to the invention of all kinds of synthetic chemicals for killing bugs and weeds. Chlordane, dieldrin and aldrin are three chemical relatives of DDT created in the 1940s to target various insects such as termites, moths and grasshoppers. The patent for 2,4-D was issued in 1945,[6] laying the cornerstone of present-day weed science.[7]

Though synthetic pesticides were the talk of the town, the potential perils of DDT use were recognized early on. Scientists began to express concern regarding the human health and biological hazards of the chemical in the mid-1940s, calling DDT "the atomic bomb of the insect world," with "possibilities for evil as well as what seems to the human race good."[8] As far back as 1949, the U.S. Food and Drug Administration commissioner, Paul B. Dunbar, was worried that people exposed to small amounts of DDT and other chemicals over long periods of time might be in greater jeopardy than the soldiers who were briefly exposed to higher levels amid wartime spraying of Agent Orange.[9] The manufacturers of DDT went to great lengths to sell the benefits of DDT to the American public. Witness the 1947 *Time* advertisement "DDT is good for me-e-e!" Creating "meatier" beef, "healthier" homes and apples with no "unsightly worms," DDT was held up as the solution to many problems. But by 1949 the bloom was coming off the rose. DDT began to lose some of its insecticidal effect. Mosquitoes became resistant and required ten times the dose before they would die. And as DDT's intended victims became more immune to its killing power, the impact on its unintended victims became impossible to deny. In 1972, less than thirty years after its first commercial application, all uses of DDT were banned in the United States and in many other countries. Two years later the U.S. banned the use of DDT's toxic cousins aldrin and dieldrin. Unused, yes. Gone, no. Decades later DDT still exists at measurable levels in the environment, and its persistence ensures that its toxic legacy will continue for the foreseeable future. (DDT use continues in countries where malaria is prevalent.)

According to a 2008 study, men with DDE, a byproduct of DDT, in their bodies are 1.7 times more likely than those without DDE to develop testicular cancer.[10] Studies also show that DDT compounds contribute to breast cancer development by blocking the actions of natural hormones that slow down the growth of cancerous tumours.[11] It seems incredible that DDT was used widely in North America for only three decades but is still causing cancer more than forty years after it was banned. This is a powerful lesson in the dangers of highly persistent toxic substances.

2, 4-D, the Hormone Herbicide—and Me

As DDT's fortunes waned, those of 2,4-D waxed.

Short for 2,4 dichlorophenoxyacetic acid, 2,4-D is a synthetic chemical herbicide. More importantly, it is one of the earliest "hormone herbicides." Working its magic by disrupting a number of hormone processes in plants, 2,4-D causes them to grow uncontrollably and keel over dead. It was designed primarily to kill broadleaf weeds (think dandelions), weedy trees and aquatic weeds (seaweed that gets in the way of oyster farming, for example). It is especially valued because it kills selectively, targeting flowering plants and trees but sparing grasses and their

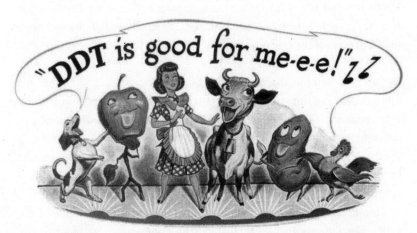

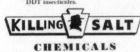

The great expectations held for DDT have been realized. During 1946, exhaustive scientific tests have shown that, when properly used, DDT kills a host of destructive insect pests, and is a benefactor of all humanity.

Pennsalt produces DDT and its products in all standard forms and is now one of the country's largest producers of this amazing insecticide. Today, everyone can enjoy added comfort, health and safety through the insect-killing powers of Pennsalt DDT products . . . and DDT is only one of Pennsalt's many chemical products which benefit industry, farm and home.

GOOD FOR FRUITS—Bigger apples, juicier fruits that are free from unsightly worms . . . all benefits resulting from DDT dusts and sprays.

GOOD FOR STEERS—Beef grows meatier nowadays . . . for it's a scientific fact that—compared to untreated cattle—beef-steers gain up to 50 pounds extra when protected from horn flies and many other pests with DDT insecticides.

Knox-Out FOR THE HOME—helps to make healthier, more comfortable homes . . . protects your family from dangerous insect pests. Use Knox-Out DDT Powders and Sprays as directed . . . then watch the bugs "bite the dust"!

Knox-Out FOR DAIRIES—Up to 20% more milk . . . more butter . . . more cheese . . . tests prove greater milk production when dairy cows are protected from the annoyance of many insects with DDT insecticides like Knox-Out Stock and Barn Spray.

GOOD FOR ROW CROPS—25 more barrels of potatoes per acre . . . actual DDT tests have shown crop increases like this! DDT dusts and sprays help truck farmers pass these gains along to you.

Knox-Out FOR INDUSTRY—Food processing plants, laundries, dry cleaning plants, hotels . . . dozens of industries gain effective bug control, more pleasant work conditions with Pennsalt DDT products.

KILLING SALT CHEMICALS

97 Years' Service to Industry • Farm • Home

Ad for DDT in *Time* magazine, June 30, 1947.

relatives. That is why we can spread 2,4-D all over our lawn and kill the weeds but not the grass. Since corn, grains and rice are in the grass family, 2,4-D was the perfect chemical to kill weeds and plants that grow between rows of these crops. But 2,4-D was hardly perfect.

The list of known or suspected health effects of this herbicide reads like an inventory of the worst possible things that could happen to a human. And I'm not even referring to the nausea, headaches, vomiting, eye irritation, difficulty breathing and lack of coordination that can occur from accidentally spilling 2,4-D on your skin. I'm referring to the long-term effects of exposure to 2,4-D: non-Hodgkin's lymphoma (a form of blood cancer), neurological impairment, asthma, immune system suppression, reproductive problems and birth defects.[12]

This pesticide enjoys particular notoriety because it was one of the active ingredients in Agent Orange, the chemical spray used in the Vietnam War to clear jungle foliage. Agent Orange remains at the centre of ongoing medical and legal battles initiated by soldiers seeking compensation for cancers and other ailments they attribute to wartime exposure. The United States government recently allocated $13 billion in Agent Orange–related health funding for exposed veterans. The people of Vietnam dealing with the aftermath of massively contaminated land have no such recourse.[13]

Given all these deleterious side effects, Rick and I weren't enthused at the prospect of experimenting with 2,4-D, but low-level, short-term exposure is at least less damaging than long-term exposure. So we thought long and hard about the best experiment to increase and then measure 2,4-D in my blood. An obvious test was for me to spray some 2,4-D–laced herbicide on somebody's lawn and measure the 2,4-D in my blood before, during and after the spraying. Remarkably, just as we started laying our plans, the Government of Ontario decided to ban the cosmetic use of lawn herbicides and pesticides throughout the province (not just Toronto, where the cosmetic use of pesticides was banned in 2004). So we decided against trying to measure an increase in my 2,4-D levels. Instead, we did a one-time test for a variety of pesticides in my blood.[14] Because about 50 percent of my diet is organic, and it's been shown that people with organic diets, especially children, have lower pesticide levels in their bodies (see chapter 8), I assumed that my results would be pretty clean.[15]

There was good news and bad news, as it turned out. The bad news was that—like every other person tested by Environmental Defence—I had pesticides coursing through my veins that had been banned for years (see table 5). Hexachlorobenzene, a fungicide used mostly on grain, was phased out in Canada and the United States by the early 1970s, but in 2008 it was still present in me at a level of 1.2 ng/mL (nanograms per millilitre). This was somewhat higher than the U.S. average.[16] At 2.9 ng/mL, my DDE levels were very similar to the U.S. mean of 3.5 ng/mL.[17] Though DDT has been banned in the United States and Canada since I was a child, this telltale sign of chemical pollution still lingered in my bloodstream. Chlordane, a pesticide commonly used on crops like corn and citrus fruits and on home lawns and gardens right up to the late 1980s, was detectable in me in the form of two breakdown products: oxychlordane and trans-nonachlor. Finally, traces of the agricultural pesticide and louse treatment lindane, still in use in North America until the mid-2000s, were also found in my body. And not just mine. All of these pesticides are found in a large percentage of the US population.[18, 19]

Table 5. Bruce's pesticide levels.

Pesticide	Bruce's Levels (ng/mL)*	Health Effects
Hexachlorobenzene (HCB)	1.2	Recognized: carcinogen, reproductive/developmental toxin Suspected: hormone disruptor
Beta-BHC (lindane)	0.5	Recognized: carcinogen, neurotoxin Suspected: hormone disruptor, reproductive toxin
Oxychlordane (chlordane)	0.4	Suspected: hormone disruptor
Trans-nonachlor (chlordane)	1	Suspected: hormone disruptor
DDE	2.9	Recognized: carcinogen, reproductive/developmental toxin Suspected: hormone disruptor, respiratory toxin

* Measured in serum

The good news was that 2,4-D was not found in me at detectable levels. There are a couple of possible reasons for this. 2,4-D is water soluble, not fat soluble like many other pesticides, so it does not accumulate in the body's fatty tissue. In addition, your average 2,4-D molecule has a half-life in the environment of a few months at most, and Toronto's ban on the stuff had been in place for over four years at the time my blood was tested. Many of my fellow North Americans have not been so fortunate. In a 2005 report, for instance, the U.S. Centers for Disease Control measured 2,4-D in a subsample of the U.S. population between the ages of six and fifty-nine and found that one-quarter of Americans who had their blood tested in 2001 or 2002 had detectable levels of 2,4-D in their bodies.[20] However, the real issue is not so much the amounts of 2,4-D found in Americans but the fact that researchers found any quantity of the possible cancer-causer at all. Frustratingly, the U.S. Environmental Protection Agency rejected a petition from the National Resource Defense Council for a countrywide ban of 2,4-D in 2012.[21]

Spray, Baby, Spray

Despite the enormous growth in organic food production over the past two decades, pesticides continue to be used in extraordinary quantities. According to the U.S. Environmental Protection Agency, worldwide pesticide expenditures totalled more than $32 billion in 2000, and this figure grew to $58 billion in 2015.[22] The evident dangers notwithstanding, Americans now spread roughly four million kilograms of 2,4-D on their lawns every year.[23, 24]

One of the most powerful challenges to environmental progress is inertia. The chemical industry works hard to maintain continued pesticide use and thus protect the status quo. The entire procedure works like a game, but the rules are written by the companies that manufacture pesticides. The winners sell more chemicals, but the losers may have much more at stake: cancer and neurodevelopmental disease, for example. The rules of the game are simple. First is the notion that chemicals currently in use are safe, de facto, so companies fight hard to keep existing products on the shelf, and product bans are almost always followed by lawsuits initiated by the manufacturer. As a result, governments are much less likely to restrict or ban an existing product than a new product. In Canada, as with many countries, the onus is on public health advocates to prove that a product is harmful; toxic pesticides are therefore used for years or even decades before enough evidence emerges to have them banned. Thankfully, after years of effort, Canada now leads the world in restrictions on the use of residential lawn and garden pesticides.

The second rule of the game is never to question the fundamental purpose of a product and certainly never to introduce alternative means of reaching the same end. Take lawn care and 2,4-D, for example. The perceived need for smooth green, weed-free lawns is essential to pushing 2,4-D in the market. Many scientists whose studies are financed by the pesticide industry intentionally or unintentionally reinforce the status quo. For example, in a study on environmental persistence and human exposure to 2,4-D conducted by the University of Guelph's Centre for Toxicology, the study begins with the line "Pesticide use can be an important component in well-designed programs to maintain turf grass."[25] This study could also have started with the line "Turf grass is a largely nonessential ground cover requiring the application of toxic pesticides."

Happily, better lawn management has progressed at a rapid pace, and municipalities in Canada now lead the world in their efforts to restrict pesticide use on lawns. What has now become a substantial grassroots (no pun intended) citizens' movement to ban lawn pesticides in hundreds of municipalities across the country first started in the quaint town of Hudson, Quebec, on the outskirts of Montreal. In 1991 Hudson passed a bylaw restricting the cosmetic use of lawn pesticides. This was an innovative move, the first of its kind in Canada. Predictably, a number of chemical companies took the little town to court, claiming that it did not have the legal jurisdiction to ban pesticides. (It is noteworthy that the safety of pesticides was not their primary point.)

A decade passed before the Hudson lawsuit was settled after going all the way to Canada's Supreme Court. But in 2001 the town won the legal right to maintain its bylaw. This paved the way for the dramatic, and rapid, passage of municipal pesticide bans across Canada. What's more, the Supreme Court case was won in part on the precautionary principle. That is, although it was not definitively proven that pesticides on lawns cause specific cancers in people, it was known that many pesticides are linked to health problems, and as the Court ruled,[26] the "weight of evidence" leaned in favour of taking preventive or precautionary action to protect human health and therefore to support the pesticide ban.

In 2003 Quebec became the first large jurisdiction in North America to ban the cosmetic use of pesticides on public lands, when the provincial government consolidated all the individual municipal bans into one province-wide ban. The legislation was extended to cover private and commercial lawns in 2006. As of August 2016, over two hundred Canadian municipalities and seven provinces have enacted cosmetic pesticide bans in varying degrees.[27] And a ban on the cosmetic use of pesticides effectively translates into a 2,4-D ban, since 2,4-D is the primary pesticide used for cosmetic purposes in Canada.

Watching 2,4-D use decline was, of course, highly troubling to the chemical industry. So disturbing, in fact, that in 2008 Dow Agrosciences, a manufacturer of 2,4-D, launched a $2 million lawsuit under the North American Free Trade Agreement (NAFTA), claiming that Quebec's provincial pesticide law was illegal.[28] Dow claimed that the Quebec ban was not based on science. This was a curious position, given that a number of groups representing or including physicians had supported bans on the cosmetic use of pesticides: the Canadian Paediatric Society, the Canadian Cancer Society, the Canadian Nurses Association, the Ontario College of Family Physicians, the Canadian Public Health Association and many other professional medical associations.[29] But for chemical companies facing pesticide regulations, when in doubt, sue somebody.

The moral of this story is that if you leave setting the rules of the game to chemical manufacturers, it's almost guaranteed that the future will look a lot like the present. But happily, the game itself is finally being questioned by astute community leaders and thoughtful politicians. And citizens are the winners, hands down.

Double Exposure

You do not want to spill 2,4-D on yourself. But spills do happen. Based on numerous studies on the effects of toxic substances, there are three fundamental categories of exposure: accidents; ongoing, non-accidental exposure through use at work; and the day-to-day exposure everyone around the world faces. Accidental exposure refers to cases where people using pesticides have spilled them onto their skin or clothes. Studies and clinical assessments of people who have experienced this show that 2,4-D causes nasty immediate effects, such as headache, nausea, vomiting and eye irritation. The chemical is easily absorbed into the body through the skin and the lungs. In a number of cases, it has also disrupted an individual's ability to walk, and these debilitating effects have lasted for three years or more. But the industry will claim only that a chemical is safe under "approved uses" or "when used according to directions." Because these incidents are considered accidental when risk assessments are conducted, in the eyes of the pesticide industry, they don't count.

"Workplace exposure" refers to the regular direct exposure of farmers and pesticide applicators (including people who spray pesticides on lawns for a living). In addition to being much more likely to encounter a spill, they breathe it in and get it on their clothes and possibly their skin if they are not adequately protected. Numerous studies point to a wide range of health problems for this group. The most serious is that they are two and a half times more likely to get non-Hodgkin's lymphoma, a form of blood cancer. People who work with pesticides also have more difficulty having healthy babies. In farming families in North America, for instance, there is a higher incidence of miscarriages and birth defects than in the general population. Farmers in Ontario who use pesticides also have lower sperm counts and poorer-quality sperm than non-farmers.[30]

In addition to exposure through accidents and ongoing everyday use at work, everyone throughout most of the world experiences chronic low-level exposure to pesticides. We encounter pesticide residues on food and in dust and, in some jurisdictions, pesticides sprayed on our own lawns or neighbours' lawns. Sadly, infants are also exposed to pesticides—through their mothers' milk.[31] The potential health effects associated with chronic low-level exposure are the most difficult to identify and understand, but hormone mimicking and other forms of endocrine disruption can result in neurodevelopmental and fertility problems. In these disorders, chemicals interfere with and confuse the development of critical functions related to the brain, the nervous system and/or the reproductive system.

There is a clear link between pesticide exposure and many forms of cancer, and this has doctors concerned. New research suggests that home pesticide use may increase the risk of children developing lymphoma or leukemia.[32] A recent examination by a team of doctors and scientists of more than one hundred studies on pesticides and cancer concluded that most studies on non-Hodgkin's lymphoma and leukemia showed positive associations with pesticide exposure. Children's and pregnant women's exposure to pesticides was positively associated with the cancers examined in some studies, as was parents' exposure to pesticides at work. The most consistent associations were found for brain and prostate cancer.[33]

When the team of doctors looked at research studies on non-cancer health effects of pesticides, the results were even more disturbing and the conclusions more direct. After reviewing 124 studies, doctors found consistent evidence that pesticide exposure increases the risk of neurological, reproductive and genotoxic effects. They found strong evidence linking pesticide exposure and birth defects, fetal death and altered growth. Exposure to pesticides generally doubled the level of genetic damage as measured by chromosome aberrations in white blood cells.[34]

According to the chemical industry, pesticides are safe and there is no science to suggest otherwise. According to doctors, hundreds of studies link pesticides to neurological problems, cancers, birth defects and many other disorders and diseases. This brings two questions to mind. First, what would motivate doctors to publish a research paper showing that pesticides are a problem? Let's hear from the doctors themselves: "Family physicians need evidence-based information on the health effects of pesticides to guide their advice to patients and their involvement in community decisions to restrict use of pesticides."[35] And second, in the face of this evidence, what would motivate a corporation (Dow Agrosciences) to manufacture pesticides in the first place and to sue a jurisdiction (the Province of Quebec) in opposition to a ban on the cosmetic use of pesticides?[36]

After reading dozens of industry-funded studies and learning about the Dow Agrosciences lawsuit, it's easy to see why people wonder who is right. Are doctors fearmongers? Are pesticides actually safe? Is it possible that chemical companies have a point and concerns are overstated? I asked Gideon Forman, who was at the time the executive director of the Canadian Association of Physicians for the Environment-

(CAPE), to tell me his opinion about the role chemical companies play in the pesticides debate.

"They claimed that there's no science behind this when, in fact, there's a huge amount of science connecting pesticides to a whole range of very serious illness. They claim that the alternatives don't work when, in fact, if you look at properties that are maintained without toxic pesticides, they're beautiful properties. I mean, some of the most high-profile properties in the province . . . have been non-toxic for years and they're beautiful. . . . Much of it is based on the sort of thinking that was used by the tobacco lobby. Much of it is word for word taken from the tobacco lobby. The first thing they say is that there's no science connecting cigarettes to lung cancer or pesticides to cancer. And then the whole thrust of what the industry does is to place doubt in the minds of legislators. So the industry doesn't have to prove anything. They just have to raise doubt, and that was exactly their game plan with tobacco."

Forman also pointed me to another group of Canadian doctors who had reviewed studies on 2,4-D specifically. Given that so many toxic studies point to the particular sensitivity of children, it is no surprise that pediatricians have a keen interest in the subject. More recently, the journal *Pediatrics and Child Health* concluded that there is a persuasive link between 2,4-D and cancers, neurological impairment and reproductive problems.[37] A significant contribution to the momentum behind municipal and provincial pesticide bans came from the vocal support and organizational prowess of the Canadian Cancer Society, a charity juggernaut with tens of thousands of volunteers across the country. I spoke with Rowena Pinto, then the senior director of public affairs for the Ontario division of the society, about why the normally conservative organization has become so front and centre on the pesticide issue. "We reviewed the research," she said simply. "We saw a lot of potential links to cancers such as childhood brain cancer, child and adult leukemia and neuroblastoma. What made formulating a position even easier for us was that the whole idea of using pesticides for the sole intent of beautifying gardens and private lawns had no countervailing health benefit." According to Pinto, the society is concerned about many cancer risk factors, but "we know that pesticides contain chemicals that are possibly carcinogenic and are one of many things that can contribute to someone developing cancer. And I'm very confident that anything we can do to reduce risk of cancer by changing the things that we can control, that aren't necessary, that have no other clear health benefit, are things we should be advocating for."

Medical researchers seem quite convinced that 2,4-D and other pesticides pose a serious human health problem. And doctors do not have a financial interest in saying pesticides are harmful. So why the controversy? Even if we accept that pesticide studies may not offer one hundred percent conclusive proof that these substances cause particular effects (as human toxicological studies rarely do), it still seems to make sense to exercise some caution. Chemical companies tell us we need all the answers before they stop selling pesticides that have been linked to cancer in so many studies. But do we really want to take that chance for the sake of stamping out a few dandelions?

Theo's Brains

Of all the potential risks associated with pesticide use, harming the brains of children is perhaps the worst. The late Dr. Theo Colborn was an influential American environmental health expert, trained as a zoologist with expertise in toxicology and epidemiology. She became known for helping define the issue of endocrine disruption, which was highlighted in the 1996 book she co-authored, *Our Stolen Future*. In January 2006, Dr. Colborn published a research paper questioning pesticide safety and summarizing the medical science research on the neurodevelopmental effects of exposure to pesticides.[38] She focused in particular on the development of the prenatal brain and the neonatal brain. One of the critical issues Dr. Colborn highlighted is the fact that pesticides attack neurons in the brain. This does not sound good, and it isn't. According to Dr. Colborn, "Neurons process information and are the signalling or transmitting elements in the nervous system." So any impairment of neurons will affect how our brains develop and function. As an aside, mercury (described in chapter 4) also attacks and destroys neurons, but risk assessments for pesticides carried out by government or industry do not factor in the potentially damaging effects of exposure to mercury, or other substances for that matter, as an additional assault on the brain.

The research on the effects of pesticides on brain development and later mental or physical impairment is extraordinary, both because of the effects observed after minuscule doses and because of the elaborate nature of the studies undertaken. Among other things, these findings suggest we need to know at least five things about early exposure to pesticides and the health problems that can occur when babies (and fetuses) are exposed to everyday products, including their mother's milk.

First, even tiny and very brief doses of pesticides, far below current safety levels, can damage infant brains. Second, with more than eight hundred varieties and approximately one billion pounds of pesticides used every year in the United States alone,[39] it is not surprising that pesticides are found in virtually every organ and fluid of every animal (including humans) on Earth. Third, neuron damage can occur when the infant brain is developing, but the neurological effects may not be seen until adolescence or adulthood. In fact, most neurological defects are not detected until later in life. Fourth, health effects linked to pesticides include everything from attention deficit hyperactivity disorder (ADHD), autism and deficits in motor performance to reproductive and hormonal defects. And finally, neurological impairments in humans are extremely difficult to test for and are therefore difficult to identify.

It is impossible to achieve the levels of proof that risk managers and government officials demand before they might deem pesticides to be unsafe—that is, unless the precautionary principle is adopted, as occurred in the Canadian Supreme Court decision regarding the Town of Hudson, Quebec. In her January 2006 paper, Dr. Colborn points in the same direction, concluding her research by saying, "An entirely new approach to determining the safety of pesticides is needed," along with "a new regulatory approach." Many people who are affected or who will potentially be affected by the damaging effects of pesticides would be the first to agree.

Rachel's Intuition

Rachel Carson's *Silent Spring* was the first major public exposé of the ecological damage caused by pesticide spraying in North America. *Silent Spring* was considered controversial at the time and some critics castigated Carson for her work, but it marked the beginning of an era in which citizens seriously questioned the pervasive use of pesticides.

At the time, nearly sixty years ago, Rachel Carson was writing largely from direct field observation combined with what one might call an ecological instinct. The evidence of declining songbird populations was strong, but the direct link to pesticide spraying had not been well established. She drew on the kind of intuition that is hardwired in many humans but these days is mostly ignored. Early humans learned to rely on clues in nature and even incorporated them directly into early warning systems. The calls, migration patterns and health of other species were all sources of information, and they were used to help direct human behaviour. The challenge today is that, unlike the obvious causes of disease and death that our ancient ancestors faced, toxic chemicals may lead to slow, insidious death from diseases such as cancer or Parkinson's, which take years to manifest themselves. In other instances toxic substances may cause neurological problems that are difficult to detect. Identifying causal linkages between the exposure of a mother to a pesticide and a learning disorder in her child, for instance, is virtually impossible. So if scientists have difficulty sorting these things out, the average citizen will have even more trouble determining the safety of a product.

But many citizens still possess an innate sense of danger, and although their observations may not be entirely accurate and are therefore not permissible in a regulatory context, this innate instinct should not be completely ignored. Rachel Carson was on to something and so was Lois Gibbs at Love Canal. So was Erin Brockovich, who won a major legal battle against Pacific Gas and Electric over chromium-contaminated water, and so is Joe Kiger in Parkersburg (chapter 2). These are citizens who observe their surroundings and sometimes their own health and sense that something is wrong. They may not always have epidemiological data or double-blind longitudinal health studies to present, but they have eyes and common sense.

Risky Business

I am often asked why we knowingly use chemicals that cause cancer and other diseases. My response, increasingly, is "risk assessment." How is it possible that the very tool designed to prevent humans from being exposed to toxic chemicals is actually responsible for their continued use? The answer is that risk assessment helps make it easy for industry to promote so-called "sound science," which often results in requests for more and more studies, thus effectively delaying regulations that would protect the health of citizens. Risk studies assess "acceptable harm" not to establish safety standards but to determine what industry can get away with, and for how long.

Here's one example of how risk assessment may be delaying necessary regulations. DuPont, for example, references Harvard University's Harvard Center for Risk Analysis (HCRA) in its defence of the safety of PFOA and non-stick coatings, the chemicals that may be harming the people of Parkersburg (see chapter 2).[40] The founding director of this agency, Dr. John Graham, was appointed by George W. Bush in 2001 to oversee environmental, health and safety regulations in the United States as head of the Office of Information and Regulatory Affairs (OIRA). According to some observers, however, Graham (no longer head of the HCRA or OIRA) intended to render powerless the U.S. Environmental Protection Agency's ability to regulate toxic substances. Graham had "an axe to grind on cancer risk assessment," said one insider.[41] In retrospect, this pales in comparison with Donald Trump's appointment of his friend the former attorney general of Oklahoma, Scott Pruitt, to head the Environmental Protection Agency—an agency he has sued over a dozen times. "Pruitt is waging an all-out assault on our environment and health," proclaims the Natural Resources Defense Council, adding that he is suspending, cancelling and repealing dozens of regulations fundamental to the protection of clean air, water and human health.[42] Thanks to Pruitt's actions, Americans will now face more pesticides, more mercury, more arsenic and more poisons of all kinds in their food, air and water.

I had the opportunity to hear Graham speak at a conference organized in Washington, D.C., by the Harvard Center when Graham was still its director. Although the conference was about the precautionary principle (which I'll come back to in a moment), it seemed apparent to me that efforts were being made to convince lawmakers in Washington that the precautionary principle was unworkable and therefore of questionable value. In his opening remarks Graham made some remarkable assertions. He talked about the potential benefits of global warming and how nitrous oxide emissions from coal plants may be good for our farms. He also suggested that too little research has been done on the potential health benefits of dioxin, one of the world's most notoriously deadly substances.

The main financial sponsors of the Harvard Center for Risk Analysis are chemical, pharmaceutical, petroleum and other large industrial

companies, the U.S. government—and Health Canada. The list of con-
tributors to the Harvard Center reads much the same as the list of the
world's top chemical manufacturers.[43] Some risk managers question
the assumption that health effects in lab animals such as rats and mice
also have the potential to appear in humans. But for years scientists
have used mice and rats for experimental purposes because the genetic
variation among all animals, including humans, is remarkably small.
Humans, for example, share 97 percent of the genetic makeup of an
orangutan. Rats and mice share more than 80 percent of the genetics
of a human and for decades have been part of an accepted and well-
established research methodology for testing chemicals, including
toxins. Rats also breed rapidly and live relatively short lives. This
makes it possible to test many variations of substances and different
doses on genetically similar animals. Because they age rapidly as well,
the process of developing tumours or other health effects takes place
within a compressed time frame.

Major corporations go to great lengths trying to convince the public
or government regulatory bodies or courts that their products are safe.
When it comes to scientific research using rats or mice, one of the first
lines of argument corporations use is that rats aren't humans. Their
claim, ironically, is that rats are probably more sensitive to the effects
of various toxic substances than humans. So, unlike a toughened and
self-sufficient human baby, the science-lab relatives of poor little
sewer-dwelling, garbage-eating rodents are actually quite sensitive to
what they put in their furry little tummies. Who'd've thought?

It's the Dose

Here's a favourite line of risk managers: "The dose makes the poison."
In other words, a small amount of a substance can be perfectly harm-
less, or in fact necessary to life, whereas a large amount can be lethal.
Salt is one example of such a substance. Humans require salt in their
diets, yet a large quantity of salt over a short period of time can be
lethal. Some risk managers have even used water as a demonstration of
this point: no water and you die, too much and you drown.

There is some truth to this, and it certainly conforms to a basic early
understanding of toxicology, whereby the goal of researchers was to
identify a "threshold," or level below which a substance is deemed to be

safe. According to modern environmental toxicology and endocrinology, however, in the case of some toxic substances, it has been determined that there simply is no safe limit. This means that any amount greater than zero may cause harm. Mercury (see chapter 4) is a perfect example. For years medical researchers focused on finding a "safe level" of mercury in humans. But over time, as in the case of many toxic substances, the level at which some form of human harm was detected kept getting lower. Finally, the most sophisticated mercury studies determined that the safe level is zero. That is, there is no safe level.

Risk management systems don't work well when the answer is zero, because they're designed to find a safe level that can be measured. Zero in risk management terms is portrayed as an impossibility both to achieve and to quantify. It is for this reason that risk managers oppose environmental concepts such as "zero discharge" and "virtual elimination." They prefer the term "safe level." Furthermore, the whole concept of zero is antithetical to the risk profession because, as risk managers like to say, there is no such thing as zero risk.

Fortunately, there is a thoughtful alternative to the rigid risk assessment approach: the precautionary principle. In a nutshell it means "better safe than sorry." The most widely agreed-upon formulation of the concept is contained in Principle 15 of the Rio Declaration on Environment and Development, passed in 1992 at the United Nations Conference on Environment and Development in Rio de Janeiro, Brazil: "Where there are threats of serious or irreversible damage, lack of full scientific certainty shall not be used as a reason for postponing cost-effective measures to prevent environmental degradation." Though not always easy to implement, because it disrupts the status quo, the precautionary principle is finding its way into more and more environmental statutes and regulations—including the Canadian *Environmental Protection Act* and the recently adopted U.S. *Consumer Product Safety Commission Reform Act*, which banned a variety of phthalates (see chapter 1) already on the market until such time as the chemical industry could demonstrate their safety.

In the case of 2,4-D, it is the precautionary principle that Canadian municipalities and provinces are successfully invoking in order to ditch the chemical once and for all. Simply put, citizens in communities of all shapes and sizes right across the country overwhelmingly support pesticide bans.[44] "Better safe than sorry" makes sense to people, and loudly and clearly, they are choosing the safety of their children over weed-free lawns.

It seems we may have our priorities right after all.

SEVEN: MOTHERS KNOW BEST

[RICK DRINKS FROM A BABY BOTTLE]

MR. MCGUIRE: *I just want to say one word to you. Just one word.*

BENJAMIN: *Yes, sir.*

MR. MCGUIRE: *Are you listening?*

BENJAMIN: *Yes, I am.*

MR. MCGUIRE: *Plastics.*

BENJAMIN: *Exactly how do you mean?*

MR. MCGUIRE: *There's a great future in plastics. Think about it.*

—*The Graduate*, 1967

THE MOMENT I KNEW we were going to win arrived on a typically overcast Tuesday morning in November 2007.

I was standing on a stage outside Queen's Park (the Ontario provincial legislature) in Toronto with my colleagues from Environmental Defence. For weeks we had been advertising a "Baby Rally"—a demonstration of children—for this morning. We had urged people to come out with their kids to pressure the Ontario government to ban bisphenol A (BPA).

I was very nervous. "Don't worry! They'll come," said our talented organizer, Cassandra Polyzou. The Baby Rally was an idea we had brainstormed at Environmental Defence as a way to kick the BPA debate into high gear. We had been generating good media attention in Canada with our call for a ban on this hormone-disrupting chemical in food and beverage containers. The fact that it was the main ingredient in all the market-leading baby bottles just horrified people, and the baby bottle had quickly become a powerful icon for our campaign.

But we needed to create a "happening" in Toronto, Canada's media capital, to really engage Ontario politicians and elicit a commitment from the premier to act. So we asked ourselves what politicians really like to do. What would really pique their interest? Someone jokingly said, "Kissing babies." And the Baby Rally was born.

Polyzou was right. I shouldn't have worried. As the sun finally peeked through the clouds and across the paths leading to the front doors of the legislature, where our stage was set up, the strollers started arriving. Nearly three hundred people with their newborns, toddlers and school-aged children streamed onto the legislature's grand front lawn. Some people spread out picnic blankets. Volunteers distributed specially made "baby pickets"—small pieces of cardboard stuck to Popsicle sticks bearing the messages "Don't Pollute Me" and "Toxic Free Ontario."

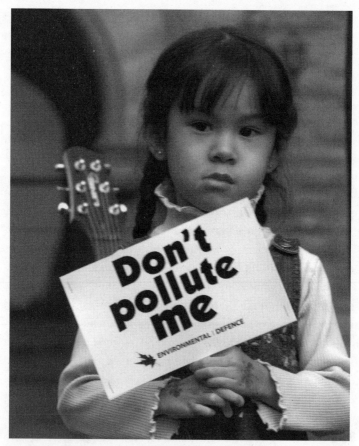

Young girl at BPA rally with her "baby picket"

The world's first (and, I believe, still the only) rally against BPA was ready to roll.

My Mother Joins In

Considering the rally's finicky participants, we'd planned it to be short and sweet.

Andrea Page, the well-known founder of the exercise program "Fitmom," was our dynamic emcee and held her young son on her hip throughout. She really was the perfect spokesperson for this issue, powerfully chastising industry and government for not taking the health of children seriously.

A couple of other powerful women spoke: a mom who runs a business selling "green" products for babies (who remarked on the increasing consumer demand for these items) and a representative of the Ontario Coalition for Better Child Care (who talked about why daycares had started ditching their BPA-filled baby bottles).

I was up next, and spoke as both an advocate and a parent. I told the crowd that, like them, I was there for my kids. "Because I want my two boys to grow up in a world full of possibility and hope, not a world where pollution is rampant and invisible toxins threaten their health." My four-year-old son Zack, who was with me on stage, made it onto the evening TV news by hollering "That's right" into the microphone at key moments.

Dr. Pete Myers, co-author of *Our Stolen Future*, the best-selling book on hormone-disrupting pollution and an expert on BPA, flew up from Virginia for the occasion. He started off by asking the crowd, "How many of you have a relative or friend who has been touched by breast or prostate cancer?" A sea of hands went up. "What about learning disabilities?" More hands. "How about type 2 diabetes or infertility?" Even more. "Well, that's what we're talking about," continued Myers. "That's why we're here. The link between BPA and these diseases is strong enough scientifically to think we may be able to prevent some portion of the burden of these diseases. From everything we know about this chemical, exposure in childhood increases the likelihood of kids having health problems later in life. And the good news is that if we act on this science, we can help make people healthier."

Myers told us that no country in the world, until then, had taken strong action on BPA. The chemical companies loved to hammer home this point in order to dissuade anyone from becoming the first. "The world is watching Canada closely," Myers said. "What you are doing today matters a heckuva lot."

I looked over at my mother, who'd taken a commuter train down from the suburbs to lend a hand with childcare. Over the years she'd never seemed terribly impressed with my rally-going, but there she was, hooting and stomping. When the convoy of strollers started to disperse, it was time for a few of us to hike over to one of the many surrounding government buildings for a previously arranged meeting with the Ontario premier, Dalton McGuinty, and the minister of the environment, John Gerretsen.

Baby Lobbyists

Now, meeting politicians and asking for stuff was a big part of what I did for a living in 2007. Most often, such encounters follow a template. They're usually a bit formal. You present your case the best you can, and the politician in question looks at you in all sincerity and gives an oblique and puzzling answer that only partly addresses the topic at hand. You come away shaking your head.

I am delighted to report that this was not one of those meetings. In fact, it was one of the funniest lobbying experiences I've ever had.

Things started out on an embarrassing note. As you might expect, the premier was protected by a phalanx of police officers and his "advance" staff, whose job it was to make sure his schedule ran smoothly. One of the advance guys, in what was likely the most uncomfortable thing he had to do all day, asked all the moms (and their babies!) to turn over their five-inch-tall Popsicle pickets.

A few of the moms blinked in surprise. The babies gurgled. The guy shuffled his feet. Just standard procedure that people meeting with the premier couldn't be carrying pickets, he said. Even if the people in question were six months old. The moms took pity on him, and the babies were duly stripped of their weaponry.

Three city blocks, a few elevators and stairwells and several long corridors later, the moms and their tired, hungry infants arrived at the foodless meeting room around lunchtime. A possible meltdown loomed.

We sat at a large boardroom table, the premier and the minister of the environment on one side and about eight moms and their kids arrayed on the other. The media cameras, which were allowed to stay for the beginning of the meeting, contributed the occasional popping flash.

One of the moms breastfed. Some of the older kids ran laps around the table. A few diapers were changed on the floor. A little girl sat directly opposite the premier in her mother's lap and would occasionally punctuate the conversation by locking eyes with him, leaning forward and slamming her glass baby bottle on the table. Kids were laughing. Kids were crying. It was minor mayhem. Despite the distractions, or perhaps because of them, the meeting worked. The moms, who were certainly not going to take no for an answer, emerged smiling. And the premier made a commitment that all the parents in the room wanted to hear: Ontario would move to establish Canada's first *Toxic Pollution Reduction Act* and would immediately seek advice from experts as to what to do about bisphenol A. No need to wait for action from the federal government, the premier announced to the assembled moms. If the advice from the experts was to ban it, he'd ban it.

When I interviewed McGuinty a few months later and asked why he'd made the BPA commitment so quickly that day, he said that the government's best scientific advice was pointing in that direction. He went on to say, "Though in an immediate sense, a lot of this new stuff is helpful to us, makes our lives more comfortable and adds to the level of convenience associated with living in the twenty-first century, I've always had this sinking feeling that we haven't really fully explored the potential downsides associated with using these new materials and chemicals in consumer products." He told me how he and his wife were already trying to use more glass and fewer plastics in their kitchen at home.

The premier's announcement did indeed kick the bisphenol A debate into high gear. Queen's Park had just put Ottawa on notice that it would be a race to the finish line, with the Ontario and federal governments competing to be the first to protect Canada's kids.

Content with a good day's work, the babies went home for their afternoon naps.

Getting to Know Them

To say in 2006 that the environmental movement didn't have much of a relationship with the Conservative federal government would be an understatement. But it hadn't always been that way. In fact, the last

Progressive Conservative prime minister, Brian Mulroney, was awarded the honour of "Greenest Prime Minister in Canadian History" by a panel of environmental experts (of which I was one) for his work on parks, pollution and biodiversity. After his government was defeated in 1993, the Progressive Conservatives shattered into three parties—the continuing Progressive Conservatives, the Reform Party and the Bloc Québécois. The dominant one of these—Reform—was based in oil-rich Alberta and seemed little interested in Mulroney's environmental legacy. Throughout much of the subsequent thirteen-year Liberal government, environmentalists became convinced that Reform was a puppet of the oil patch and Reformers were grumpy that environmentalists were too close to the Liberal Party. And to be honest, there was some truth to both of those perspectives.

Things didn't really improve when the Conservative Party patched itself back together again in 2003. You could cut the mutual suspicion with a knife. And so there we were in 2005, the Tories likely about to regain power and most environmental leaders not having even so much as a Tory e-mail address to ask them out for a coffee at Tim Hortons.

It was in this context that Environmental Defence Canada launched the Toxic Nation campaign (see the introduction).

Toxic Nation

When the Conservatives won office (albeit with a tenuous minority government) in January 2006, we started meeting up a storm. We sat down with senior Environment Canada bureaucrats during the critical transition period that shapes any new government's initial priorities. We introduced ourselves to the new minister of the environment and to the officials in the Prime Minister's Office (PMO).

Around this same time, on the nation's airwaves and in the newspapers, Toxic Nation was getting a lot of play. There was something about it that appealed to politicians of all stripes, including Conservatives. "Toxic Nation fitted with the mainstreet ethos" of the new government, explained Tim Powers, a conservative commentator and government relations consultant we worked with. "You can see a plastic water bottle; you can't see a greenhouse gas."

At the provincial level, Premier McGuinty of Ontario felt that Toxic Nation contributed to a changing public perception of environmental issues: "The environment is no longer an abstract, esoteric, ephemeral and romantic notion," he told me. "It's no longer just about the quality of a distant stream or the health and vigour of a remote forest. It's about the air that I'm breathing into my lungs right now. It's about the quality of the water that I give to my child at seven-thirty in the evening, just before she goes to bed. It's about the container that my food has been heated up in—and that I'm about to eat from. It's become part of human health."

By demonstrating that contaminants come from many parts of our lives, Toxic Nation paved the way for the bisphenol A decision. Pollution again became a live discussion at the federal level.

In early 2006, on the same day the Conservatives took office, I had an opinion piece in the *Globe and Mail,* co-authored by Adam Daifallah, a prominent Tory activist. The column was titled "It's in Tory Genes to Go Green" and it made this strong case: "In a minority 'pizza Parliament,' where cooperation between parties will be a prerequisite to getting anything done, there exists at least one priority common to the Conservative, Liberal, NDP and Bloc platforms. . . . The issue is pollution. An area where Prime Minister—designate Stephen Harper can not only find common ground with other parties, and make a real difference in the lives of ordinary Canadians, but one where there exists an impressive Conservative tradition just waiting to be dusted off and rehabilitated."[1]

Thankfully, at least some in the new government were listening.

Chemicals Management Plan

After the media exposure from our first Toxic Nation studies, our office started to get spontaneous phone calls from people wanting to have their personal levels of pollution tested. All sorts of people, young and old. Moms and dads. Plumbers and physiotherapists. And politicians. Politicians of all stripes. All of a sudden elected officials were approaching us to donate their blood and pee in a cup for Toxic Nation.

We were happy to oblige. In June 2006 we released the test results for Rona Ambrose, then the federal minister of the environment; Tony Clement, federal minister of health; Jack Layton, leader of the New Democratic Party; and John Godfrey, the Liberal Party's environment critic. All of them were good sports. All of them used the opportunity of their testing to garner national headlines about how seriously they were taking the pollution problem and why they wanted to solve it.

For her troubles, Ambrose was savaged in some traditionally supportive Conservative media. A "classic piece of environmental horrorism, a sort of updated take on Bram Stoker's *Dracula*" was how one commentator framed our campaign while assailing "Rona Brockovich" for her part in volunteering for it.[2] Apparently, in the minds of some conservatives, a comparison to the famed California pollution fighter Erin Brockovich is supposed to be unflattering. It's a point of view that still leaves me scratching my head, but I know that this criticism left some Tory strategists smarting.

In December 2006 the federal Tories introduced their "Chemicals Management Plan," a dramatic overhaul of the way in which Canada assesses and regulates two hundred high-priority chemicals used commonly in everyday life. Bisphenol A was at the top of the list.

A few months later the very first people to be tested for BPA in Canada were Ontario premier Dalton McGuinty and the two provincial opposition party leaders. All three gentlemen had levels of the chemical at concentrations found in some studies to potentially affect health. "I always knew you guys were out for my blood in a figurative way—but literally?" McGuinty joked later.

John Tory, the Conservative Party leader in Ontario at the time (and now mayor of Toronto), even allowed media cameras to film him as he donated blood for our tests. With a ring of six or so TV cameras surrounding him, flashes popping, reporters completely focused on the needle sticking out of his arm, I thought the poor nurse who was drawing the blood was going to pass out with the stress of it all. "I'm disappointed my blood is Liberal red and not Conservative blue," Tory said as he winked at the cameras.

The Rise of BPA

Before we continue with the BPA story in Canada, let's take a step back for a second and talk about BPA 101: what it is, where it comes from and why it should concern us all.

Though the levels of this chemical in the three Ontario political leaders became the first BPA data publicly available in Canada, the Centers for Disease Control and Prevention (CDC) in the U.S. had already done extensive testing. A stunning 93 percent of Americans tested had measurable amounts of BPA in their bodies.[3] Canadians are almost certainly polluted at similar levels. The fact that virtually all of us have measurable levels of BPA all the time is even more astounding when you consider that BPA is rapidly metabolized by the human body—in just a few hours. The only possible conclusion to draw is that we are all being re-exposed on a constant basis. We're marinating in BPA every day.

Where does BPA lurk in our daily lives? In a great many places. BPA is one of the most commonly produced chemicals in the world, with industry pumping out 3.6 billion kilograms in 2010 versus 45 million kg in 1970—an astronomical increase in just over thirty years.[4] In the U.S. today, it is estimated that about 70 percent of BPA is used to manufacture polycarbonate plastic (the hard, clear plastic often marked with recycling symbol #7) and about 20 percent is used in sports equipment, medical devices, dental fillings, household electronics, eyeglasses, foundry castings and water pipe linings.[5] Manufacturers of the chemical include some of the largest companies going: Bayer, Dow, Hexion, SABIC Innovative Plastics (once known as GE Plastics) and Sunoco.[6]

A typical house is chock full of BPA. Polycarbonate plastic is used to make CDs and DVDs, water bottles, drinking glasses, kitchen appliances and utensils, eyeglass lenses (like the ones I have on at the moment), bottled water carboys (the big water jugs used in office water coolers), hockey helmet visors, baby bottles, medical supplies and the screens of my laptop and mobile phone. Polycarbonate is also extensively used in cars and trucks for things like headlights, and it's right there in my kids' toy bin—in the windshields of their tiny cars, for example. Epoxy resins are used as adhesives in sporting equipment, airplanes and cars. They're also commonly found in dental filling materials, protective coatings around wire and piping and what is likely the primary avenue of exposure for most people: the interior lining of virtually every tin can found in every home and grocery store.

The explosive growth of BPA-laden products is a fairly new phenomenon. Though BPA was first synthesized way back in 1891 and its hormone-disrupting properties discovered in the 1930s, it was a while before the true commercial worth of BPA was appreciated. Large-scale production of epoxy resins began in the 1950s. Researchers also discovered at about this time that if you polymerize BPA (link the molecules together into long strings), you can make a hard and durable plastic—polycarbonate (polycarbonate plastic is mostly 100 percent

BPA). With increasing demand for plastics in the 1960s and 1970s, production of BPA took off. And now it's everywhere.

Now I bet at this point you're asking yourself the obvious question: What in God's name were manufacturers thinking when they started making household plastics out of a chemical that has been known for over seventy years to screw up the human body's hormone system? The short answer is that they weren't thinking about that at all. And to the extent that any brain synapses were firing, the assumption may have been made that BPA would remain bound in the plastic or come out at such low levels that it wouldn't cause any harm. Wrong, as it turns out, on both counts.

Low Dose

Anyone who works on the question of BPA very quickly comes across Dr. Fred vom Saal, professor emeritus of biological sciences at the University of Missouri. Unlike many university researchers, vom Saal doesn't shrink from the public eye, seeming quite content to take, head-on, the double-barrelled invective that the chemical industry levels at him. For nearly twenty-five years, vom Saal has been at the eye of the BPA tornado.

In many ways the tornado was started by vom Saal himself. It was the late 1990s, and for a number of years he had been looking at the effects of hormones on the behaviour of mice. He studied "a phenomenon that people found very interesting, that we now know occurs in human twins, and that is that babies transfer hormones to each other when they're in the uterus together." Despite the fact that the amount of hormone transferred is "just stunningly small," these exposures have specific and dramatic effects seemingly independent of the genetic makeup of the animals involved.

In one of his experiments, vom Saal observed that male mice, when exposed to tiny amounts of an estrogen hormone called estradiol, developed enlarged prostates. The result met with skepticism; at the time, prostate cancer patients were given estrogens on the assumption that it would suppress testosterone and bring their prostate growth under control. Vom Saal's results, if correct, ran entirely counter to this approach. In a series of trials, he gave progressively greater doses of estradiol and the synthetic hormone diethylstilbestrol (DES) to mice. He found the same phenomenon again: high doses blocked prostate growth and low doses dramatically stimulated prostate growth. His research contributed to new approaches in the use of antiestrogens to treat prostate cancer.

At the same time that vom Saal was undertaking these important experiments on estradiol and DES "low-dose" effects, he started looking at other synthetic chemicals that might have similar properties. In 1997 he published his first work on BPA. "In that study we demonstrated that a dose of BPA twenty-five thousand times lower than had ever been tested also stimulated prostate development, exactly like low doses of estradiol. This had been missed in the high-dose [BPA] studies." If the reaction to his estradiol study was lively, the chemical industry's reaction to this BPA work was textbook crisis management. "They came after us like a freight train," said vom Saal.

From the industry's point of view, the stakes couldn't have been higher. If BPA was so toxic at such low levels, billions of dollars in profit were at risk. In an unusually candid comment at the time, John Waechter, a senior scientist with Dow Chemical and the Society of the Plastics Industry, admitted that should vom Saal be proven correct, the margin of safety for BPA in consumer products would be less than previously thought.[7]

According to vom Saal, the industry's efforts to get him to back off began even before his study was published. The chemical companies first became aware that something was up when he presented his results at a conference, and "the first thing they did was to send John Waechter down here to ask us, and this is a direct quote: 'Is there a mutually beneficial outcome we can arrive at where you delay the publication of your findings until the chemical industry approves them for publication?'" Vom Saal says he felt like a bribe was being offered and he was being asked to name his price. The industry claims that this was all a profound misunderstanding.

In any event, what is beyond dispute is that the industry has spent twenty years commissioning research that might torpedo the "low-dose hypothesis." The only problem is that more and more researchers are buttressing vom Saal's findings with their own low-dose discoveries. Recent evidence, for instance, suggests an association between "increased incidence of breast cancer" and BPA exposure at levels below commonly accepted "safe reference doses."[8]

Accidental Discoveries

When I asked Dr. Pat Hunt, a prominent geneticist and a professor at Washington State University, how she first became aware of BPA, she laughed loudly.

"We did it by pure accident," she said. "We were in the midst of some other studies. We were studying eggs from some normal mice and some mutant mice, and suddenly eggs from normal animals just went completely crazy and the data suddenly switched. . . . We went from seeing an abnormality rate of 1 to 2 percent to 40 percent in the 'normal' animals. So we knew something was up, and it took us weeks to figure out exactly what had happened." She and her colleagues looked at everything and finally concluded it was the animals themselves. "We started looking down in our animal facility," she explained. A worker had started washing the cages and water bottles with floor detergent, corroding the polycarbonate plastics and allowing them to leach BPA.

Hunt and her colleagues published their study five years later, in 2003. "We didn't rush. We wanted to make certain we had the story correct, because we realized that what we were coming out in the press and saying was that exposure to this chemical could cause miscarriages. This was sufficiently worrying that I wanted to make sure that we had all our t's crossed and i's dotted." Hunt continued her BPA research and says, "Everything we've done with this chemical since has only made me more concerned." Her latest discovery is that BPA exposure can cause damage to multiple generations at the same time. For this experiment, she exposed pregnant mice to BPA just as the ovaries in their developing female fetuses were producing a lifetime supply of eggs. When the exposed fetuses became adults, 40 percent of their eggs were damaged. "With that one exposure," Hunt explained, "we're actually affecting three generations simultaneously." In 2012, scientists found additional evidence to corroborate these observations, noting that "BPA produces transgenerational alterations" in the genes and behaviour of mice.[9]

As I interviewed people for this chapter, I realized that Pat Hunt's story is not atypical in the field of BPA research. Dr. Ana Soto, a medical doctor at the Tufts University School of Medicine in Boston, is another prominent researcher who started working on BPA unexpectedly. She and her colleagues became quite famous in the late 1980s when they became the first to discover an estrogen-like chemical, nonylphenol, leaching out of plastic. In fact, they discovered this after another laboratory "accident" like Pat Hunt's. Their new plastic test tubes started causing weird things to happen in their experiments until they isolated the estrogen-mimicking chemical in the plastic. This discovery launched her laboratory into investigations of other hormone-disrupting chemicals, including BPA; her recent research has focused on prenatal exposure to BPA and its impact on reproductive development.[10] "What we observed in animals is that even with low doses of this chemical, we saw the development of precancerous lesions. It logically follows from this that human exposure to BPA increases the likelihood of developing breast cancer later in life."

Soto made the larger point that "all these artificial estrogens are producing in animals the effects of some of the current human epidemics. I mean breast cancer, attention deficit disorders, prostate cancer. . . . It's scary, I would say." In fact, the number of studies linking tiny amounts of BPA—amounts well within the range currently found in human bodies—to various illnesses have increased dramatically since Soto first began her BPA work.

As Fred vom Saal explained it, "We have reached a critical mass of studies that take us through the exact molecular details of the response systems in human and animal cells that allow these cells to respond to staggeringly low doses of BPA. We understand now what happens at the molecular level." More recent research on the impact of BPA exposure on human health has found worrying links to adverse perinatal, childhood and adult health outcomes, including reproductive and developmental effects, metabolic disease and a variety of child-specific pathologies.[11]

Low Dose and Paracelsus

So how could one chemical be responsible for so many ailments? For centuries, the basic tenet of toxicology has been Paracelsus's sixteenth-century observation that "all things are poison and nothing is without poison; only the dose permits something not to be poisonous." This is generally shortened to "the dose makes the poison" and taken to mean that the higher the exposure to a certain chemical, the greater the impact (Bruce delves into this concept with respect to pesticides in chapter 6). The chemical industry is fond of quoting Paracelsus, as are many toxicologists who have never been educated in the concept of hormonally active chemicals.

Although this sixteenth-century logic makes intuitive sense for things like beer consumption or the amount of sugar I put in my wife's coffee every morning (which I regularly screw up), it increasingly does not make sense for hormone-mimicking chemicals like BPA. The simple reason for this is that humans (and all other animals, for that matter) have evolved over time to be sensitive to even very small amounts of hormone. It stands to reason that our bodies will be similarly sensitive to synthetic chemicals that act like the real thing. And a huge number of our internal workings are driven by subtle proddings from hormones. They bind to cell receptors and turn genes on and off—and so do hormone mimickers. A little hormone goes a long way.

The key to this is that hormones and compounds that behave like hormones stimulate different genes at different concentrations. And at high concentrations, they can be overtly toxic. That means that at a low dose you get one set of genes being turned on, with one or more effects, while at a high dose you get another set of genes, with effects that can be completely different. At very high doses genes get shut down because of the over-toxicity.

Pete Myers, co-author of *Our Stolen Future,* once got this concept across to me in a particularly evocative way. "Picture a drop of water in which BPA is present in a concentration of one part per billion," he said. "Now tell me how many individual molecules of BPA would be in that water drop."

"A few thousand?" (Have I mentioned I'm a zoologist and not a chemist?)

"Nope."

"A few hundred thousand?"

"Not even close. Try 132 billion. And each one of those molecules is able to turn cell receptors on and off just like hormones do."

The implications of BPA having such major low-dose effects are profound. Government regulators, who have been focused for years on setting the so-called safe level of exposure to various chemicals, have royally screwed up by overestimating the levels for hormone-disrupting chemicals. Because BPA has completely different effects at low levels than it does at high levels, there's no such thing as a "safe" level.

As Fred vom Saal put it, "The traditional approach of just testing high doses of BPA completely got it wrong. This is the chemical that proves that the chemical risk assessment process is absolutely invalid for hormonally active chemicals. With Ana Soto's group at Tufts now showing effects [from BPA] at levels two million times lower than the lowest dose ever tested by a toxicologist, we're talking about a scale of error that's horrifying beyond belief."

In the United States the debate about low-dose effects and BPA came to a head in 2007 with the publication of two reports. In the first, an advisory committee to the federal government's National Toxicology Program expressed "some concern" about the neural and behavioural impacts of fetal exposure to low doses of BPA. The report was made public under a cloud of accusation that some of the key contractors hired by the federal government to research and write it had links to the BPA industry.

The second report is the real blockbuster. The product of a remarkable U.S. National Institutes of Health–funded meeting of thirty-eight of the world's top BPA researchers, the so-called Chapel Hill Consensus Statement is very strong in its warning: "The wide range of adverse effects of low doses of BPA in laboratory animals exposed both during development and in adulthood is a great cause for concern with regard to the potential for similar adverse effects in humans."[12] Specific human illnesses these experts believe may be linked to rising levels of BPA include increases in prostate and breast cancer; urogenital abnormalities in male babies; a decline in semen quality in men; early onset of puberty in girls; metabolic disorders, including insulin-resistant diabetes and obesity; and neurobehavioural problems such as attention deficit hyperactivity disorder.

The Chapel Hill statement makes for chilling reading. Still, the debate over BPA rages on. In February 2018 the U.S. Food and Drug Administration released a report stating that—as currently regulated—BPA produces "minimal effects" in rodent test-subjects.[13] Groups of dissenting scientists immediately objected to this language, characterizing the FDA studies as "incomplete" and calling for further testing and research.[14]

Toxic as Tofu

Now back to Canada to finish our story.

Sometimes, during a campaign, manna falls from heaven. You can't plan for these surprising moments. You just need to be ready to run with them when they happen.

For many years Martin Mittelstaedt was an environment reporter at the *Globe and Mail*. He had begun doggedly pursuing the story of BPA's toxicity in early 2006. In June 2007 he broke a story about Mark Richardson (the scientist Health Canada had appointed to head up its investigation of BPA) giving a speech to a medical group in Tucson, Arizona, in which he endorsed continued use of the chemical. Richardson did so using colourful language, saying "Yes, bisphenol A is estrogenic—it interacts with estrogen receptors—but a myriad of other things do as well, including proteins in tofu." He also said BPA exposures were "so low as to be totally inconsequential, in my view." Unfortunately for him, Richardson made these comments in front of a camera filming the meeting proceedings and Mittelstaedt was able to buy the DVD online for a few bucks. Pretty good investment for the *Globe and Mail*. Pretty bad day for an embarrassed federal government, which promptly yanked Richardson from the BPA file.

When Mittelstaedt first phoned me for a comment on the story, I couldn't believe what I was hearing. Not only was it exceedingly rare that a bureaucrat as experienced as Richardson would be so indiscreet, it was also a minor miracle that anyone had found out about it.

We had just been handed a heaven-sent opportunity to confront the chemical industry's pro-BPA lobby machine.

The Perfect Storm

By the time of the Baby Rally, as I mentioned at the beginning of this chapter, I had a feeling the tide was turning in our favour. Both the Ontario and federal governments had started signalling that they were going to take action. The Chapel Hill statement was released and widely circulated, and it provided the most powerful summary to date of BPA's damaging effects.

In December Canada's largest outdoor retailer, Mountain Equipment Co-op (MEC), announced publicly that it would remove BPA-containing products from its shelves until such time as the federal government had rendered its determination of BPA's toxicity. Lululemon, the large active-wear retailer, soon followed suit. Shortly thereafter, the Environmental Working Group produced a report revealing that the tins of every major brand of infant formula leached BPA into the contents of the containers, and in early 2008 we released a study with U.S. colleagues measuring levels of BPA leaching out of the market-leading baby bottles.

By this point there was a prominent media story nearly every day about some aspect of BPA. Seemingly overnight, stainless-steel kids' canteens and glass baby bottles became the standard.

Then things really went nutso, on April 15, 2008. This was the morning when Martin Mittelstaedt broke a story in the *Globe* confirming that the federal government would be declaring BPA a toxic substance within a few days and banning it in certain products, such as baby bottles. Even Mittelstaedt wasn't prepared for what happened next. "I've never seen anything like it," he said.

When the government didn't deny Mittelstaedt's story, major retailers started lining up to jettison BPA products from their inventory. On the 16th it was Wal-Mart Canada, Canadian Tire, the Forzani Group (owner of several chains of sporting goods stores) and the Hudson's Bay Company.

In another dramatic development, the U.S. National Toxicology Program chose that day to release its own assessment of BPA. For the first time a U.S. government agency raised concerns regarding BPA's links to early puberty, breast cancer, prostate effects and behavioural problems, and highlighted that pregnancy and early life are especially sensitive periods, given higher exposure to the chemical and limited ability to metabolize it. The U.S. media promptly started their own BPA frenzy, matching the one that was already going on north of the border.

"It's like the perfect storm," said an elated Pete Myers when I spoke with him later in the afternoon.

On the 17th, Sears Canada, Rexall pharmacies, London Drugs and Home Depot Canada joined the parade. Our office was overwhelmed with media interest, large retailers phoning to apprise us of their plans and general calls from concerned members of the public. We usually work on many issues, but that week it was all BPA all the time. Later that day, I finally got the call from Ottawa I had been waiting for. "We're having a press conference to make an announcement on BPA tomorrow. We'd be glad if you could make it."

Anticipating a good announcement, I asked the environment minister's office if we could do anything to help them. Silence for a second. "Actually, yes," was the reply. "Could you bring some moms and babies out for the occasion? It would be great to have them there, but if we do it ourselves the national media will make a story about our cynicism."

Better Safe Than Sorry

I flew to Ottawa early that morning. By the time I landed, my cellphone voicemail was already full of media calls asking for confirmation of what the government was about to do. On the way to the press conference, I gave radio interviews from the cab.

My colleague Aaron Freeman and I waited in the hotel lobby for our friends, five good-natured moms who'd agreed on short notice to bring their babies to the press conference. A few minutes later we were all downstairs in a basement room, the moms and babies and their strollers taking up most of the front row, waiting for the health minister, Tony Clement, and the environment minister, John Baird, to make their entrance. Finally the two ministers entered the room and, after the requisite amount of goo-gooing with the kids, took the podium.

As the health minister started to speak, I could feel the tension leaving my shoulders: "Based on the results of our assessment, today I am proposing precautionary action to reduce exposure and increase safety. . . . We have concluded that early development is sensitive to the effects of bisphenol A. Although our science tells us exposure levels to newborns and infants are below the levels that cause effects, it is better to be safe than sorry. . . . It is our intention to ban the importation, sale and advertising of polycarbonate baby bottles."

Success! I looked at one of the babies hanging over her mom's shoulder and winked. At that moment Canada became the first country in the world to take action to limit exposure to bisphenol A. "Toxic" was now the legal term applied to BPA by Canada's federal pollution legislation. With such a label, I told the media in my interviews, it was only a matter of time before BPA disappeared from many products. I didn't care what justifications the chemical industry tried to come up with, no parent in their right mind was going to put up with their child being subjected to a toxic substance. The Canadian announcement was, in Fred vom Saal's words, "a bombshell." It deprived the chemical industry of their best self-fulfilling prophecy (no country has banned this substance yet, so why should anyone start now?) and reverberated around the world. As of 2018—and despite the stonewalling by the Trump administration of any progress on toxic chemicals at a national level—BPA bans have gone into effect in a dozen U.S. states. As we noted in the introduction, great progress has occurred in countries around the world. All those initiatives cite Canada as having shown the way.

Back-of-the-Envelope Planning

As I waited for Tony Clement's announcement in that hotel basement, I was also wondering what my own BPA results were going to look like. Sure, there's been testing for BPA in people's blood before. But no one had been dumb enough to deliberately raise their BPA levels. With BPA—unlike phthalates, triclosan and mercury, where we had at least some scientific experiments to guide us—we were breaking completely new ground.

In designing our experiment I'd first called up the BPA guru himself, Dr. Fred vom Saal, to pick his brain. After laughing out loud when I told him my intentions, he started musing with me about how it could be done. I filled him in on what we already had in mind for the phthalates experiment: an initial period of "detox" to depress my phthalate levels, urine collection of this lowered level twenty-four hours later, and then a second collection twenty-four hours after that, to see the effect of my phthalate exposure.

"Sounds okay," vom Saal responded. "The BPA experiment will be similar, and you can probably do it at the same time. Because the half-life of a BPA molecule in the human body is relatively short, give yourself eighteen to twenty-four hours to try to flush it from your system. The other thing you should do to get rid of the BPA in your system is to avoid showering. It's in surface waters and you want to avoid inhaling the steam."

No shower for two days? No problem, I thought. That's more common on busy, kid-filled weekends than I care to admit.

"Then you should move into the deliberate exposure phase of the experiment. You're going to want to eat foods that are as rich in BPA as possible. Canned foods are ideal." Vom Saal told me he could help prepare a shopping list, based on the relative levels of BPA in different canned goods that he has measured—the makings for a Meal from Hell (as I came to call it).

Coffee Troubles

As I explained in chapter 1, I decided to go two whole days eating food that had not come into contact with plastic, to try to depress the levels of BPA and phthalates in my body. I won't duplicate that explanation here, but let me tell you that the cruellest blow came when the no-plastics rule disrupted my daily coffee intake. My original plan was to forgo my morning coffee from coffeemakers both at home and at work. They're standard drip machines and are both made largely from plastic. Instead, what I thought I'd do was load up on double Americanos—made fresh in a giant, expensive stainless-steel cappuccino machine at my favourite café.

I'm in the place often enough that the owner knows me, and I asked him to show me how he made my coffee—from the moment the beans came in the door of the café to the minute the cup hit my lips. I followed him around the tiny shop. First the beans arrived in bags. Then the bags were poured into the bean grinders, which look like classic grocery store bubble-gum machines—storage tank for the beans up top, grinder on the bottom.

Problem no. 1: The storage tank, where the beans could sit for hours on end, was made of polycarbonate.

Next the beans were dropped down into the grinder.

Problem no. 2: The receptacle that caught the crushed beans was made of polycarbonate.

From there on in, the beans seemed to contact only metal before the beverage was poured into the paper cup. But the possibility of some serious BPA contamination had already occurred in the grinding process.

I felt snookered. Grumpier by the second, I muddled through until the early afternoon, when I was saved by a glass Bodum-style French press coffeemaker. One problem solved.

The one-litre jug of urine in the fridge quickly filled up.

Enriched with Delicious BPA

During our time in the condo test room, there's no question that Bruce ate better than I did. While he was chowing down on expensive, tasty, mercury-laden tuna steaks, I ate nothing for a day and a half but canned foods heated in a polycarbonate Rubbermaid container in the microwave.[15] Campbell's chicken noodle soup, canned pineapple, Heinz spaghetti, and tuna casserole made with a variety of canned ingredients were the highlights. I drank a few Cokes (the cans are lined with BPA), and made my coffee in a polycarbonate French press coffeemaker purchased at Starbucks. I then drank my coffee from an old Avent polycarbonate baby bottle that Jen and I had used with our eldest son, Zack.

"Aha!" I can hear the supporters of bisphenol A crowing. "He drank his coffee out of an old baby bottle. Who does that? Smith broke his own cardinal rule of experimentation by doing something abnormal."

Not true. Most parents I know who used baby bottles heated them in the microwave. The hot coffee drunk from the bottle mimics the warm milk that babies receive. Also, until recently, the Starbucks near me sold a wide variety of polycarbonate travel mugs. Drinking coffee from a polycarbonate bottle is well within the bounds of normal.

"Holy Mackerel!"

So what was the outcome of this strange diet? I increased my BPA levels more than sevenfold from before exposure to after exposure (see figure 8). In addition to the twenty-four-hour samples, I took three spot samples throughout the two-day test period. These show my BPA levels at a moment in time and, as you might expect, show a dramatic spike in BPA levels and then a decrease as my body gradually rids itself of the toxin (see figure 9).

Figure 8. Levels of BPA in Rick's urine (in ng/mL) measured in two 24-hour urine collections before and after deliberate exposure.

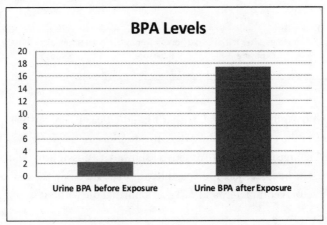

"Holy mackerel!" were Fred vom Saal's first words when I sent him the numbers. He zeroed right in on the implications for babies. "This is really scary. . . . Babies are essentially doing all day, every day, what you did for one day."

Vom Saal explained that babies have a very different metabolism than adults and that the rate at which they are able to flush the BPA out of their systems and into their urine is much slower. This means that in addition to receiving high levels of BPA in 100 percent of their food (formula from BPA-leaching cans delivered in polycarbonate bottles warmed in the microwave), any given hormone-mimicking BPA molecule is bound to stick around in a little baby body much longer than in my six-foot-six frame.

"Remarkable," said Pete Myers. "You managed to pull yourself from just below the median BPA level for the U.S. to way on top of the curve by these manipulations. But interestingly, the low levels are still reflecting some exposure, and the question is: Where is that coming from?"

Figure 9. Levels of BPA in Rick's urine sampled 3 hours, 10 hours and 28 hours after initial exposure (μg BPA/g creatinine).

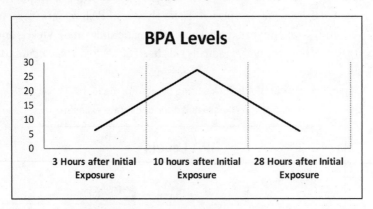

One possibility, of course, is that I handled cash register receipts in advance of the experiment (see the introduction, re the potency of these as a BPA source in daily life). Although I showed it's possible to reduce BPA levels in the body, it's just not possible (unfortunately!) at the moment to eliminate BPA completely and carry on a normal life without it.

BPA and Me

As you can probably tell, I take BPA personally. It's hard not to when I look at my two fantastic little boys and remember that Zack was raised on an Avent BPA bottle and sippy cup, because Jen and I didn't know any better, and Owain was not. I worry about the effects of Zack ingesting all that BPA. And the more I learn about this substance, the more my worries grow.

As my father is fond of reminding me, I'm also personally responsible for polluting *him* with BPA over the past two decades. "Do you think it's responsible for my hair loss?" he once asked me with a wink. My dad is an avid canoe tripper. And sometime in the early 1990s (at Christmas, I think it was), I replaced all his beat-up stainless-steel and aluminum camping plates, bowls, mugs and utensils with a brand-spanking-new matching polycarbonate set.

You shouldn't have to be a chemical engineer to shop for your dad for Christmas, or to supply your child's baby needs. So what we saw with bisphenol A in North America was parents waking up to the fact that their governments were not doing enough to protect their children's health. Together they are working to do something about it.

In North America, the term "soccer mom" was coined in the 1990s to describe a demographic of middle-class women who spend a significant amount of time transporting their kids to activities like soccer practice. Politicians and marketers were particularly anxious to reach them because they're an influential group that has considerable disposable income and votes in large numbers. The significance of the BPA debate is that the soccer moms and the slightly younger parents— let's call them the "sippy cup moms"—started biting back. The founder of SafeMama.com explains it this way: "I am a mother of a two-and-a-half-year-old little boy, a working mom, an author and woman of many trades. I found it completely overwhelming spending so much time researching safety issues for my child. I spent hours looking up bisphenol A or looking for the latest toy recalls. I had an aha! moment and thought that I must not be the only parent scouring the Internet for information about things that affect our children. So I started this website to keep it all in one place."[16] SafeMama.com, together with other blogs like MomsRising.org (co-founded by Joan Blades, she of MoveOn.org fame), mobilized over a hundred thousand letters to

Congress in support of the *Children's Safe Products Act*, which was passed in August 2008.

The power of moms clearly had an impact on the Canadian Conservative Party. The very first thing that Conservative environment minister John Baird mentioned when I asked him why his government had moved against BPA was this: "I had two mothers come up to me sometime last year in a grocery store to raise this issue with me. You can see that while you have large issues like climate change, like smog, this is an in-your-face, frontline environmental concern for Canadian families."

And what companies are only beginning to understand is that this new parental community can damage or benefit brands. As one blogger put it, "The word is out—none of my friends will buy these products, nor will I. These companies risk their reputations and their profits. Mothers are networked together around the country. If they don't change—they'll see it in their bottom line." The final word goes to Agatha Christie. Because, well, Miss Marple is a fount of knowledge about human nature: "A mother's love for her child is like nothing else in the world. It knows no law, no pity; it dares all things and crushes down remorselessly all that stands in its path."

EIGHT: ORGANIC TEA PARTY

Life expectancy would grow by leaps and bounds if green vegetables smelled as good as bacon.

—DOUG LARSON

"CAN I ANSWER 'ALL OF THE ABOVE'?" the young mother wearing yoga pants and a stylish purple barrette asked, her little daughter peeking out from behind her legs.

"Naw. That won't really tell me much," I replied, and tried again. "Even if you agree with all these statements, which is most important to you?"

She looked at the multiple-choice question displayed on my clipboard as we talked in the middle of east-end Toronto's organic food mecca, the Big Carrot. With busy shoppers flowing past, we occasionally had to stand on our tiptoes to let them by.

"I guess it would have to be number one, then. I'm really concerned about toxic chemicals."

I had come to the epicentre of sandal-wearing culture in my city on this busy Saturday afternoon, survey in hand, with one simple question: Why do you buy organic food? Over the course of a few hours, my co-worker Rachel Potter and I spoke with almost 250 people, and the results were clear.[1] More than 60 percent of those we quizzed identified their concern with toxins in non-organic food as their main reason for shopping at the Big Carrot—a finding similar to those of other studies that have looked at this question.[2]

The Big Carrot itself is a testament to the increasing interest in organic food. Founded in 1983, "the Carrot," as it's affectionately known, was the first one-stop-shopping natural and organic food store in Toronto. It survived for a number of years in a cramped 185 square metres of space: a far cry from its current palatial digs in the sprawling "Carrot Common" complex, which includes sundry retail outlets such as a juice bar, a wholistic dispensary and an independent bookstore. On average, the store now services about 2,500 people every day and the cooperative that runs it has just opened a second retail location.

Comparing Apples to (Organic) Apples

So let's drill down to the main concern of Big Carrot shoppers. Sure, people want to avoid toxins. But is there any proof that organic food can deliver on this?

I'll put my cards on the table. Though I've long been a consumer of organic food, I'd always assumed that empirical evidence of its worth was lacking. In that case, why did I buy it? you ask. Out of faith, I guess. A sort of nutritional Hail Mary pass, a hope that it was sort of, kind of better—if not for me, then for the planet.

Not everyone is so casual about this, however. Judging by the vehemence in his voice coming through the phone line, Chuck Benbrook has little time for such vague thinking. Organic food has hard science on its side, he tells me.

An agricultural economist and former research professor in Washington State University's Center for Sustaining Agriculture and Natural Resources (CSANR), Benbrook has had a long career in the agricultural sector. He worked for nearly twenty years in a variety of senior roles with the U.S. federal government and has published widely on pesticide use and residue levels in food, as well as on the relative nutritional merits of different types of produce. After a 2012 article that was played by the media as torpedoing the value of organic food (discussed further below), Benbrook dryly rebutted this assumption, noting that he was among a small group of people who had actually *read* the hundreds of food studies the article cited.[3] No two ways about it: "There is absolutely no way to escape the conclusion, based on a mountain of data, that consumers who seek out organic food to reduce their own personal or family's exposure to possibly risky pesticides are getting a significant return on their investment. They're lowering their risk by approximately eighty-fold."

Benbrook has focused on pesticides in food because of the evidence that much of a typical person's pesticide exposure comes from the residue of agricultural chemicals on fresh fruits and vegetables. He is particularly concerned that certain highly vulnerable segments of the population—including children and pregnant women (especially during the three months before conception and the first trimester of pregnancy)—are being exposed on a daily basis to pesticide levels that have the potential to trigger developmental problems. His argument rests not only on the presence of pesticides in certain types of produce, but also on their toxicity.[4] Benbrook's research team undertook what he characterizes as an "extremely excessive" analysis of the U.S. Department of Agriculture's pesticide programme database, which encompasses 15,000 to 25,000 food samples a year, including an increasing number from organic food. They analyzed these figures back to 1993 and created the Dietary Risk Index (DRI), which takes into account the frequency of residues, average residue levels and toxicity of the pesticide in question.

For example, Benbrook and his team compared conventionally grown varieties of eleven tree-fruit crops with the same produce grown organically and found that there was, on average, an 84-fold difference. That is, the pesticide residues that typically appear in conventional tree-fruit crops in the U.S. food supply make that produce 84 times riskier (to cause harm as defined by the United States Environmental Protection Agency) to consume than organic fruit. Benbrook has done the same sort of head-to-head comparison for many vegetables and concludes that the DRI difference is typically between 50-fold and 150-fold.

To boil this down further, Benbrook calculated that on an average day an American consumer of conventionally grown produce will be exposed to seventeen pesticide residues: a combined DRI value of 2.0. Now, if this consumer replaces twelve foods or ingredients in his diet with organic items, the number of residues will drop from seventeen to five, and his combined DRI value will drop by over two-thirds, to 0.62. This finding fits well with one of the key points of this book—that is, the first thing to do in order to get toxins out of your body is to avoid them in the first place.

One interesting phenomenon that has Benbrook increasingly concerned is the change in the relative contribution to consumers' pesticide risk of domestically grown versus imported produce. "In 1996, when the *Food Quality Protection Act* (FQPA) passed in the United States," he noted in an interview with me, "by our calculations about 75 percent of the dietary risk from pesticides came from domestically grown fruits and vegetables and about 25 percent of the risk came from imported foods. Today, the ratio has flipped to 75 percent from imports and only 25 percent from domestically grown foods." His conclusion is that though the U.S. Environmental Protection Agency (EPA) is using the 1996 law to reduce pesticide levels in U.S.-grown food—undeniably good news—this has no effect on how pesticides are used overseas. As a result, most of the exposure of American (and, we can assume, other) consumers to pesticides like malathion and chlorpyrifos comes during the winter months, when we rely on imported fresh produce. "If this trend continues, another five years down the road, we might have 90 percent of the risk to consumers from pesticides happening in three months, virtually all from imports," Benbrook concluded grimly.

So, according to Benbrook's evidence, the answer to my initial question is clear, and unfortunate: most North American consumers are being exposed, on a daily basis, to pesticide levels that can hurt them. And others share Benbrook's view. More scientific evidence of this problem is accumulating by the day (see table 5). Exposure to many commonly used agricultural pesticides is linked to a variety of health problems, particularly in kids.

It turns out that the Big Carrot shoppers have reason for concern after all.

Table 6. Recent science points to negative health effects from pesticide exposure.

Health Effects	Study Description	Year of Study
Non-Hodgkin's lymphoma	Elevated levels of organochlorine (OC) pesticides years before cancer develops increase risk of non-Hodgkin's lymphoma later in life.	2012
Endocrine disruption	Thirty out of 37 widely used agricultural pesticides blocked or mimicked testosterone and other androgens.	2011

Health Effects	Study Description	Year of Study
General developmental problems and cognitive deficits in infants and children	Prenatal exposure to chlorpyrifos is associated with decreased IQ and working memory scores. Increased levels of prenatal dialkylphosphates (DAPs) are associated with lower neurodevelopment scores at 12 months. Increased urinary dimethyl organophosphate (OP) pesticides are associated with increased odds of ADHD.	2011, 2016[5]
Low birth weight, smaller brain	Higher levels of OP pesticides in umbilical cord plasma are associated with lower birth weight, shorter length and smaller head circumference.	2011
Asthma and poor respiratory health	Any exposure to pesticides is associated with an increased risk of asthma, while living in a region heavily treated with pesticides presents the highest risk.	2011
Increased risk of obesity and diabetes	Low-dose pesticide exposure predicts incidents of type 2 diabetes and future adiposity, dyslipidemia and insulin resistance.	2010, 2011
Infertility	Increased concentration of DDT in maternal milk is associated with an increased risk of infertility.	2009

The Birds and the Bees and the Kids

If pesticide residues in organic produce are significantly lower than in conventional produce, the next question to answer (given the vagaries and variability of the human metabolism) is whether the transition to organic food will result in measurably lower pesticide levels in the body. Like Ray and Jessa's experiment with cosmetics in chapter 1, does the notion of "detox by avoidance" work for pesticides in food as well?

Of the surprisingly few studies that have explored this area, the most convincing is that of Alex Lu, a professor in the Harvard School of Public Health in Boston.[6] I sat with Dr. Lu in his sunny office in the beautifully restored art deco Landmark Center as he gave me a short history of pesticides. "Every thirty years or so we start using a different kind of pesticide," he said. "There are a couple of reasons for this: one

is because of resistance—the more you use a pesticide, the more toler-
ant of it the insects become. The other reason is that negative effects on
human health or the environment start to surface." Qualitatively
speaking, Lu continued, our grandparents were exposed to different
pesticides than we are today. Theirs was the generation that got bom-
barded by hazardous organochlorines—the family of compounds that
includes DDT. "After the banning of DDT we started using organophosphate pesticides," Lu said. "And around 2000, the U.S. started
taking action to reduce organophosphates because evidence of health
effects began to surface. History repeating itself."

Though the U.S. Environmental Protection Agency had dramatically
reduced most indoor uses of organophosphate pesticides by the early
2000s, the use of chemicals like malathion and chlorpyrifos on food
crops was still allowed. Lu decided to investigate the effect of this practice on the human body with a simple but elegant experiment. "At the
time nobody knew whether eating organic produce would have any beneficial effects, specifically for pesticide exposures. So we designed a
crossover study with a group of kids lasting fifteen days. For the middle
five days, they ate nothing but organic produce, and they ate their regular
conventional food before and after the organic feeding days." After com-
pletion of the study, Lu and his colleagues found that not only did the
organic food they provided reduce the kids' pesticide exposure, it largely
eliminated the residues of malathion and chlorpyrifos in their bodies.
The study demonstrated that an organic diet provides almost immediate
protection against exposure to organophosphate pesticides that are commonly used in agriculture. It also showed that children are most likely
exposed to these particular chemicals exclusively through their diet.

Interestingly, when Lu tested the same group of kids for another class
of pesticides—pyrethroids—he found no similar reduction in levels as a
result of eating organic food.[7] Pyrethroids are synthetic chemicals similar to those found in chrysanthemums. Because of their effectiveness
in eating away at the hard external skeleton of various bugs, they are now
the most commonly used pesticides in the average home. Though the
levels of pyrethroid pesticides in the urine of Lu's test subjects didn't
diminish as a result of eating organic food, kids whose parents reported
using pesticides at home (both in the house and in the garden) did have
significantly higher pyrethroid levels. From this Lu concluded that

residential pesticide use represents the most important risk factor for children's exposure to pyrethroid insecticides.

Lu is also a pioneer with another family of pesticides that have—infamously—started to replace some organophosphates: neonicotinoids.[8] Synthetic chemicals similar to nicotine, neonicotinoids are "systemic insecticides": rather than sitting on the surface of the crops, they are actually slurped up by a plant through its root system. As Lu explained, Monsanto has teamed up with Bayer AG to coat their GMO corn seed with neonicotinoids. The claim is that, for the farmer, it will be one-stop shopping: you buy GMO corn pre-treated with insecticide and you don't even have to spray. You just put down the seed and it will grow. The downside is that in the past when farmers sprayed with pesticides, consumers hoped that the residue on, for example, the surface of a tomato would dissipate over time because of sunlight, rainfall and so on. But with this new technology, Lu pointed out, there's no way that you can remove the chemical prior to eating it.

Luckily for tomato eaters (and eaters of any other conventionally farmed fruits and veggies), there is currently no evidence that neonicotinoids are hazardous to human health.[9] A good thing, given that one chemical from this family, imidacloprid, is the most commonly used pesticide in the world today.[10, 11] It's not so lucky for one group of insects, though: the bees. There is now considerable evidence that imidacloprid causes "colony collapse disorder," or CCD—the mysterious global trend whereby bees up and desert their hives, never to be seen again. Given that bee pollination is involved in foods that comprise one-third of the U.S. diet and that commercial pollination is valued at about US$217 billion a year globally, this is a bit of a problem, to say the least.[12] There are many competing hypotheses being put forward to account for CCD, which has now manifested itself in many places around the world. Some have theorized that colony collapse disorder may result from mite and virus infestations, bee malnutrition or even cellphone radiation. Alex Lu, however, provides convincing evidence that very small doses of imidacloprid can produce the CCD effect. In his carefully constructed experiment, fifteen of sixteen imidacloprid-treated hives were abandoned in four different apiaries twenty-three weeks after imidacloprid dosing. The survival of the "control" hives—those not treated with insecticide and managed alongside the treated hives—buttresses this conclusion.

In a serious bummer for them, honeybees don't have the option of relying on organic food sources. They're stuck buzzing around crops that, it is now fairly clear, are slowly poisoning them to death. Luckily for them, governments started to step in to protect the bees (or at least their economic value). In late April 2013, the European Commission passed a proposal to restrict the use of three types of neonicotinoids (including imidacloprid), effective December 2013 for a period of two years. The Commission took action in response to what it identified as "high acute risks" for bees when exposed to these pesticides.[13] As of May 2018, the commission voted to "completely ban . . . outdoor uses" of these neonicotinoids, again citing their pernicious effect on bee populations.[14] The U. S. Department of Agriculture initially rejected the EC's claim that pesticides played an important role in colony collapse disorder, but eventually called for further investigation of the problem.[15] As of December 2017, the EPA had scheduled a review and risk assessment of five neonicotinoid pesticides.[16] In Canada, meanwhile, the CBC reported in December 2017 that the federal government had proposed "tighter restrictions" on neonicotinoids but stopped short of "an all-out ban."[17] Sub-national governments, however, have acted more assertively. Ontario has regulated a reduction in neonicotinoid use[18] and Montreal and Vancouver have both banned neonicotinoids within city limits.[19] Given the evidence of sky-high levels of neonicotinoids in honey right around the world—a fact that spells serious trouble for bees everywhere— this regulatory scrutiny is long overdue.[20]

The Hundred-Year Diet

Firestorm. That's the word I'd use to describe the reaction to what became known as the "Stanford study" (reflecting the study's institutional origin).[21] The title —"Are Organic Foods Safer or Healthier Than Conventional Alternatives?"—tells you everything you need to know about the question it posed. And the screaming headlines that ensued— "Organic Food Isn't Healthier and No Safer," "Little Evidence of Health Benefits from Organic Food" and "It's Official: Organic Food Is a Waste of Cash"—were the organic industry's worst nightmare.

When I asked him for his reaction to the furor, Matt Holmes, who was then the executive director of the Canada Organic Trade Association (COTA), let out an exasperated sigh. Holmes is generally optimistic.

After he started at COTA, Canada implemented the first-ever national standard and labelling system for organic products and signed major agreements with the E.U. and the U.S. to increase exports of Canadian organic food. Still, he admitted to some frustration. "I don't think there's an evil conspiracy against organic," Holmes told me as we shared a drink overlooking Baltimore harbour's historic warships. (We were both in town to attend Natural Products Expo East—one of the biggest organic industry conventions and trade shows of the year.) "I just think there's a human tendency to assume organic should be a solution to everything, and it's not. It can't be. But the media, in particular, love to pull the 'gotcha' routine."

Holmes told me about a recent incident involving a TV story about pesticide residues on organic apples. No matter how many times Holmes tried to explain that pesticides are ubiquitous (and therefore it's no surprise that even organic apples have a bit on their skin), the journalist was determined to run with an "exposé" angle: "Revealed: Pesticides Found in Organic Produce!" "The levels they found were similar to those in unborn children and Arctic sea ice," Holmes said. "The reality of today's world is that this stuff is absolutely everywhere. Organic doesn't promise to be completely pesticide-free—it can't escape the random pesticides that are floating around. It promises to be an alternative system that doesn't contribute to the problem."

Holmes pointed out that the Stanford study set up a straw man that was further torqued through the extensive media coverage: that organic food is primarily desirable because of the claim that it has a higher nutrient content than conventional food. "It ignored or downplayed the other benefits of organic production. I like to describe organic agriculture as the hundred-year diet. It's a system of agriculture that perpetuates itself, that creates a healthy ecosystem that will in turn continue to support plants in the long term, so you're not in this deathly cycle of creating short-term nutrients—which then can contribute to pest infestations that need to be counteracted by immediate and short-term chemical pesticides, which then kill the life in the soil, which then requires another synthetic input. Holmes underlined that, despite the media hype, buried in the Stanford study are tepid admissions of the worth of organic food: a finding that organic produce has a 30 percent lower risk of containing pesticides than does conventional produce (a number that Chuck Benbrook believes is closer to 90 percent[22]) and another finding that conventional meats have a 33 percent higher risk of contamination with bacteria resistant to antibiotics than do organic meats (a figure that Benbrook calculates as being far too low).

Even if you accept the Stanford study's contention that evidence for the nutritional superiority of organic food is lacking (which, by the way, flies in the face of other, more compelling studies that have concluded that organic foods are more nutrient-rich[23, 24]), it strongly reinforces the argument that organic food is better for the consumer when it comes to levels of pesticides and disease-causing bacteria. This from a study that was widely trumpeted by the media as being a disaster for the organics industry.[25]

Post-Niche

"In Organic We Trust" read the placards of the crowd milling outside the front doors of the Baltimore Convention Center.

As I pushed through the picketers to get inside, someone thrust a small envelope into my hand. It was a package of tea, a determined Uncle Sam staring out at me from one side and the Organic Tea Party's "platform" emblazoned on the other: "The Organic Tea Party is a non-partisan celebration of people, planet and pure tea. Our aim is a healthy and happy planet where our food chain and tea farmers are free from pesticides, chemically-enhanced fertilizers and genetically modified organisms (GMOs) . . . Declare Your inTEApendence and Vote Organic!" In the 2012 U.S. presidential election season, this fun gimmick by the Numi tea company was the first of many indicators at Natural Products Expo East that the organic industry was feeling pretty pleased with itself. One might say even cocky.

During the conference in Charm City, I heard a keynote speech by Kathleen Merrigan, who was deputy secretary of the U.S. Department of Agriculture at that time; more than ten years earlier she had been one of the lead authors of the USDA's organic labelling rules. In her upbeat remarks, Merrigan at one point said that the "USDA as a department is really owning organic," which caused the assembled organic industry leaders to look at each other and murmur in delight—no doubt thinking that only a few years earlier, such a powerful validation from a government leader would have been utterly unthinkable. Another surprise, a made-in-Canada one this time, occurred at the gala dinner of the Organic Trade Association (OTA; affiliated with Matt Holmes's COTA), the organic industry's lobbying arm. In a sea of (charming) Americans, I sat at a table with a number of fellow Canucks, including a guy from Export Development Canada (EDC). EDC is the Canadian federal government's export credit agency, and it's a big deal, providing financing to Canadian exporters and investors in more than two hundred markets worldwide. In 2009 alone, EDC facilitated over C$82 billion in investment, export and domestic support. Every few years EDC picks a new batch of strategic areas on which to focus its largesse—areas the agency believes will prove winners on the international stage. And guess what? Organic agriculture is now one of those areas. As of 2017, the Canadian organic sector generates annual sales of $5.4 billion and the EDC frequently provides financing to organics-focused companies as part of a larger effort to cultivate "new markets for Canada's agrifood companies."[26, 27]

Another organic expert I chatted with in Baltimore (over a delicious cup of organic tea) was Katherine DiMatteo. The energetic, grey-haired DiMatteo was for sixteen years the executive director of the OTA, leading the industry through the critical years that culminated in implementation of the first U.S. National Organic Program (NOP) standards in 2002. DiMatteo still remembers the excitement of that time. "It was a very unified effort. It was initiated by environmental and consumer activist groups, then the farmer organizations came on, and the Organic Trade Association—which was little bitty at the time—with our small group of processors and retailers also joined in. It was multi-stakeholder and multi-interest, but we knew this was *the* moment to get a breakthrough at the national level." The results of the new standard have been truly impressive. In 1990, the year that DiMatteo joined the "little bitty" OTA, U.S. sales of organic food were US$1 billion annually. In 2002, the year the NOP standards were implemented, that number had grown to US$8.6 billion. In 2017, U.S. sales stood at $49.4 billion.[28]

Despite this astounding growth (which shows no signs of abating anytime soon) and the generally positive mood in the Baltimore Convention Center, DiMatteo confessed to fretting about some storm clouds on the horizon. I asked her about a recent article in the *New York*

Times that detailed infighting between organic advocates. The dispute has centred on the actions of the National Organic Standards Board (NOSB) in approving some food additives—like carrageenan, a seaweed-derived thickener—as being okay to include in certified organic products.[29] "Absolutely benign and consistent with organic principles," say the majority of those on the NOSB. "A sellout to big business and a betrayal," retort some organic purists like the Cornucopia Institute, publisher of the provocative report *The Organic Watergate—Connecting the Dots: Corporate Influence at the USDA's National Organic Program*.[30] Looking at me over the top of her glasses as she nursed her steaming tea, DiMatteo observed that the organic industry is often its own worst enemy. "Certified organic is a rigorous adherence to now nationally required standards," she explained. "It's costly in terms of certification, inspection, paperwork and all these other things, and the regulations constantly get tightened. Our movement wants continuous improvement, quickly—and we're not patient."

DiMatteo is concerned not only that this "constant tightening" of the NOP standards dissuades potential new entrants to the organic market, but also that the constant push to expand the meaning of "organic" is making the concept too unwieldy and undeliverable. "Other agendas are beginning to be played out in the organic regulations," she told me. "Like allergies. Our standards aren't about allergenicity. We're supposed to be about environmental protection and biodiversity. Now all of a sudden we have to talk about things like 'Is it an allergen?' The organizations that have the energy to push and work on these things are now using organic as a platform for moving towards an agenda that is making it very difficult for both the people already in organic to stay in and new people to get in." DiMatteo wonders whether some organic advocates are really trying to drive processed foods out of the organic certification system entirely. In her view—and I have to say I agree with her—this would be entirely counterproductive. "At least here in the U.S., we still buy an awful lot of processed food. That culture isn't going to change," she said. "The way to mainstream consumers is not by telling them you have to *only* eat fresh fruits and vegetables and whole grains."

It falls to DiMatteo's successors at the OTA to work through these complicated issues. Clearly, they have their plate full. The way Laura Batcha, the OTA's current CEO, sees it, the organic industry is at an exciting but vulnerable moment. "A lot of the conventional agriculture industry has been annoyed hearing the USDA endorse and recognize organic across the whole agency. Even though the institutions and the dollars and a lot of the change haven't happened yet, they just don't like the talk of it," she told me as we tried to find a quiet corner on the noisy convention floor. "There's been a much more coordinated pushback on us from the conventional industry, and we're at a vulnerable spot in our growth because we're no longer under the radar."

"So you're not niche anymore," I offered.

"We're not niche. We're post-niche! And it's a vulnerable place to be because we're between. We're increasingly mainstream but we're still operating from a minority position."

"Everywhere Food Is Sold"

Whether you're Apple or a small organic food store, the pressures and complications that emerge from expanding your business are often difficult to manage. Given the organic sector's very rapid emergence into the consumer mainstream, it's perhaps not surprising that there are some growing pains. Many organic companies are experiencing year-over-year double-digit increases in their revenue. Some of their stories are quite spectacular.

Here's an example. At its founding in Vancouver in 1985, Nature's Path sold just one product: Manna Bread, a dense and nutritious sprouted-grain concoction that quickly became a health food store fixture. Still privately held and run by Arran and Ratana Stephens and their children, Nature's Path is now the largest organic cereal company in North America, with annual sales in excess of C$200 million and distribution in 42 countries.[31] As I munched my way through the overflowing basket of samples sent to me by Maria Emmer-Aanes, at the time the company's director of marketing and communications, I didn't find this terribly surprising. Their cereal is delicious: I now keep a pack of Love Crunch Apple Crumble granola on my desk. Emmer-Aanes told me that Nature's Path has bought nearly three thousand acres of farmland in Saskatchewan to supply many of their whole-grain needs and continues to invest in social causes like the Prop 37 battle (described below). "The company is fiercely independent," she says. "We feel that it's socially responsible to make sure that everyone—no matter your economic status—has access to chemical-free food. This is a company that decides what its margins are going to be, decides what it's going to put back into the world and isn't afraid to make unconventional financial decisions. The strategy has paid off. When you give, it comes back to you!"

Another story of success is that of possibly the most ebullient champion of all things organic: Gary Hirshberg, chairman and former "CE-Yo" of Stonyfield, an organic yogurt maker in Londonderry, New Hampshire. A tagline on Stonyfield's website reads "Environmentalists turned yogurt makers"—a succinct summary of the company's DNA. Hirshberg joined what was a tiny business in 1983 hoping to turn the cottage industry into a profit centre that would fund a local farming school dedicated to teaching sustainable agricultural practices. That year, the first fifty-gallon batch of yogurt was made and annual sales totalled US$56,000.[32] The demand for their yogurt soon outpaced Stonyfield's nineteen cows' ability to supply the milk, and the company began buying product from local dairy farmers. By 1988, the company had expanded so much that they were able to build a large industrial facility in Londonderry with sophisticated dairy-processing equipment that could handle the increasing demand.[33] As of 2012, Stonyfield Farm had production companies in the United States and Canada and ventures in France and Ireland—and was valued at US$400 million.[34] Choosing a different growth strategy than Nature's Path, Stonyfield partnered with food product multinational Danone Group in 2001, and in 2014 Danone purchased a controlling stake in the company.[35] The transaction helped to propel the company to its current position as the largest organic yogurt producer in the world and the third-largest yogurt brand in the United States.[36] In July 2017, however, Danone sold Stonyfield to Lactalis for $875 million, largely because of anti-trust pressure from the U.S. Department of Justice.[37]

Stonyfield's affiliation with a larger global food company is typical of a wider consolidation trend in the organic sector. Multinational food companies have got into the business of not *going* but *getting* organic: acquiring successful smaller organic companies. Those delicious, all-natural Naked fruit juices and smoothies? Since 2006 these beverages have been brought to you by PepsiCo. General Mills, the makers of such staples as Betty Crocker, Lucky Charms and Pillsbury, actually entered the organic business pretty early on, with their 1999 acquisition of

Small Planet Foods, adding the likes of Muir Glen organic canned tomatoes, juices and sauces to their already humongous stock list. And what better example of granola going corporate than the buyout of Kashi by the Kellogg Company in 2000?[38]

For Hirshberg, a wiry and intense guy who admits to preferring peppermint tea because no one could handle him on caffeine, there's no time to waste. "We've got to become part of the mainstream. It's got to happen. We're on a chemical time bomb as a species." Hirshberg's perspective is simple: "Everywhere food is sold there should be organic. Walmart, airlines, airports. I've worked very closely with Walmart—I think I was the first mainstream organic company to be in Walmart. I have gone down and given lectures at their infamous Saturday morning town hall meetings. I've met with heads of Walmart in other countries. I think a lot of activists are very troubled by places like Walmart, but I'll tell you, the nail in the coffin of synthetic growth hormone was driven by Walmart." In Hirshberg's view it was Walmart's refusal to buy products containing synthetic growth hormone that spurred other companies, such as Danone and Yoplait, to change (food sales account for over half of Walmart's total revenue, totalling $200 billion in 2016).[39] "A big player like that can move mountains."

Given that Bruce and I have the primary objective of reducing levels of synthetic chemicals in people's bodies—as many people as possible as quickly as possible—I tend to agree with Hirshberg's logic. After chatting with him, I actually phoned up Walmart to find out more about their sales of organic products. Just by dint of its enormous size (accounting for about 26 percent of all groceries sold in the U.S. in 2017), Walmart moves more organic food than any other retailer. I spoke with Ron McCormick, then Senior Director of Sustainable Agriculture for Walmart U.S. He told me that after a very public commitment in 2006 to double sales of organics, the retailer has now zeroed in on those areas where organic sales continue to grow. "If you look at where organic is really selling, you have big dollars in dairy and big dollars in organic baby food and big dollars in fresh produce."

Local vs. Carbon

I was surprised when McCormick told me that, these days, Walmart sees more interest in local food than in organic. The retailer committed to increasing local's share of its total produce sales to 9 percent by 2015—and in 2018 local produce represented 10 percent of the total sold in U.S. stores.[40] McCormick foresees further great opportunities to increase the amount of local production across the country, and in this sense Walmart is simply responding to what is clearly a pervasive trend. "Locavore" was named 2007 Word of the Year by the Oxford American Dictionary, and I now stumble upon farmers' markets selling local produce in virtually every city I visit. Locally sourced ingredients are now *de rigueur* on restaurant menus everywhere, and the "100-Mile Diet" is ensconced in the vernacular.

This rise in the prominence of local food clearly irks some organic advocates. The Canada Organic Trade Association, for instance, has published a hard-hitting postcard enumerating the advantages of organic food: it's subject to a rigorous, government-regulated labelling and certification system; it's guaranteed to have been produced without the addition of pesticides, synthetic fertilizers or growth hormones or antibiotics; it's made without artificial preservatives, colours, flavours or chemical additives; and animals providing organic meat are raised in accordance with humane standards. Meanwhile, COTA gives "local" a failing grade across the board. Unlike the term "organic" on food, which now in many other parts of the world is subject to government oversight, the term "local" can be slapped on any food with wild abandon. What does it mean? How local is local? Who checks up on whether a given item was really produced locally?

One potential comparative advantage that local has over organic is its generally smaller carbon footprint. Logically, if a product comes from the local vicinity, transporting it to your table should create fewer greenhouse-gas pollutants than the amount created when a similar item is brought in from abroad. This raises the question of whether organic food is simply trading one type of pollution for another: carcinogens for global-warming gases. Andre Leu, president of the International Federation of Organic Agriculture Movements (IFOAM until 2017), has thought a lot about this issue, not only because this Bonn, Germany–based global umbrella body for the organic sector represents over 1,000 affiliates in 120 countries,[41] but also because he's an organic tropical fruit farmer in a remote area of Queensland, Australia. Shipping organic produce to buyers halfway around the world is what he does for a living. I met Leu at Natural Products Expo East in Baltimore.

"When it comes to carbon dioxide, there are really two issues," Leu began. "In terms of the amount put into the atmosphere during the life cycle of a crop, the transport from the farm to the market is very minimal compared to other inputs. For instance, there's some wonderful work done in New Zealand: it's actually better for the environment for England to air-freight all its organic products from New Zealand every day as opposed to the way they're producing it conventionally now, particularly in winter, when you have hothouses and heating." Leu argues that the amount of carbon dioxide and other greenhouse-gas pollutants like nitrous oxide that are given off by chemical fertilizers, along with the amount of carbon dioxide used to actually produce the pesticides, means organic has a much lower carbon footprint than conventionally produced "local" food.

The other significant carbon advantage of organic, according to Leu, is the amount of carbon sequestered in the soil by organic agriculture. "The word 'organic' actually comes from the fact that we recycle organic matter in the soil through composting and the like," Leu said. "As a primary practice, our focus has been building up soil organic matter—in other words, organic soil carbon. And now we have very good data showing that organic practices not only emit less carbon in the growing than conventional, but also, when we factor in the amount of carbon dioxide we can strip out of the atmosphere and sequester in the soil when we build up the organic soil matter, we are actually not just greenhouse-neutral. We mitigate more than we put out." Leu became more animated as he described new data indicating that a more wide-spread adoption of organic agriculture could have a huge impact on the reduction of greenhouse-gas pollution. Leu claims that with organic we could remove up to 20 percent of all current global greenhouse-gas output. Call this "atmospheric detox."

I can think of no one who shows more passion for food issues than Sarah Elton. Sarah is a friend, a prominent journalist and author of the bestselling *Locavore: From Farmers' Fields to Rooftop Gardens—How Canadians Are Changing the Way We Eat.* She eschews packaged food, preferring instead to make all her family's meals from scratch, and she worries aloud that she wasn't able to can as many vegetables this past autumn as she usually does. I figured if anybody was prepared to eloquently and aggressively defend the moral superiority of local over organic it would be Sarah. Turns out I was completely wrong.

For starters, in terms of her personal buying habits for her husband and two young daughters, she regularly shops at the Big Carrot and is "one hundred percent behind organic. We definitely need to be pushing in that direction," she told me emphatically. I told her about the COTA postcard and its criticisms of local food's lack of rigour or definition, and she agreed with it totally. "I was just chopping my pear this morning and remembering the sign about low-spray pesticides at the Brickworks [a farmers' market in downtown Toronto], where I bought it. What the heck does 'low spray' mean? Who decides what's low and what's high? What happens if you have pests one year? Are you going to tell me that you've gone high spray? I don't think so. So I agree, local is not the be-all and end-all. It's a piece of the sustainable food system."

Elton defines her number one concern as "sustainable food," by which she means food that's good for people and good for the planet. "There's no question that organic is better for the environment, because organic agriculture nurtures the soil. If you're worried about carbon emissions, it sequesters more carbon than conventional agriculture. It doesn't rely on toxic chemicals because it sees agriculture as ecology rather than a war against the earth. On the other hand, local food economies are so good on so many levels for rural and urban communities. So local plus organic equals sustainability: socially, culturally and environmentally."

Even though she figures her own family eats 80 to 90 percent organic, Elton isn't too fussed if, for the time being, local is stealing some of organic's buzz. "I see local as a first step in the learning process and the first step towards building a more sustainable food system. Hopefully, by realizing we want our local farmers, soon we'll be able to talk about why organic local is better than just local."

Nine Kids

With the exception of Alex Lu's studies on pesticides and food, few efforts have been made to evaluate whether organic food results in lower levels of toxins in your body.[42] So Bruce and I set out to see whether we could duplicate Lu's then-decade-old work. The task at hand for our big experiment was a pretty strange one—we needed a bunch of kids to agree to eat lots of vegetables over the course of twelve days during their summer break, *and* they had to collect their pee each day. To find these kids, we did what any good twenty-first-century researcher does: we took to Facebook. Our call outlined the following: the word on the street is that an organic diet might be better for the environment and our bodies, and eating organic could mean reduced exposure to the harmful chemicals that are in conventional food—something we wanted to show with their help. After a few days of interviews, we found nine really great kids from five Toronto-area families who were excited to participate in our experiment. They included five girls and four boys, ages three to twelve. These families were all different in a lot of wonderful ways, but they had two important things in common: they didn't at present eat any organic food *and* they were willing to spend twelve days of their summer holidays helping out with our experiment.

Here's what the 12 days looked like for these nine kids:

Phase 1: Days 1–3

8 a.m. collection of urine sample each day, conventional diet

Phase 2: Days 4–8

8 a.m. collection of urine sample each day, organic diet only

Phase 3: Days 9–12

8 a.m. collection of urine sample each day, conventional diet

We were very lucky to have that wonderful grocery store, the Big Carrot, offer to donate all the organic food for the organic portion of the experiment. And I'm not just talking apples and oranges. I'm talking organic applesauce, organic zucchini bread and all that falls in between: olive oil, flour, canned tomatoes and—unanimously appreciated by our participants' moms and dads—organic ice cream for those hot summer days. So the night before the organic phase of their experiment, whether by car, streetcar or bike, each of these five families made the trek to the Carrot on Danforth Avenue to pick up their supplies for the next five days.

By now I'll bet a lot of you are wondering what happened with all that pee. The families kept each day's samples in their freezers until the end of the experiment, at which point our intrepid research assistant, Rachel, collected the samples from each kid—all 108 jars. The urine samples were shipped off to a lab in California for testing and then we waited for the results. Several anxious months later, we received the results table with a daunting 1,800-plus pieces of data on urinary pesticide levels. It was quite a dramatic hour as we oh so carefully entered the lab results into a spreadsheet for our analysis, eager to see what they would demonstrate.

Our objective was to compare the organophosphate (OP) pesticide metabolite levels in the urine of the children. OP pesticides were chosen because of their widespread use, their reported presence as residues on foods frequently consumed by children and their acute toxicity.[43] Check out figure 10 for a graph of the results (and the endnotes for an explanation of our calculations).

Figure 10. Average of dimethyl dialkylphosphate (DAP) levels for nine children over the three phases of the experiment (units are ng/L).

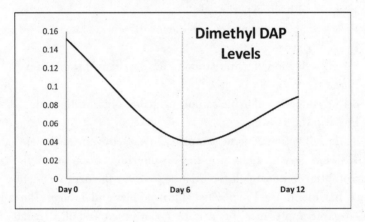

The graph, you'll see, shows average concentrations, for all the children together, of dimethyl dialkylphosphate (DAP) metabolites (which are common to OP pesticides) over each of the three phases of the experiment (conventional, organic, conventional). Notice the significant drop in dimethyl DAP levels during phase 2 (the organic phase) and the increase again once the kids started eating conventional food in phase 3. In scientific parlance, the organic and conventional results are "significantly" different. What does this mean to everyone in general? *Eating organic really can lower your pesticide levels!* A particular comment stuck with me when we did our follow-up interviews. One mother told me that she was initially interested in the study because her father, following some health issues, had become an "organic/ vegan freak" but that she didn't really believe all the hype about organics and being chemical-free. As a single parent, she was also wary of organics' cost (though the cost difference between organic and non-organic food is rapidly shrinking as the organic industry grows).[44] "Now," she said, half-laughing, half-sighing, "I've got some real numbers proving my dad is right." She said she didn't know what was more annoying: admitting that her father was right or that those chemicals were in her daughter at all.

I think we can all guess what she really believes.

NINE: STRAIGHT FLUSH

[BRUCE DETOXES]

Kick back in the back, get the phantom to drop. Bass blarin' outta my system, that's how I detox.[1]

— JAY-Z, "REHAB (REMIX)"

IS DETOX THE "MASS DELUSION" that at least one doctor has called it?[2] Surely something can be done to reduce our toxic burden and the various nasty diseases that may ensue from inadvertent exposure to or ingestion of the poisons around us—and that's without touching on exposure that is absolutely intentional. Rick and I have been asked many times, "Did you use any special detox treatments to lower your chemical levels after the *Slow Death* experiments?" The answer is no, so here is our opportunity to dig into what we could have done.

Step one is understanding detoxification. And to do that, in this chapter we'll unpack and assess the multibillion-dollar detox industry[3] through the experiences of individuals and health experts who have devoted years of their lives to the complex, often expensive and sometimes painful journey of personal detoxification.

Detox Man

I first met Peter Sullivan following a San Francisco speaking event in Haight-Ashbury, the 1960s hippie hangout. Rick and I were on our book tour, and we had an amazing conversation with Peter over dinner following our talk. We were both struck by his matter-of-fact approach to his intense focus on detoxing his life and the lives of his family members. Peter wanted to tell his personal story—including his devotion to self-experimenting with virtually every detox technique that exists.

In late spring of 2012 I travelled to Silicon Valley to meet with Peter. I thought Rick and I were good at self-experimentation, but compared to Peter we are mere amateurs.

Peter is able to devote the necessary time and financial resources to test hundreds of detox strategies in a way that nobody else in the world has likely done. With a graduate degree in computer science from Stanford, Peter designed and ran the web interface for Netscape. That may sound quaint now, but at the time it was the second-largest Internet portal in the world. Peter is a genuine and easygoing guy who, despite his success, doesn't set himself apart from the rest of us. But the real difference between him and the general populace who are concerned about the effect of synthetic chemicals on their health is this: as a lifelong allergy sufferer who is mindful of the recent rise of peanut and other lethal allergies, he's spent the better part of twenty years seeking answers to the basic question "What is going on?" Visiting with him not only helped me understand the stunning breadth and diversity of detox techniques currently on the market, it also helped me identify what are probably the most effective techniques to use if—like Rick and me—you have more modest means.

In addition to allergies, in the late 1990s Peter began to face acute health issues. One night in 1998 he passed out and had difficulty waking up. Later he suspected that episode had been caused by something to do with food, but the experience was nothing like food poisoning. The fainting episode became the trigger for Peter's research into what was going on with his body and his life.

Irritable, stressed out, unhappy and feeling generally unwell, he was under tremendous pressure at work and feeling burned out. Strange and unpleasant things were happening to his family too: one of his young sons was diagnosed with "sensory integration" and was experiencing emotional breakdowns, night tremors and autistic behaviours—including headbanging. Peter's other son, at five years of age, was expelled from kindergarten for his antisocial behaviour.

Peter turned his sharp, analytical mind to the problems he and his family were facing and started to connect a few dots. Food was an obvious place to start. Were he and his family experiencing undiagnosed food allergies? Intolerances to lactose or gluten perhaps? Mercury also came to mind. Although at the time Peter was largely unfamiliar with the health problems associated with high levels of mercury, it didn't take too much digging around for him to discover that stress and irritability are among the many symptoms. If mercury was indeed part of the problem, what was the source of the mercury?

Fish and dental amalgams (mercury fillings) are the primary sources of mercury in most people. Peter ate a lot of fish and had many amalgam fillings. What's more, his dentist had informed him that he was grinding his teeth when he was sleeping—as many people do. He found the idea of grinding the mercury in his teeth and ingesting that highly poisonous neurotoxin (a toxin that affects the brain) to be literally sickening. And what about his kids? They didn't have mercury fillings, but they ate fish and likely received vaccines with mercury in them (mercury was used as a preservative in vaccines). Peter began asking health professionals whether he needed to be concerned about mercury and its possible relation to his health problems and those of his kids—especially the autistic behaviours. One doctor had no advice to give, another indicated that mercury was not used in dental fillings and another said that ideas about links between mercury and the problems Peter's family was experiencing were "fringe." All these were typical of the responses traditional doctors would give, especially two decades ago. Doctors today are better informed.

But Peter did not give up. As a search-engine designer, he did the obvious thing and went hunting for a new doctor online. He found a local doctor who specialized in "integrated medicine." One of the first things his new doctor did was correct the misinformation regarding mercury fillings: Peter's mouth was *filled* with them. When he was tested for mercury, the results were shocking. His mercury level was 23 micrograms per millilitre—nearly three times higher than what is considered to be safe. He decided to have his sons and his wife tested too, and it turned out that they all had elevated mercury levels. This was the beginning of Peter's first dedicated foray into personal body detox.

He followed what is now a familiar procedure for heavy-metal detox. Step 1: he had his mercury fillings removed. Step 2: he embarked on chelation (pronounced *ke-layshun*) therapy. Put in simple terms, chelation is a medical treatment that involves introducing specialized solutions into a patient, either orally or intravenously, that bind to heavy metals and cause them to be eliminated from the body via urine.[4] I tried this treatment as well (as you'll read later).

Peter underwent two and a half years of intravenous chelation treatments with DMPS (2,3-dimercapto-1-propanesulphonic acid), and he also tried chelation using DMSA (DL-2,3-dimercaptosuccinic acid, the oral solution). At the end of the treatment period Peter's mercury levels had declined and he felt better—his mind was clearer and he could think faster, although he still had problems sleeping.

We talked about the dozens of cleanses and diets that Peter tried as part of his detox quest. Rick made sure that I asked Peter about colonic irrigation, for instance. Peter said he'd tried it three or four times, the last time in Hawaii, where it made him feel quite good. Some of us go to Hawaii for the scuba diving and surfing; Peter goes for the colonic water sports. He cautioned me, however, that colonic irrigation can destroy the flora in the body (I managed to avoid the topic of fecal transplants, a bizarre but apparently effective means of replacing body flora).[5] Others go much further in their critique of the resurgence of colonic irrigation, stating that it is not only quackery but is associated with potentially serious health risks.[6] If there is a product, potion or procedure with a detox claim, chances are Peter has tried it.

Electromagnetic Personalities

After our lengthy conversation earlier in the day, Peter and I met for dinner in Palo Alto at a fine restaurant that serves local organic food and has an on-site drinking-water filtration system. We each savoured a glass of the water as though it were a fine California Zinfandel and jumped through several topics, including ion balance, heavy-metal toxicity, the effects of electromagnetic fields (EMFs) and his experience with chelation.

One of the things that Peter is particularly preoccupied with is EMF radiation. Electrical currents create electromagnetic fields, so any electrical device in our homes can emit EMF radiation, as do the increasing number of mobile phones, wireless modems, cellphone towers and, of course, microwave ovens. Electromagnetic radiation is invisible, and most people experience no symptoms during or after being exposed to it. But others find that certain EMFs are almost paralyzing. The ambiguity surrounding the effects of this type of radiation is only intensified by the fact that it seems as many studies have been carried out concerning the inconclusiveness of EMF research as concerning EMFs themselves. According to one of the basic tenets of risk—that risk of harm equals hazard times exposure—the possibility of harm appears to be increasing, because exposure to EMFs is increasing exponentially as the number of electronic devices increases. At the end of 2011 there were six billion mobile phone subscriptions worldwide.[7] Since then, curiously, estimates have fallen back to roughly five billion—still, five billion![8] With all of these mobile phones emitting direct, close-range EMF doses, risk by its very definition is increasing.

If you are an avid mobile phone user you may have experienced a warm sensation on the side of your head after a lengthy phone call—this is caused by microwave radiation and can actually cause localized heating up of your brain. In 2011, the International Agency for Research on Cancer classified mobile phones as possibly causing cancer in humans, despite the fact that numerous studies on large numbers of mobile phone users have not found increases in cancer rates. Research and regulatory bodies are taking a precautionary approach. The California Department of Public Health, for instance, recently issued guidelines that recommend keeping phones away from one's head (where and when possible) and carrying phones in a "backpack, briefcase or purse" as opposed to a "pocket, bra or belt holster."[9]

After dinner we went to check out Peter's EMF-proof Faraday cage, named after Michael Faraday, the nineteenth-century English scientist who discovered how electromagnetic fields work. I could see that getting to Peter's house was going to be half the fun: parked outside the restaurant was his white Tesla electric sports car. With some effort I squeezed my six-foot-two frame into the tiny passenger compartment, and off we sped out of Palo Alto into the misty hills of Los Altos at dusk. Peter's house was a large, modern three-storey structure with fabulous views down the valley. Much of the structure was unused or under construction because of the extraordinary efforts he has undertaken to replace wiring to eliminate "dirty electricity," clean up mould, add high-end air filtration systems and remove toxic materials. ("Dirty electricity" is unwanted electromagnetic energy that can be produced by dimmer switches, compact fluorescent light bulbs—yet another reason to move on to LEDs—or poor wiring. It is measured in Graham-Stetzer [GS] units.)

The Faraday cage was what I had come to see and Peter took me to an upstairs bedroom to check it out. Turns out the bedroom *was* the Faraday cage. I had somehow imagined that there would be steel mesh involved, and that it would be a solitary cage sitting in the middle of a dark room, perhaps suspended from the ceiling in true Batman style—ideally in a dank, windowless basement. But no, it was a pretty normal-looking bedroom with a small mattress on the floor, a desk and a table.

Peter took me to his office—a room down the hall—where a bizarre measuring instrument was sitting on his desk, looking as if it had sprung from the imagination of Jules Verne. It resembled some sort of Victorian weather instrument made of glass and brass, attached to a metal box and featuring various switches and readout screens. A regular blip kept appearing on the screen, and I asked Peter what it was measuring. He explained that it was EMF radiation coming in from the rotating military radar perhaps five miles down the valley from where we stood. "And that is a bad thing?" I asked, knowing the answer. "Very bad," said Peter. Hence the Faraday cage.

Having worked in software design and electronics all his life, Peter is now convinced that electrical devices have been the cause of tremendous suffering for him, his family and millions of others. We walked into the Faraday bedroom, Peter carrying the EMF device, and sure enough, the radar signal ceased to blip. The cage was working.

It was nearly time to turn in and experience first-hand a night in the Faraday cage. Before leaving, Peter wanted to do a quick check of the house to make sure there was no EMF contamination to disturb me. He grabbed the Graham-Stetzer Stetzerizer Microsurge Meter and turned it on. This instrument measures "dirty electricity," and much to Peter's dismay the readout showed a measurement of more than 100 Hz. Peter raced around the house, turning light switches on and off, trying to find the dirty electricity offender while I held the microsurge meter. "That's the one," I yelled out to Peter when I saw the readout suddenly plummet. The kitchen pot lights, very near the Faraday room, were the culprits. Peter was happy that we'd isolated the source but dismayed that the wiring in that location was still bad after all the time and money he'd spent trying to clean up his electricity.

Sleeping in Palo Alto was far more pleasant than being locked in a room in Toronto breathing stain-repellent perfluorinated compounds, as Rick and I had done. I lay in bed in the Faraday cage, handwriting my experience, free of the electromagnetic field my computer would have generated. The painted surfaces of the room concealed a coat of dark graphite paint, one of the main features of the cage. Since it's a soft metal, the graphite provided a shield against the incoming radiation, as did the metallic film covering the windows. The entire room was also grounded. And as if that was not enough, at the foot of the mattress was a special sheet with grounding built into it and a wire going to one of the grounding points in the room. I started humming "Good Vibrations." With the various instruments at my disposal, I knew that I was 774 feet above sea level, the barometric pressure was 941 millibars, the temperature was 70.7 degrees Fahrenheit (21.8 degrees Celsius), the humidity was 55.3 percent, dirty electricity was 40 GS and EMF was almost nonexistent, at 5 Hz. No need to worry.

I strapped a monitor onto my wrist to record my sleep quality and download the data onto Peter's iPhone, which he would check in the morning. I was ready to sleep.

Peter's Purification Potions

Well rested and free of any electromagnetic contamination, I chatted with Peter in his large, sparsely furnished living room. We delved into the various cleanses, supplements, waters and ionic cellular hydration drinks that he had tried over the years. We shared a bottle (glass, of course) of water containing "Zeta Aid" crystals. "Helps the brain connect the dots," Peter said.

He then handed me an antioxidant supplement to take with the water. I took one capsule of Phyto 5000, described as "a Powerful Anti Oxidant" with "an incredible 42,000 units of anti-oxidant power (or ORAC value) in one capsule." "It's to protect against free radical damage," Peter explained. Free radicals are those nasty molecules blamed for the majority of cellular damage that causes aging.

I was curious to try first-hand some of the detox potions Peter had told me about, especially after hearing how his health, and that of his sons, had improved so dramatically following their detoxification regime. Peter explained how his eldest son—the one expelled from kindergarten—was now excelling at school and no longer exhibiting antisocial behaviour. He rummaged through his kitchen cabinets, gathering dozens of boxes, packets and measurement tools, explaining how to use them. Peter wished me good luck and zoomed off in his Tesla, saying he'd be back at the end of the day. I used the handy litmus paper kit to test the pH of my saliva. It measured 6.3, or slightly acidic—I didn't know if that was good or not (I found out—see below).

It was nearly noon and I was starting to feel a bit sluggish from my commitment to fast prior to dinner, plus I had an aching neck and head. Peter had said to me before he sped away that if I started to get a headache (I'd mentioned to him that I'm headache-prone), I should take a swig of oxygenated water and "Zap," he declared with a Zorro-like gesture, it would be gone. I was not really in the mood for more water, since I was heading to the washroom every fifteen minutes. But I opened a bottle of the locally produced O2Cool and glugged a third of it down, then stopped and assessed the state of my head. Amazingly, it did feel better!

By early afternoon I had consumed nearly one hundred ounces of water (distilled or reverse osmosis, and some with Zeta Aid). This was the equivalent of six pints. My energy level was dropping because of missing out on lunch, but I found an energy enhancer on the counter called Vison Present, with "ionic cellular hydration . . . nano-clustered." The instructions called for an eighth of a teaspoon of the fine white powder to be added to eight ounces of water—just what I needed! The mere thought of it made me run to the bathroom one more time.

After a while I tested the pH of my saliva again and, wonder of wonders, I had become a basic person. My pH reading had jumped five categories and now read 7.6. *What is this all about?* I asked myself. I did a little research and discovered that being basic (a pH above 7) is a good thing. In fact, a pH of 7.6 is in the optimal range (7.2 to 7.6) for good health. A cancer patient will sometimes have a pH of 3.5 or lower, and usually the older you are, the lower your pH will be, because of free-radical damage associated with declining health. Was it possible that my day-long consumption of Zeta Aid and other supplements had taken me into a pH zone of better health?

Peter picked me up at the end of the day, and after another delicious and much-needed dinner, delivered me to my hotel in Palo Alto. The next day I awoke in my no doubt EMF-filled hotel room after another outstanding sleep. I wish I'd been wearing the sleep meter. I gazed into the lush, palm-tree-filled courtyard of my hotel, reflecting on my two days with Peter. He had used the image of a compass to demonstrate that in the end it was all about balance and that some of the detox products and routines seemed to work for him, notably chelation, hydration, avoiding EMFs and eating an organic diet, while others did not.

Let's be honest: scientific proof that these remedies are making us healthier is decidedly elusive. Nonetheless, it seems clear that proper nutrition, hydration and exercise and adopting a non-toxic lifestyle are the backbone of good health. But could hard science prove what anecdote (and our bodies) seemed to be telling us about achieving the balance Peter was talking about? I was about to find out.

Detox Docs: From "Quackery" to Convention

Armed with a reasonable understanding of detoxification, I felt it was now time to speak with some medical experts. There was no shortage of personal testimonials about the fantastic recoveries experienced by individuals, nor of "health experts" whose research supported the claims, but there didn't seem to be many statistical studies by medical doctors evaluating detox treatments.

My first serious conversation about detox medicine was with Dr. Stephen Genuis, a well-known authority on the subject based in Edmonton, Alberta. I wanted to learn more about his expertise in using different detox treatments. Detox medicine, Dr. Genuis said, is "in its infancy." He explained that medical testing for detoxification is not common and is expensive, and that it is difficult to measure chemicals because they move in and out of the body so rapidly. He also emphasized the fact that different people have different genetic makeups, including varying personal biochemistry. All of these factors make toxicological research and diagnostics challenging. He went on to explain that not only are people different, but the chemicals we are exposed to are different, and each one has its own nature.

How a particular chemical behaves depends on many variables, including the biochemistry of the individual. "So when I see a patient," Dr. Genuis said, "I'm trying to assess what toxins I think they have in them. Then I come up with a detoxification strategy or plan that is tailored to what I think they have." Dr. Genuis's approach addresses one of the main criticisms of detoxification: the fact that it is often not specific enough. Exactly which toxins are being targeted for reduction or elimination, and how are the before-and-after levels being measured?

Dr. Genuis noted that there are tens of thousands of chemicals in use, and the more toxic compounds that a person accumulates, the more those compounds will disrupt the biochemistry of their body. He first advises patients to find out where and how they are being exposed to toxins so they can adjust their habits, products or living situation. As he pointed out, "In order to get stuff out of people, you've got to stop putting it in" (an idea fundamental to our own experiments). To identify the toxins entering his patients' bodies, Dr. Genuis conducts an inventory of potential exposure points with his patients. He goes through everything they are doing in their lives and then identifies where they can reduce or eliminate that exposure.

"When you remove what's going *into* the pail," Dr. Genuis says, "then their body is able to devote its efforts to dealing with what's *left* in the pail." The idea that chemicals are not only harming our bodies but are in fact preventing our bodies from detoxifying properly is critical. If toxic chemicals are compromising our immune systems, our bodies are constantly fighting just to *stay* healthy, and our major detox organs, such as the liver and kidneys, can't focus on their main job of removing toxins. So Dr. Genuis typically runs a battery of tests on all his patients. "I get the specific molecular makeup of their body so I see what they have and don't have [i.e., levels of essential vitamins, nutrients, heavy metals and toxins], so I can get their biochemistry to work properly." Toxic chemicals can disrupt our biochemistry, and the more toxins a person bioaccumulates, the greater the chance that the toxins will disrupt our bodily functions.

Dr. Genuis is one of the few medical doctors who write about clinical detox experiences in medical journals. He's also undertaken a detailed review of different detox therapies and has created a handy table that I have modified slightly for simplicity (see table 7).

Table 7. Detox treatment evaluation.[10]

Type of Detox Therapy	Alleged Detox Mechanism	Detox Effectiveness
Fasting	Breakdown of body's fat cells and their stored chemicals, which are then released into circulation and available for excretion	*Limited* Some evidence showing caloric restriction can increase circulating concentration of some toxicants[11]
Chelation	Use of chelating agents (certain molecules and ions) known to chemically bind specific heavy-metal toxins, which allows for excretion of toxic compounds	*Proven* Recognized treatment for some types of heavy-metal poisoning[12]
Ionic foot baths	Feet placed in a bath that sends a current into the body, generating positive ions that then attach to negatively charged toxins, which are excreted through foot pores.	*None* No evidence in scientific literature. Clinical studies have confirmed no toxins are released.[13]
Colonic cleansing	Flushes encrusted material from the colon, which diminishes absorption of toxins and allows for improved excretion of body's waste	*None* Some research about benefits[14], but empirical evidence lacking in scientific literature
Exercise	Breakdown of fat cells and their stored toxins, which are then excreted through lungs and perspiration and/or enhanced enzyme activity in detox pathways	*Limited* Some evidence confirming enhanced excretion of some toxic compounds through exercise.[15] (General health benefits of exercise make it important for overall health.)
Prebiotics and probiotics	Through dietary ingestion, restore damaged germ environment of intestines, which assists with gastrointestinal removal of certain toxic compounds	*Limited* Limited research associates prebiotics and probiotics with excretion of some toxic compounds.[16]

Type of Detox Therapy	Alleged Detox Mechanism	Detox Effectiveness
Sauna therapy	Inducing perspiration results in toxins being excreted into sweat.	*Proven* Some clinical studies have shown release of selected toxins.[17]
Food and drink cleanses	Specific dietary interventions or restrictions stimulate excretion of body's stored toxins.	*None* No consistent confirmation found in scientific literature
Leeching	Leeches suck toxins from blood.	*None* No confirmation in scientific literature
Herbal supplements	Certain supplements facilitate excretion by enhancing body's natural detoxification processes.	*Limited* Evidence suggests selected supplements may work,[18] but majority have not been confirmed in scientific literature.
Hot springs	Immersing body in natural hot springs facilitates absorption of natural compounds that can enhance the excretion of toxins.	*None* No confirmation in scientific literature of enhanced excretion through this method

Chemicals Get Stuck Inside Us

Not all chemicals are flushed out of our bodies quickly or fully. In fact, one of the properties that make some of these chemicals particularly dangerous is their ability to attach themselves to organs, fatty tissues and cells—or even to reside in our bones. This idea fascinates me, but it also scares me. Rick and I demonstrated in our experiments that we could rapidly alter the levels of synthetic chemicals in our bodies, but I'm concerned that we may have been cavalier in our assumption that all the chemicals we absorbed or ingested left our bodies as quickly as they entered.

Heavy metals bind to proteins and tend to migrate into our major organs, such as the brain, liver, heart and kidneys. Among these heavy metals are mercury and lead, which are linked to heart and liver disease; cadmium, a potent neurotoxin; and lead, which builds up in our bones.

As if that weren't enough, Dr. Genuis explained that toxins can travel around inside us, moving from organ to organ, thanks to our body's internal recycling mechanism, called enterohepatic circulation. Enterohepatic (intestine-liver) circulation essentially describes the flow of bile (and bile salts and acids) from our liver to our intestines. It is an efficient mechanism for reusing and recycling bile.

Our liver can remove toxic substances from our blood and discard them, via bile, in the intestines or the kidneys. These organs then eliminate the toxins from the body. But because bile recirculates through the body and because it is effective in carrying hormones and lipophilic (literally "fat-loving") chemicals, it is one of the means by which harmful chemicals can recirculate through the blood and then the liver and be reabsorbed in fat or organs. Dr. Genuis maintains that this cycle can be damaging to our health because destructive chemicals don't remain stuck in one part of the body; they travel from organ to organ, finding a spot where they prefer to hang out. One of these chemicals might make its home in a fat cell in your brain or it may become embedded in cells of your small intestine—and it's impossible to know what kind of damage it may cause once lodged in those areas.

The propensity of toxic chemicals to move around also explains why measuring levels in our bodies is not always straightforward. Doctors take samples from blood, urine, hair or feces, and in some rare cases from sweat. Depending on the time of day, our drinking and eating habits and other, metabolic factors over which we have no control, a toxic substance that we are trying to measure may be more concentrated in the blood, liver, bile, urine, intestines or kidneys—or it may be stuck in a fat cell where we cannot measure it. This indicates that simple "one-off" test results may not provide an accurate picture of toxicity, and it also explains why Dr. Genuis uses a variety of detox treatments with his patients in an effort to mobilize and remove toxins by using all of our body's natural detox pathways.

Dr. Genuis has conducted what may be the first study of its kind that looks simultaneously at the levels of toxic chemicals in the blood, sweat and urine of the same individuals. His research demonstrates that we sweat out certain toxins, notably cadmium and lead, at levels many times greater than what is measured in our blood or urine. Individual body biochemistry, state of hydration and the location of stored toxins in our body may contribute to the differential excretion rates of toxins.

A comprehensive detox must take into account lifestyle, work history, diet, toxic chemical levels and an individual analysis of body chemistry. Dr. Genuis believes an assessment of all these factors is particularly important for people who are suffering from one or more ailments and are looking to detoxification as a prescribed medical therapy.

Synthetic chemicals are often lipophilic ("fat-loving," as just mentioned), and they include hundreds of cancer-causing agents such as some pesticides, PCBs and compounds in household items like nonstick frying pans. They are notorious not just for being absorbed into fat cells but also for building up in fatty tissue. That's why weight loss, as well as personal detoxification, is vital to the removal of toxic chemicals. As long as we're walking around carrying a chemical storehouse of blubber, we'll never adequately detox; reducing fat limits the toxic storage capacity of our bodies. "[These chemicals] don't leave our bodies easily," Dr. Genuis said. "They deposit themselves in fat-loving organs like the thyroid, the adrenals or the brain." Not only do different chemicals prefer different organs, Dr. Genuis said, certain toxins may like to hang out in your flabby gut fat while others prefer the fat in your butt.

Breasts, one of the fattiest parts of our bodies, are a primary repository for toxic chemicals—hence the association between synthetic chemicals and breast cancer. They "soak up pollution like a pair of soft sponges," says Florence Williams, author of *Breasts: A Natural and Unnatural History*.[19] Our bodies do their level best to isolate and eliminate unwanted toxins, and in this instance the body releases the toxins in mother's milk. So, through the most natural act of breastfeeding, poisons are passed on to our newborn children, which Rick has noted is also the case with phthalates.

Semper Fi: Always Faithful, a documentary film about male breast cancer, is an eye-opening exposé of the direct causal link between contaminated water, childhood exposure and breast cancer. For thirty years marines and their families living at Camp Lejeune, a U.S. Marine Corps base in North Carolina, were exposed to volatile organic compounds (VOCs) in their drinking water, which resulted in hugely elevated rates of male breast cancer, miscarriages among women who drank the water and many other diseases, including cancers.[20] Camp Lejeune is now infamous for having and allegedly hiding the worst case of drinking water contamination in American history.[21]

I had the opportunity to meet Mike Partain, one of the Camp Lejeune breast cancer survivors and an advocate for the affected families. Mike was not a typical candidate for breast cancer. He didn't drink or smoke and there was no history of cancer in his family. In fact, he wasn't even a marine and had spent very little time at Camp Lejeune. But he was born on the base and lived the first few critical years of his life there as the son of a marine. The water that Mike drank as a child caused his breast cancer more than thirty years later.

Mike has joined the outspoken advocates and survivors tired of being ignored by various authorities who have been pretending that chemical contamination is not a problem.[22] In August of 2012 they won a small victory when President Obama signed into law the *Janey Ensminger Act*, named after the daughter of a Camp Lejeune marine who died of cancer at age nine. The law provides medical coverage for the marines and their families who were poisoned at Camp Lejeune. But that was only a small remedy, and it came rather late.

Fear of cancer is one of the motivating factors behind the exponential growth in healthy living and detox programmes. Over 40 percent of kids born in the United States today will be diagnosed with cancer at some point in their lifetime[23]—in short, nearly one out of every two children born today will be diagnosed with cancer. If that doesn't scare the crap out of us, I'm not sure what will. Perhaps the fact that over 550,000 Americans,[24] 75,000 Canadians[25] and 40,000 Australians[26] die of cancer every year. That's nearly 2,000 people dying every day in these three countries alone. Admittedly, cancer is still largely a disease that afflicts older populations, but if half of us are going to develop cancer at some point, wouldn't it be worth finding every possible way to prevent it? We know that ingesting animal fats, eating a poor diet, smoking and not exercising enough may contribute to cancer, as well as to obesity, stroke and heart attack. And we know that many synthetic chemicals cause cancer. Recent thinking led by the Halifax Project underlines the notion that the creation of cancers is likely due to the mixture of chemicals in the body—many of them in very low doses—and highlights the urgency of tackling the toxic-chemical problem once and for all.[27]

How exactly do our bodies expel toxic chemicals? There are seven main pathways for detoxification: the lungs, liver, colon, kidneys, skin, blood and lymph system. In some cases these are simply the reverse routes of toxification. For example, we exhale toxic chemicals through our lungs, just as we inhaled them. We ingest toxic chemicals in food and water and expel them as solid and liquid waste. And our largest organ, our skin, can play a helpful role in eliminating toxic waste, even as it absorbs the synthetic chemicals in lotions and creams.

The most important part of detoxification is to provide your body with the tools it needs to detoxify itself.

Liver, Kidneys and Lungs

Virtually all detox experts focus on our two main detox organs: the liver and the kidneys. That's because the first detox process that our body manages is the liver-kidney-bladder connection. Blood produced in the liver is filtered through the kidneys, where impurities and excess minerals are removed and carried away by urine, which is manufactured by the kidneys. Urine is stored in the bladder prior to being expelled. It is this highly efficient toxic-waste elimination process that Rick and I rely on when we test the levels of toxic substances in urine.

The second elimination pathway is the liver-bile-gallbladder-intestine connection, which can be described as the "highway of fat." If you've ever wondered where all the grease and fat from those yummy French fries ends up, here's the answer: it goes to the liver, which sends it to the bile, where it's broken down and then sent through the gallbladder to the intestines. It's digested further in the small intestine before being expelled by the colon.

Suddenly, understanding this process starts to provide explanations for some of the many health problems plaguing the populations of industrial nations. We consume too much fat, making it impossible for our liver and gallbladder to keep up, and this results in fatty residues entering our colon that have not been sufficiently processed by our body. Add to that the lack of fibre in most Western diets and we are further impairing the ability of our intestines to digest, process and eliminate fat and waste. We also know that so many of the toxic substances we need to avoid are fat-soluble—and are therefore stored in the fat that our body can no longer process effectively. As if that wasn't enough, the triple threat of poor diet (excessive fat and lack of fibre), pervasive toxic chemicals and lack of exercise means that our livers have even *more* difficulty doing their primary job of ridding the body of toxins. The more toxic chemicals we ingest, the more we reduce our body's natural cleansing ability. Is it any wonder that we have a nightmarish epidemic of fatty livers, high cholesterol, diabetes, gallstones, liver cancer, bladder cancer, colon cancer and generally poor health? The importance of a well-functioning waste-elimination system cannot be overstated. Colorectal cancer alone is the second leading cause of cancer death in North America.[28]

How is it that breathing air can result in toxic chemicals damaging our heart, our liver or a developing fetus? When we inhale polluted air—for example, air contaminated by the off-gassing plastics in the interior of Rick's car or by a phthalate-filled home air freshener—our lungs transport not only oxygen to our blood (their primary function) but also the toxic chemicals we breathe in. Anytime that we can detect a strong chemical smell—think turpentine or gasoline—we are inhaling the toxic chemicals in those products.

Though it's generally well known that the lungs filter out particles before they enter the bloodstream, its other detox functions are more obscure. However, there's one prominent volatile organic compound that is readily expelled through our lungs—alcohol. In fact, we can use the alcohol levels in our breath to estimate exactly how much is in our blood. It makes me wonder how we so readily accept the court-tested precision of a Breathalyzer in measuring blood-alcohol levels while industry and government agencies still question the validity of measuring toxic chemicals directly from our blood or urine. Rather than using nasty and invasive blood, sweat and urine sampling techniques in our self-experimentation, could Rick and I have just blown into some device to measure the levels of toxic chemicals in our bodies?

Using our breath to analyze our health is not too far-fetched a notion. Breath tests are being used to detect cancer. Researchers have also found that chemicals absorbed by our skin can be found in our breath, and in some cases chemicals or medications used in the past can be detected in the breath many weeks later. Doctors are already measuring toxins in our breath as part of their environmental testing. They can detect not only toxins but also female birth control drugs in the breath of . . . men. A substance that is manufactured as a pill, ingested by a woman, eliminated through her urine, processed in a water treatment facility, dumped into a lake or ocean, subjected to more water treatment and then consumed in drinking water can show up in the breath of anyone who drinks that water.[29]

Breathing, sweating, peeing and pooing are the natural processes that flush toxins from our bodies. For the most part these mechanisms do a good job. So we'd be well advised to keep them healthy and functioning optimally, especially given the growing number of chemicals we take in every day.

Chelate This

It was time to test one of Dr. Genuis's "proven" detox therapies first-hand. I hopped a plane to Houston, Texas, to meet up with my first cousin Dr. Peter Erickson, a well-established environmental physician and a specialist in chelation therapy. I wasn't looking forward to having my arm poked with a needle and lying around for three hours with an intravenous solution of chemicals coursing through my veins. But that is what chelation therapy is all about, and it's the most specific and well-researched detox treatment available—and the one with the clearest demonstrated effectiveness, particularly for heavy-metal detoxification.

Doctors use chelation to treat a wide range of conditions, among them arthritis, arteriosclerosis (hardening of the arteries), fibromyalgia (a condition characterized by chronic pain and fatigue, with unknown cause), Parkinson's disease, and autism associated with mercury (a connection disputed by some doctors and therefore making its treatment with chelation controversial). A study with more than a thousand registered participants concluded in 2012, and its results showed that chelation (as opposed to a placebo) offers modest benefits for recovering heart patients.[30]

Not all of the controversy around chelation has to do with autism. There have been cases where chelating agents have been too aggressive in the removal of essential elements, especially calcium, resulting in a number of deaths in the United States due to heart failure (calcium in the blood plays a critical role in maintaining a heartbeat).

Given that chelation is an invasive medical treatment and not without risk of complications, only trained medical doctors should administer intravenous chelation. This is a requirement in some jurisdictions but not all. Chelation is essentially an application of chemistry, so I felt some additional relief that Dr. Erickson has a degree in chemical engineering on top of his medical degree.

Lazy Boys and Dogs

The chelation therapy I received can best be described as a "demonstration project." My earlier tuna-eating experience had shown quite vividly that the mercury from the tuna was piling up in my blood at a rapid rate, nearly tripling in forty-eight hours. The goal of the chelation therapy was to do a "reverse tuna" experiment: I wanted to find out whether chelation could remove mercury from my body and whether I could measure the amount of mercury being removed. I wasn't convinced it would be possible with only one session.

The experiment was divided into two parts. Day 1 was called "preprovocation," meaning that I would undergo a baseline assessment of how much mercury I peed out in a normal day. Day 2 was treatment day, when the chelation chemicals would scavenge my body for heavy metals, literally grabbing on to the toxic molecules and removing them via my kidneys and urine. The term "chelate" comes from the Greek word for a lobster claw (*chela*), referring to the pincer-like action of the chelation chemicals.

When the big day arrived, I was more than a little anxious. After I ate a bowl of organic fruit, Dr. Erickson and I headed to his medical clinic in the small, dusty town of Boling. He pointed out that the slightly sagging clapboard clinic was itself one of the oldest buildings in Boling and had housed the town's first doctor's office and pharmacy.

Chelation is the opposite of most medical experiences. It is a peaceful, relaxing, unobtrusive procedure (apart from the IV insertion—I really don't like needles) where you basically sit back in a comfy chair, feet up, reading, listening to music and letting the little chelation lobsters run around your bloodstream catching their toxic metal prey. One of Dr. Erickson's Yorkshire terriers decided to keep me company and lay on my lap for most of the time that the needle was in my arm. On both day 1 and day 2, I consumed large quantities of water, which allowed for the collection of nearly four litres of urine over each of the two six-hour urine-collection periods.

Back in Toronto several weeks later, I received a large envelope delivered by courier. I tore open the package from Doctors Data Inc. (a lab in St. Charles, Illinois), anxious to see my test results, and plain as day I could see that chelation had done its job. The graph showed a striking contrast between the amounts of aluminum, lead, mercury and tin that were removed from my body during chelation and the amounts of those same toxic heavy metals that had been detected in my urine pre-provocation (my normal state; see figure 11). More than four times as much aluminum was pulled from my body during chelation, over five times as much lead and mercury, and twenty times the tin. The first three metals are serious poisons, and it's not safe to have *any* amount of lead or mercury in our bodies.

Figure 11. Bruce's urinary heavy metals: levels of removal before and during chelation (ng/g).

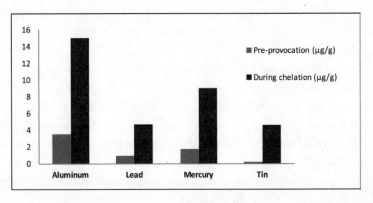

The chelation procedure had a similar effect on fundamental (and essential) elements in my body, such as sodium, calcium and magnesium, with levels removed during the intravenous treatment that were between two and fifteen times the level that my body would normally excrete (see figure 12). This not only demonstrates the effectiveness of chelation but also points to one of the risks that must be managed.

Figure 12. Bruce's urinary essential elements: levels of removal before and during chelation (ng/g).

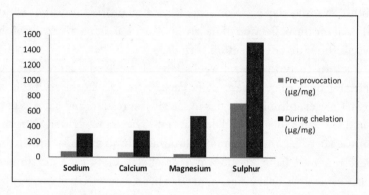

Detox Debunked

Some detox remedies are helpful and some are hokum, and certain elements of the multibillion-dollar detox industry have figured out how to prey on people who are unwell and vulnerable. To defend yourself against iffy or entirely useless treatments, take another look at Dr. Genuis's advice, summarized in table 7. There is no point in paying for treatments that don't work, and specialized therapies such as chelation are meant for people with serious, medically diagnosed toxicity.

On the other hand, practitioners of conventional medicine are often too quick to dismiss the potential benefits of various approaches to detox, and the doctors who are most skeptical end up chasing their patients away and into the world of alternative medicine anyway. We need to seek a healthy middle ground. This means shifting the emphasis so that health expenditures and cancer research dollars reflect the medical and ethical importance of not just curing but also preventing disease. Alternative medicine and personalized detox treatments can play a critical role in this shift.

We are all full of toxins. There's no question about that. The issue is how to figure out the most effective course of action for each individual, based on their specific health circumstances. First and foremost, we must avoid toxic chemicals in our food, homes, workplaces and lives in general. If there are no toxins, we won't need toxouts!

Most of us aren't going to spend many of our waking hours figuring out how to detox, nor are we going to build Faraday cages or undergo chelation. So what about the easier and cheaper detox approaches? Herbal formulas, supplements and all those off-the-shelf cleansing diets? That's the subject of the next chapter.

TEN: SWEAT THE SMALL STUFF

[BRUCE PERSPIRES HEAVILY]

Don't sweat the petty things and don't pet the sweaty things.

—ANONYMOUS

I DON'T GET SICK OFTEN. I exercise modestly (though I need to do more) and eat a healthy diet (though I need to eat less). So entering the detox world for me is very different than for many who are suffering from serious, sometimes debilitating symptoms for which they are not finding remedies through conventional medicine.

I asked my friend Bryce Wylde, who is a homeopath and author, where he stood on the detox industry. "Craziness," he said. "You get people running out and taking things because the Kardashians are." In terms of the natural products on the market, he maintains that "50 percent are junk and 50 percent are hidden gems worthy of further research." Two of the gems are fatty acids and vitamin D—natural supplements with tremendous, well-researched, proven and medically accepted benefits. "There are lots more of those out there," he said. We just need to continue exploring and researching them.

My Google search for "detox diet" turned up over 5.8 million references, including everything from relatively reasonable nutrition and lifestyle approaches to thousands of cleanses and diets of questionable value. If you want to play a fun game, Google "detox diet" in quotations, then type in your favourite fruit or vegetable and see what happens— the lemon detox diet, the grapefruit detox diet, the avocado detox diet, the African mango detox diet, kiwi detox recipes, to name a few.

What seems to happen with diet fads is that somebody takes a basic idea—eat more fruit—and turns it into a gimmick that they then profit from. So rather than focusing on fresh fruit as part of a healthy life-style, we end up with the "insert favourite fruit here" detox diet.

Clearly, one of the downsides of the Internet Age is that anyone with a computer can create a diet, design a web page and make stuff up. Take one "lipid detoxification diet," for example: the recipes include eggnog, potatoes fried with bacon, steak ("eat as much of the fat as you can") and whipped cream. The recipe for a baked potato suggests that it be eaten with "at least half a stick of butter and a quarter cup of sour cream." Wow, now that is a detox diet I could live with! Or maybe die by! And judging by the ever-increasing girth of North Americans, perhaps there are a few too many people who have discovered the lipid detoxi-fication diet, whether they know it or not. My advice, if you happen to be one of them: it's time to switch!

As the number of detox products and treatments grows, so does the number of critics who emphasize the lack of scientific evidence that these methods actually work. The Australian consumer products watchdog group Choice reviewed seven detox kits available at pharma-cies and health food stores. Their conclusion, based on their expert panel review, was that most of the detox programmes (typically ten- to fifteen-day special diets) were of little or no value—and one of the detox diets they tested was considered to be dangerous because of the low levels of protein and nutrients a dieter was allowed to eat during the course of the regime.[1] Other studies confirm the lack of evidence regarding the benefits of detox and cleansing diets.[2]

There are three main reasons why most detox kits are of little value:

1. They provide users with a false sense that consuming juice or various herbs over ten days can somehow eliminate toxins that have accumulated over a much longer period of time. They therefore ignore one of the foundations of the detox process—namely, that detox is a continuous lifestyle shift, not a short-term diet.

2. They often recommend accompanying diets that restrict the intake of protein and other nutrients to such an extent that people unfamiliar with basic nutrition may suffer.

3. The most restrictive diets can lead to rapid and unsustainable weight loss, and much of that weight is

regained after the cleanse. This can lead to unhealthy
"yo-yo" dieting.

Detox kits do have some positive aspects, though. First, detox kits
may be an "appetizer" for people who want to begin following a healthy
lifestyle. We all need support mechanisms and tools to guide us. Using
a detox kit may be the first step that someone takes on a longer pathway
toward a sustainable detox lifestyle. Second, virtually all cleanses recommend avoiding junk food, caffeine, tobacco and alcohol, all indul-
gences that should be enjoyed only in moderation—or not at all.

A person who typically drinks four cups of coffee a day, eats a dough-
nut in the morning and then a burger, fries and a Coke for lunch, followed by a dinner of canned spaghetti, will almost certainly feel better
after two weeks of water, vegetables, legumes and a high-fibre diet. But
for a diet like that, they won't need a detox kit.

I asked Wylde what the future holds for detox medicine, and again
he gave an instant, very specific answer: "Genomic diagnostics." Huh?
"Genomics are used to evaluate personal impairment and our ability to
detoxify naturally," he explained. Genomics is the field of measuring
and evaluating the genome, and the genome is the complete DNA
sequence that determines who we are. It is distinguished from genetic
research, which focuses on individual genes, not the entire genome.
Genomic diagnostic tools combine what researchers and medical
practitioners know about genomic and clinical data to better understand the basis of disease to assist treatment and prevention.[3]

Genetic research into individual genes has helped identify those
associated with diseases like breast and ovarian cancer. In the spring of
2013 the Hollywood star Angelina Jolie made headlines with her decision
to have an elective double mastectomy to reduce her chances of developing breast cancer. Jolie has a mutation in the breast cancer 1, or BRCA1,
gene—the same mutation her mother and aunt had. Jolie's mother died
of ovarian cancer at the age of fifty-six. Her aunt succumbed to breast
cancer just two weeks after Jolie's surgery. She was sixty-one.

The BRCA1 gene plays a critical role in fighting cancer. If the gene is
damaged, it fails to protect the person with that gene, leaving them
with a 65 percent lifetime risk of developing breast cancer.[4] By choosing a proactive double mastectomy, Jolie has reduced her chances of

developing breast cancer to less than 5 percent.[5] Her decision was important, given her genetic predisposition to the disease.

However, 90 to 95 percent of breast cancer cases cannot be attributed to BRCA1 or other inherited gene mutations.[6]

There's a need for more research into environmental exposures that contribute to cancer, and the emerging field of epigenetics is doing just that. Epigenetics is the study of "gene expression"—how genes can be turned on or off by external, non-genetic influences—and it is at the heart of endocrine-disruption research. Studies show, for example, the epigenetic effects of bisphenol A (BPA) on reproductive function. Male rats exposed to BPA during the first five days after their birth had impaired fertility when mature.[7] The research demonstrates how developmental exposure to endocrine-disrupting chemicals can alter gene function much later in life.

The point is that our genes themselves may not be the determinants of cancer or other health problems. It's how our genes are expressed (turned on or off) and the extent to which synthetic toxins play a role in switching gene functions on or off that may trigger genetic disruption or disease such as cancer.

And now back to genomic diagnostics, the tool that Bryce Wylde described. "With genomics," he told me, "we can identify individuals who are more likely to have a negative reaction to toxins based on SNP factors." SNPs (pronounced "snips") are single nucleotide polymorphisms in our DNA that may, for example, predispose us to disease or influence our response to a drug. Bryce used the example of certain patients who may have serious negative reactions to chemotherapy because their bodies are not well adapted to detoxifying harsh cancer-fighting chemicals. Others, however, may be so good at detoxifying that a standard chemotherapy dose may be ineffective in treating their cancer.

Genomics and SNPs may therefore be able to tell us which person has a predisposition to detoxifying and which one does not, so the proper treatment can be administered. If genomics really delivers, we'll be able to discern with laser accuracy which people need to be examined, which need to be treated, and precisely which therapies are best suited to an individual's genetic makeup. We're not there yet, though, so for now we'll have to do our best by using effective methods of contemporary detox medicine.

Free Radicals and Antioxidant Rebels

Dr. Stephen Genuis, the detox medicine expert based in Edmonton, Alberta (my interview with him is in chapter 9), discussed one detox treatment that has some merit: supplements.

The world of vitamins and herbal supplements is huge, with global sales estimated at over US$68 billion. When I was young, Linus Pauling, the father of orthomolecular medicine (an alternative practice that focuses on achieving health through nutritional supplementation to compensate for inadequate dietary nutrition) and perhaps the best-known chemist of the twentieth century, published a number of controversial books on the benefits of taking high doses of vitamin C. Pauling took 10,000 mg per day of vitamin C and up to 40,000 mg when he wasn't feeling well. The latter is 400 times more than the typical recommendation for a daily dose.

Anything more than 250 mg is now thought to be of questionable value, because vitamin C is water-soluble and large doses are therefore easily removed in urine. Pauling may not have got the doses right, but a growing number of conventional medical doctors believe Pauling was on to something, and orthomolecular medicine is seeing a resurgence.[8]

Vitamins A, D, E and K are also important for detoxification, but they need to be taken with greater caution because they are fat-soluble, and high doses may result in dangerous levels of these vitamins lodging themselves in fatty tissues, in the same way that toxic chemicals do. If there is one simple health supplement that virtually all people would benefit from, it is vitamin D. Throughout the globe, people are deficient in vitamin D, especially those who spend a lot of time indoors or in northern regions and therefore do not receive enough natural vitamin D from sunlight.

We should be able to meet our minimum daily requirements of most minerals and vitamins (other than vitamin D) by eating sufficient quantities of organic fruits, vegetables and whole grains. But it's a practical challenge to measure our intake and to know that we are meeting our daily requirements. That's why it's smart to take a multivitamin every day that delivers minimum requirements of most essential nutrients.

When I asked what he sees as the central health issue that we're facing today, without hesitation Bryce Wylde said, "Free radicals." Free radicals aren't Greenpeace volunteers; they're atoms or molecules that contain unpaired electrons. Free radicals are basically unstable, itinerant atoms that rove through our bodies, hooking up with unpaired molecules and causing indiscriminate damage to our cells. "They are without doubt the most gnarly and dangerous toxins inside us," Wylde stated, as though he held a personal grudge against them.

Free radicals are charged atoms that are highly reactive. They steal electrons from other molecules in our cells, a process called oxidation, which can trigger chain reactions resulting in rapid and extensive cellular damage—even to our DNA. Free radicals are blamed for chronic diseases that appear as a result of aging. Chief among these are heart disease, Alzheimer's disease and cancer.

The goal of eliminating free radicals has spurred the antioxidant craze, including blueberry smoothies, pomegranate juice and broccoli drinks. Luckily, it is relatively easy to make antioxidants part of a healthy detox lifestyle. The general rule is to eat more dark-coloured berries and fruits (blackberries, raspberries, plums, prunes, etc.) as well as colourful beans (black beans, kidney beans, pinto beans, red beans), dark cruciferous vegetables (kale, broccoli) and whole grains. Garlic and tomatoes are also high in antioxidants—great news for lovers of Italian food like me. Diets that are high in antioxidant foods help us to detox, protect us from cancer and improve cardiovascular health.

When healthful fruits and vegetables are hard to come by, melatonin, known mainly for aiding sleep patterns, is an important antioxidant supplement.[9] And all the health experts I spoke with recommended taking N-acetylcysteine (NAC) supplements. NAC works by helping our body produce glutathione, a powerful antioxidant that neutralizes free radicals. Glutathione (GSH) is manufactured in our liver as a natural detox agent, and low levels can prevent us from detoxifying effectively. Glutathione, in sufficient quantities, even protects our cells from mercury damage.[10]

The use of manufactured pharmaceuticals is a relatively recent phenomenon in medicine. The active ingredient in the ubiquitous Aspirin (salicylic acid) occurs naturally in willow trees, codeine and morphine come from poppies, and the pain-relief ingredient capsaicin is found in chili peppers. About 40 to 60 percent of modern pharmaceuticals are derived from natural plants and/or synthesized plant derivatives. So I'm always surprised when conventional doctors discredit herbal medicine outright as hocus-pocus.

Ground Zero Detox

Ayurveda is one of the oldest forms of herbal medicine, originating on the Indian subcontinent. In 2012 I heard that Ayurveda was being used as a detox treatment for the 9/11 first responders in New York, and I popped down to New York City to learn more. There I met with two of the co-founders of Serving Those Who Serve (STWS), a volunteer organization created to help first responders to the 9/11 World Trade Center attack of 2001. (In the years since its founding STWS has also served Iraq veterans and others, including people affected by Hurricane Sandy and the BP oil spill.)

I met the two men, José Mestre, the son of Cuban political prisoners who fled to Miami when he was a child, and Marshall Stackman, a jovial New Yorker with a solid build, a greying ponytail and a thick Brooklyn accent, in a bright, noisy fast-food restaurant on Columbus Avenue. We drank green tea and chatted for nearly two hours.

José and Marshall recounted the tale of how STWS began after the horror and chaos of 9/11 and described the inch-thick dust that covered the cars in their Brooklyn neighbourhood. They asked me to imagine what was in that dust and smoke. "How many toxic chemicals?" they wondered aloud. "Hundreds? Thousands?" The Twin Towers attacks are considered to be among the most intense chemical exposure events in history.

Getting burned is not the main hazard connected with a modern fire. Somewhere between 50 and 80 percent of fire-related deaths are caused by smoke inhalation. When a house catches fire or when a car bursts into flames, one of the main concerns is the toxic chemicals released by the burning. The National Fire Protection Association reports that there are nearly 200,000 car fires on U.S. highways every year (that's more than 500 every day!), and close to a half a million buildings catch fire annually.[11]

Each time there's a fire in a car or modern home, a highly toxic mix of paint, vinyl, plastic, adhesive, foam, solvents and who knows what else ends up in the smoke. Look around your home and try to picture your television, computer, sofa, carpeting, cupboards, mattress, kids' toys, cleaning products, paint, wiring, insulation and roof shingles ablaze. As terrible as it would be from the standpoint of personal loss, imagine the toxic blend of fumes. This is what modern firefighters face on a daily basis. Volatile organic compounds (VOCs) are a major component of the toxic smoke and include well-known carcinogens such as benzene, toluene and naphthalene.[12]

If any group ought to be concerned about their chemical exposure, it is firefighters—especially the 9/11 first responders. The 9/11 attacks killed 2,997 people,[13] and the long-term effects of the resulting toxic debris may be more lethal. When we spoke in 2012, José claimed that an additional 2,500 people had died of related health issues in the eleven years since 9/11. Ground Zero workers are being studied constantly, and one study found that firefighters with extended exposure at the World Trade Center site have significantly increased risk of respiratory and gastroesophageal reflux disease (GERD) symptoms.[14] Studies of those present at the time of the attack have shown, within seven years of exposure, an increased risk of prostate cancer, thyroid cancer and myeloma.[15]

The U.S. Centers for Disease Control run the World Trade Center Health Program, where affected first responders and lower Manhattan survivors are eligible to receive health care. As of March 2018, 70,825 responders and 15,499 survivors had enrolled in the program; of those, 7,041 responders and 1,629 survivors were diagnosed with at least one form of cancer.[16] Cancer developing over the long term is one of the greatest scares, and firefighters know they have a "time bomb ticking" in their bodies. This was made very real for Marshall when he was told that nineteen of the thirty Trade Center rescue dogs died of cancer within just over a year of the attack. Marshall was also aware that cancers might not appear in humans for ten years or more. For the majority of cancers the latency period (the length of time between an exposure and the onset of cancer) is fifteen to thirty years.[17] A scary thought for anyone exposed to the toxic fallout at Ground Zero.

In the aftermath of the attack, several local organizations quickly surmised that there would be serious health problems due to the noxious exposures the first responders faced at Ground Zero. This was despite the official word at the time that the local air quality was not toxic, José recalled. Local churches and volunteers at Ground Zero knew this was a serious matter and immediately began setting up treatment centres for the debilitated rescue workers. Over time some of those facilities became more formalized, including Serving Those Who Serve, with their unique mission of delivering detox therapy through

Ayurvedic healing. Herbal treatments are at the core of Serving Those Who Serve, and they are combined with yoga, breathing and meditation to assist those who suffer from a wide range of health problems, including post-traumatic stress disorder.

I dug a bit deeper with José and Marshall. They described their early encounter with the doctor who developed their herbal supplement protocol, the renowned Ayurvedic physician Dr. Pankaj Naram. According to his website, "the original and authentic form of Ayurveda is based on one guiding principle: address the root cause of an ailment rather than its symptoms."[18] This seems to be pretty much in line with all forms of alternative medicine, and once again highlights the contrast between naturopathic and ancient medicine on the one hand and Western medicine on the other, with its focus on isolating symptoms and prescribing cures, mostly in the form of pharmaceuticals.

Marshall and José recounted story after story of direct experiences with first responders whose health improved dramatically after taking the herbal treatments. José maintains that the herbs "bolster the immune system and enhance the body's natural detox processes." As with so many of these "alternative" programmes, it is still difficult to find scholarly studies with conclusive results to show that herbal detox programmes remove toxic chemicals.

I asked Marshall and José if anything had been written about their programme, and José directed me to a peer-reviewed study of 9/11 responders and locally affected workers who had participated in the STWS Ayurvedic herbal supplement programme.[19] It is not a toxicology study showing the elimination of toxic compounds but a peer-reviewed survey of the participants' "post-treatment symptom impact"—meaning, Did the responders report feeling better after taking the herbal medicines?[20]

On the Likert scale of 1 to 6 for helpfulness (where 6 is the most helpful), the fifty patients participating in the study rated the herbal programme as being, on average, 50 percent more effective than conventional medicine.[21] José described what a challenge it was for those guys to take herbal supplements and undergo the Ayurveda treatments. "This is not a typical lifestyle choice [for them]." They are "tough guys," he said. "Staten Islanders, the hotbed of Republican support in New York City." Marshall added, "They eat poorly, smoke, drink, are often on prescription meds." Because firefighters historically see themselves as looking after others, they are reluctant to admit their own vulnerabilities and rarely stop to take care of themselves. However, since STWS started doing its work, 1,300 of the 2,700 people who have participated in its herbal detox programmes are firefighters, and STWS remains the only Ground Zero detox organization that is still up and running.

Canary in a Sweat Box

Armed with more information on complementary alternative medicine, body chemistry and liver function than I'd ever imagined existed, I felt ready to do some personal detox experimentation. I had been amazed when, in our own testing, we could so easily manipulate our toxic chemical intake and actually measure the toxic chemicals that entered our bodies. But the big question remained: Would the reverse be true? Could I measure the toxic chemicals *leaving* my body if I underwent specific detox treatments? My hunch was that it could be difficult to pull off and that "tox-in" testing would be more predictable than the "tox-out" version. But challenges of this nature had never stopped us before!

Results of the many detox strategies I've reviewed are not easily measurable. Most off-the-shelf cleanses are not specific enough for their effects to be measured, nor is there any evidence to suggest that they really work. Dietary changes are too subtle and incremental. Herbal detox therapies don't allow for observing the excretion of toxins either. And there is the difficulty of controlling inadvertent exposure to chemicals, a problem that Rick and I face regardless of how careful we are. One brush with a heavily perfumed individual could easily result in perceptible increases in phthalate levels that would skew the results of any experiment.

One detox strategy stood out, however: a sauna. Taking a sauna would be a reasonably accessible and proven therapy for accelerating detoxification that would allow for testing. And how unpleasant could that experiment be?

First things first. I needed to get my hands on an actual sauna unit. I contacted Rodney Palmer, an infrared sauna manufacturer I'd met at a health show. In addition to kindly lending me an infrared sauna for the experiments, Rodney provided me with a wealth of information about sauna detox therapy. What's more, like so many people immersed in alternative health, Rodney had his own story to tell.

I invited Rodney over to my house and we sat on the back deck, drinking pomegranate juice mixed with filtered, carbonated tap water.

Rodney took me back to 2003 and the SARS (severe acute respiratory syndrome) epidemic. During the outbreak he was living in Beijing with his young family, covering the story as a Canadian journalist for a major television network. One of the first things he noticed about the country was its horrendous air pollution. His family quickly started to experience health problems.

"My wife was losing weight rapidly, and there was this scaly stuff on her fingers," Rodney recalls. But his son was affected too. "My son wasn't growing properly. He had problems with his leg joints and he couldn't even hold his own weight." They were beside themselves trying to figure out what was happening. His wife had lost forty pounds and could no longer work. They were both very worried for their son.

At this point the story was becoming eerily reminiscent of Peter Sullivan's experience of extreme health issues affecting his whole family. Sure enough, Rodney described how his wife came across Sherry Rogers's book *Detoxify or Die*, which led her to have the family tested for toxic contaminants. It turns out they all had hugely elevated levels of lead in their systems. Lead is a neurotoxin that causes a variety of mental impairments, and it is also associated with dozens of other serious afflictions, including gastrointestinal problems, kidney disease, anemia and even death. The doctors they consulted in North America suspected that lead had been replacing the calcium in his son's growing bones, causing them to soften—hence his difficulty with walking. They also attributed his wife's weight loss, her anemia and her frantic mental state to elevated lead levels. Rodney had no symptoms at all despite his elevated lead levels, reinforcing the point that we all respond very differently to toxins.

Rodney's family was introduced to Dr. William Rae, a cardiovascular surgeon who is considered a father of environmental medicine. When he learned that Rodney's wife had elevated levels of lead, he administered an intensive course of sauna therapy. Within three weeks she had improved significantly.

Without easy access to a sauna, Rodney had purchased an infrared sauna kit to install in their home, but he was horrified when he turned it on and found that it smelled of airplane glue. After extensive research he discovered that most infrared sauna kits were poorly constructed and contained toxic glues and electrical components with high EMF emissions.

Rodney decided to design and build his own infrared sauna, without any glues (only screws as fasteners) and with wood and electrical components that he sourced and tested personally. And that's how his company, SaunaRay, was born. Before too long, environmental doctors were asking him about his "clean" infrared sauna, and now he sells his kits around the world.

Rodney was so convinced that sauna therapy is one of the most effective ways of removing toxins from our bodies that he took issue with one of the claims Rick and I made when we published *Slow Death*: that if people stop using toxic products they will naturally eliminate them and our levels will return to their original state. Rodney was certain that toxic chemicals do, in fact, get "stuck" in our bodies, and as proof he pointed to levels of toxins in sweat being sometimes much higher than levels seen in blood or urine. A research paper by Dr. Genuis, the detox expert I've mentioned several times, has described the same concept but in technical terms: "[Blood] serum levels of various xenobiotics [chemicals that are foreign to living things] do not necessarily reflect the total body burden of such compounds because accrued toxicants may store in tissues, and serum levels may belie actual toxicant status."[22]

Dr. Genuis also helped me design the sauna experiment described below and was invaluable when it came to teaching me the basics of sauna detox and how to create a protocol for testing and measuring my sweat. My protocol would include running, sauna therapy and the ingestion of vitamins, psyllium husk fibre and electrolytes (psyllium husk helps to absorb and bind the toxins, aiding in their removal, while electrolytes such as sodium and magnesium are critical to our health and can be depleted to dangerously low levels with vigorous sweating).

For this experiment, I undertook nearly two months of lengthy and detailed discussions about sample protocols and research parameters with several labs before I found one that was willing to perform the sweat analysis for us. At nine hundred dollars a pop for some of the samples and the complicated conversations with the labs about the chemistry behind the procedures, this kind of testing is far from routine or accessible to the general public.[23]

The Big Sweat

With the closet-like sauna installed in my basement and my sample jars and vials sorted out (no easy task), I was ready to start the first sauna sweat collection. The protocol called for two one-hour sweats per day over a three-week period, with weekly collections. This was modified to a maximum of one sweat per day over a five-week period, for reasons I'll describe below. I was also collecting urine to compare toxic levels before and after sauna sessions for the duration of the sauna treatment. And on top of that, the plan was to collect my blood to compare levels in it versus levels in my urine and my sweat. I was attempting to emulate studies that Dr. Genuis had conducted.[24]

Before entering the sauna, I drank a large glass of water (about 500 mL) with a scoop of electrolyte powder added to it. Then I collected a 100 mL urine sample and weighed in at 89.8 kilograms (198) pounds. I'd completed a twenty-minute run to get my blood circulation revved up before getting into the small wooden cubicle, and within minutes of stepping in, plenty of perspiration was flowing out of my body. The temperature was 40 degrees Celsius, and after five minutes or so, beads of sweat were dripping off my forehead and onto the floor. My run before the sauna had helped increase my internal body temperature, and that was making small, distinct droplets appear on my forearms—the first sign of a good sweat.

It turns out that medical researchers have been collecting sweat from forearms since as far back as 1934, because of interest in the relationship between sweat-gland activity and blood flow in that part of the body. Research I have read indicates that sweating happens first and then the blood vessels dilate—never vice versa—and when the blood vessels dilate, blood flow increases. So not only does the heat from a sauna provide a mechanism for certain synthetic chemicals to be excreted through sweat, but the increased flow of blood helps our livers process and detoxify a greater volume of blood. Sauna therapy therefore is a detox double whammy.

After ten minutes at 46 degrees Celsius, the sweat was streaming off me. I was pleased with the performance (based on my sweat volume) and I was feeling great. I scraped the edge of the jar along my skin, hoping that the sweat drops would find their way into the container. Before I knew it, I'd managed to collect a considerable volume. Seeing the 250 mL (8-ounce) jar nearly half full of sweat made me wonder how much I was sweating out in total.

I left the sauna, weighed myself, had a shower and drank more water with electrolytes added. According to my bathroom scale, I now weighed 88.4 kilograms (195 pounds). My one-hour sauna had sucked a remarkable three pounds of sweat out of me.[25]

After my hour of sauna therapy on day 1, I did another hour on day 2. I didn't feel so well. I had been drowsy for most of day 1, despite consuming large amounts of water, electrolyte supplements and psyllium husk powder. Day 2 was even worse: I was basically immobilized, unable to function for several hours. I started to wonder whether this was some sort of healing crisis and if saunas were even a good idea.

Day 3 and it was time for a blood sample. I'm not a big fan of giving blood, and when the nurse arrived, he began describing the blood-letting procedure in colourful detail, something I was not prepared to hear. I sat down, the nurse tightened the tourniquet around my arm, and then he began poking at veins on the top of my hand. Poke, poke, poke and still no blood. After several more attempts I started feeling very queasy. "I'm not sure what's going on, but your blood is very slow," the nurse observed. I could feel a nauseating light-headedness start to wash over me. I knew what was happening and told the nurse I was about to pass out. I went with the flow (or lack thereof) and laid my head back on the sofa as I blacked out completely.

I was conscious again when the 911 gang arrived: first the firefighters, followed by the paramedics. I was also sweating profusely. Just what I needed—more sweat. The battery of tests began. Given that I am now a post-fifty-year-old male, they were anxious to see how my heart was doing. First they checked my blood pressure: 127 over 82. "Fine," I was told. They did a full twelve-lead electrocardiogram while at the same time testing my blood for diabetes. "Not diabetic," one of the paramedics said. My dog sensed something was wrong and would not leave my side, lying against me on the sofa. "Heart looks good, heartbeat normal, beating strongly," said the guy reading a cardiogram printout on the tiny graph paper spewing out of the portable machine on my family-room floor. I thanked them and declined a ride to the hospital.

I discussed with Rodney the fact that I was feeling rather poorly after my two long sauna sessions. "I wonder if perhaps I was overdoing it,"

I said, thinking of the one-hour saunas at up to 49 degrees Celsius. "Yes, of course, you're overdoing it," he replied quickly. Rodney told me to keep the temperature lower, open the sliding glass window in the cubicle for fresh air, pull back to thirty minutes and work my way up to an hour. He also told me to make sure I was always well hydrated and to take adequate electrolyte replacements and vitamins.

The experience reminded me that, despite the incredible resilience of our bodies, we live within remarkably narrow tolerance ranges related to body temperature, hydration, salt levels, blood pressure and many other parameters. It's easier than we think to throw ourselves out of balance—beyond the defined ranges that sustain our lives—and this can pose serious health risks. Detox programmes need to be undertaken with caution and according to the advice of a trusted health practitioner.

Well, What *Was* in My Sweat?

To keep the details manageable in my blood-and-sweat sauna experiment, Rick and I decided to focus on two chemicals that we'd researched extensively: phthalates and BPA. Phthalates, as we've mentioned, are widespread in personal-care products and artificial air fresheners, and BPA is an ingredient in the plastic resin of thousands of products, from the visors of hockey helmets to the lining of food cans.

BPA (see figure 13) in both my sweat and urine was measured at 1.7 ng/mL in the first sample, which is about the mean level found in American men.[26] Over the course of the first three weeks, my BPA measurements remained fairly stable in both sweat and urine, decreasing slightly over that time period. My daily routine must have been quite consistent. But the levels found in week 4 were shocking. My BPA measurement of 4 ng/mL of urine put me in the 90th percentile of Americans, and although there are no statistics on BPA in sweat, the levels found in my week-4 sweat had skyrocketed to 14 ng/mL. A flaw in our research became obvious: I hadn't kept track of my diet or bathing routines during the experiment. Generally speaking, I avoid BPA and phthalate exposure to the extent that I can control such exposure, with one weakness: I love to cook with imported canned San Marzano tomatoes, and those cans almost certainly contain BPA in the lining. I'll bet I had a large helping of tomato pasta made with those canned tomatoes the evening before the BPA spike.

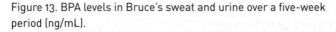

Figure 13. BPA levels in Bruce's sweat and urine over a five-week period (ng/mL).

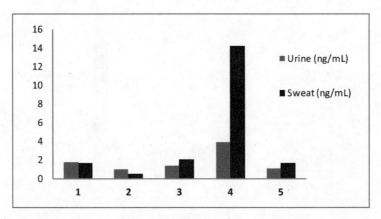

The results of my phthalate-level testing resembled those of the BPA tests, in that there was no consistency across the five-week study period. This is not entirely surprising, given that the samples are a snapshot in time. MEP and MBP, the urinary metabolites of diethyl phthalate (DEP) and dibutyl phthalate (DBP) respectively, are widespread in personal-care products and cosmetics. Though I've been steadfast about eliminating scented soaps, figures 14 and 15 show that these chemicals were still present in my body in significant amounts. My urine levels of MBP were consistent with the American mean of 33.4 ng/mL, disregarding the spike in the last week, which put me well above the 95th percentile (did I grab the wrong shampoo one day?). And my MEP levels were well below the 1,017.5 ng/mL mean, even with the significant week-3 spike (see figure 14).[27] I attribute those low MEP levels to my successful strategy of scented-soap avoidance.

Figure 14. Phthalate metabolite (MEP and MBP) levels in Bruce's urine over a five-week period (ng/mL).

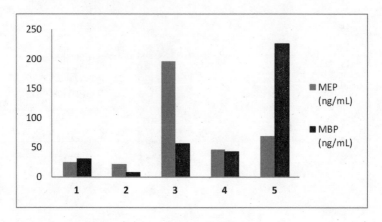

Figure 15. Phthalate metabolite (MEP and MBP) levels in Bruce's sweat over a five-week period (ng/mL).

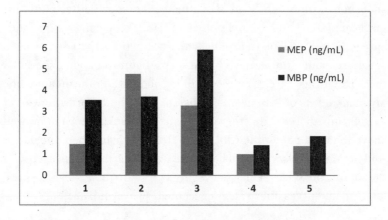

My sweat and urine levels for BPA and phthalates both followed similar curves, suggesting that testing for either urine or sweat provides an accurate indication of relative levels over a particular period of time. However, the most important information revealed by the testing is that levels of both MEP and MBP in my sweat were considerably lower than the levels found in my urine. This implies that the kidneys provide the preferred route for eliminating phthalate byproducts, whereas sweat appears to be the preferred detoxification pathway for

BPA, given that the BPA levels in my sweat were nearly five times higher than those in my urine.

Dr. Genuis's blood, urine and sweat monitoring studies[28] have looked at levels of selected toxic chemicals in sauna-induced sweat as a bio-monitoring tool for body-burden levels. It is difficult to draw a direct correlation between the quantity of chemicals found in our sweat and the overall levels in our body over time. Inadvertent daily exposures may result in levels that spike off the charts, as my test results showed. Measuring toxins in sweat confirms that we have specific chemicals in our bodies and that we can help rid ourselves of them, some more than others, by sweating them out. And that is a good thing.

Despite the little research hiccups, saunas (done the right way) make me feel great. I leave a sauna feeling clean, relaxed and serene. And my skin always feels amazing. After my intense sauna routine, people I barely knew were commenting on my skin. Given the outrageous amount of money people spend on skin and face lotions and creams, I suspect that investing in an infrared sauna and using it twice a week might actually save money, produce better results over the long term and also be safer and healthier than using personal-care products laced with harmful synthetic chemicals.

Feeling the Detox Boost

With my successful chelation results from the previous chapter in hand, along with this evidence that sweating is a great way to rid our bodies of synthetic toxins, and having consumed more water in the previous six months than in the fifty years that preceded them (or so it felt!), I was starting to understand the concept of "toxout" and could see that, in my case at least, chelation and sweating in a sauna were generally effective methods of getting synthetic chemicals out of the body. True, the chelation also took out sodium, calcium, magnesium and sulphur—elements that the body needs. And the sauna routine had its ups and downs. However, overall, they were extremely useful.

And now a final word about sweat.

Humans wouldn't spend US$18 billion per year on deodorants and antiperspirants if we liked sweat. But is perspiration getting a bad rap? Rather than thinking of sweat as disgusting, we should be thinking that *not* sweating is disgusting. Sweating helps regulate our fluid and electrolyte levels and eliminate toxins by taking waste from our blood and expelling it. Think of our pores, as I witnessed in the sauna, as little springs releasing droplets of water, salt and unwanted toxins. And we do more than sweat through our skin. Our bodies also release oils through the sebaceous glands, and these oils carry away fat-soluble toxins. Imagine if all those glands and pores were plugged with makeup, creams or, even worse, aluminum-based antiperspirants designed to shut them down. It leaves no place for anything to come out and so holds all the toxins and oils in our bodies, and this leads to irritated or inflamed skin, clogged pores, acne and other dermatological problems—not to mention preventing our body from using the full potential of this critical detox pathway.

Every minute of every day, we are expelling natural and synthetic toxins, whether we do anything about it or not. So the beauty of detox therapies is that they give our bodies a little extra help flushing out more of the nasties than we would naturally.

The critical piece of that statement is "every day." This means eating organic fruits and vegetables; cutting back on animal fats; drinking lots of fresh, filtered water; taking relevant supplements; and exercising *every day*. And if you can fit a sauna into your routine, all the better! Detoxing is not about one-off diets, cleanses or footbath fads; it's a lifestyle we need to dedicate ourselves to. So save some money and avoid the cleanse kits.

We need to push the reset button on our toxic lifestyle to keep our toxout fitness levels high.

ELEVEN: A STATIONARY ROAD TRIP

[RICK BREATHES DEEPLY]

Advertising is based on one thing: happiness. And do you know what happiness is? Happiness is the smell of a new car. It's freedom from fear. It's a billboard on the side of a road that screams with reassurance that whatever you're doing is okay.

—DON DRAPER, *Mad Men*

DON'T GET ME WRONG: Jeff Gearhart is a lovely man.

I just never want to see him again.

This is what happens when you spend a day sitting beside somebody in a car parked in a hot room with the windows rolled up, inhaling toxic fumes.

Thankfully, the stuffy vehicle of which I speak stood 3 metres (more than 9 feet) high and 5.5 metres (17 feet) long and weighed in at a whopping 3,220 kilograms (7,100 pounds). The Chevy Tahoe LT was jet black and brand spanking new. It showed just 274 miles on the odometer, and the tag on the door told us it had been built about a month before Jeff rented it. All in all, it had everything we needed for our strange day: a huge interior we could stretch out in and, most important, an overpowering, nose-tingling "new car smell."

Ahhh . . . the new car smell.

So intoxicating, yet so fleeting. Is your old beater getting you down? No problem! You now have the choice of a veritable smorgasbord of "new car smell"–scented air fresheners to give you that quick vehicular pick-me-up.[1] But that day in Ann Arbor, the Tahoe's acrid interior didn't need the boost; it stank to high heaven all on its own.

We had a hypothesis: that the new car smell would result in

measurable increases in chemicals in our body. We had an experimental design. And, very important, if anyone cares to replicate our results, we've provided enough detail that they can. Would wallowing in the SUV's pungent embrace fill our bodies with pollutants? We were about to find out.

Space Station

The cool factor of the Ecology Center's stylish walk-up office—where Jeff is research director—is seriously undermined by the shop selling "discount ugly Christmas sweaters" down below. Fortunately, we didn't linger. With his backpack stuffed full of food, we piled into Jeff's rented Tahoe and hit the road for the forty-minute drive to the Space Station self-storage facility in Petersburg, Michigan, the closest place Jeff could find that had a unit big enough for our "new car smell" experiment.

"So what are you up to again?" asked Leanne, the proprietor, who took our payment for a day's use of her large, heated garage.

"We're measuring air quality in cars," Jeff said. "We want to mimic the cabin temperature on a hot, sunny day, so don't be surprised if you come into the garage and it's a little bit warm."

"Riiighht," she said, looking us up and down, eyebrow raised, as she rang through Jeff's credit card.

Jeff and I drove the Tahoe into the middle of Leanne's garage, then cranked the thermostat on the wall to 86 degrees Fahrenheit (a common temperature on a summer's day in the Ann Arbor area). We rolled up the windows, turned off the car, tuned the radio to NPR and sat there for the next eight hours, breathing in the pungent off-gassing from the vehicle's newly minted upholstery.

Powerful memories can be triggered by smell. And I'll admit that for me, the new car smell took me right back to wondrous family holidays in Bar Harbor, Maine: the sea air, sunlight reflecting off the pink granite mountains of Acadia National Park, and watching the world go by through the window of my dad's new baby-blue 1972 Dodge Dart Swinger. On a molecular level, however, the new car smell is considerably less magical. It's nothing more than nasty volatile organic compounds (VOCs) like formaldehyde, toluene and xylenes and other chemical goodies evaporating from the adhesives, sealants and plastic bits in the vehicle's interior.

The structure of our experiment couldn't have been simpler. Before we left Jeff's office, we each banked a urine sample. And when we climbed out of the Tahoe in the early evening, we each took a second sample. We then sent the four little glass jars to EAG Life Sciences, a lab in Maryland Heights, Missouri, to measure whether the eight hours of breathing in the new car smell appreciably increased the levels of certain VOCs in our body.

If any of you have ever spent eight straight hours in a hot car with another person, you'll realize that the conversation can pretty easily go off the figurative road, but Jeff and I did manage to chat at some length about his work at the Ecology Center and the reason why we were in the car in the first place. The Ecology Center's work on cars and chemicals started at a grassroots level in the communities impacted by manufacturing plants in southeast Michigan. The center realized it could leverage broader public support by figuring in the "iconic product" of this manufacturing—the car—and tie it to their issues. So in the late 1990s they started doing report cards that examined and graded the car-manufacturing process. These reports assessed environmental factors and corporate management to determine which companies were doing better than others. Jeff told me that after a few years of preparing these report cards, they decided they had to make things more real for people. So in 2006 the center released a consumer guide to new vehicles at HealthyStuff.org—and there was so much interest that the website crashed on the first day.

The guide reviewed over two hundred of the most popular car models from that year, testing each of them for the toxic chemicals that off-gas from the interior parts. The Healthy Stuff vehicle guide focuses on chemicals such as flame retardants, plasticizers like phthalates, heavy metals and VOCs. To sample the vehicle interiors for these chemicals, Jeff and his team developed a method using a portable X-ray fluorescence (XRF) device, an impressive machine that slightly resembles a chunky phaser from *Star Trek*'s USS *Enterprise*. When you hold the XRF up to a piece of material, it identifies the elemental composition of the thing it's aiming at in less than sixty seconds. Each car is then ranked according to the results of this material analysis, with the worst cars receiving high scores due to their high chemical content.

Between 2006 and 2012, the Ecology Center released four of their ambitious consumer guides, which regularly turned up an alarming cocktail of toxic chemicals in automobile interiors. They have over one thousand cars in their database, and Jeff estimates they have data on about 90 percent of the 2006–12 vehicle models sold in North America. After years of releasing the results and naming the companies involved, the Ecology Centre drove (pun fully intended) some significant change: industry-wide, ratings started to improve, and the best vehicles eliminated some hazardous chemicals entirely. In 2012, for instance, 17 percent of new vehicles tested by the center had PVC–free interiors, and 60 percent were produced without brominated flame retardants. Jeff told me that car companies like Ford are now investing significant dollars to clean up their manufacturing act, and Honda was so delighted that its Civic was named the Ecology Center's 2012 "Best Pick"—in recognition of the company's work to make its vehicle cabins as non-toxic as possible—that it still regularly trumpets this accomplishment on social media.

When I interviewed Jeff for this tenth-anniversary edition of *Slow Death*, he told me the battle has shifted rather dramatically to global regulation of vehicle interior air quality. Interestingly, an explosion of public concern about air quality in China and south-east Asian countries has driven the creation of new regulation and caused Ford to create a crackerjack "golden nose" team to track down offending chemicals. The team's mission? Nothing less than snuffing out the new car smell. The eighteen "golden noses" work out of the company's research facility in Nanjing, China, smelling every component part of every Ford vehicle sold in every Asian country. If an armrest or air conditioning vent fails the smell test, parts are sent back to the manufacturer. And the nasal commanders take extreme precautions against infecting the parts themselves, according to *Reuters,* abstaining from smoking and even avoiding nail polish.

None of this good news applied to the Tahoe, unfortunately. In a report released around the time Jeff and I undertook our experiment, the center classified the car as of "medium concern" and found measurable levels of bromine, chlorine and other nasty chemicals in its interior.

I read this and much, much more about the Tahoe as I sat beside Jeff during the eight hours we were ensconced in its capacious interior.

Some University of Michigan graduate students took air samples from the car's interior, but they came and went in a flash, leaving Jeff and me alone, staring at the wall of the storage depot.

By hour 8 Jeff and I were hanging on to every minute as the dashboard clock clicked down to the end of the experiment. We wheeled out of the garage like bats out of hell, racing through the darkness back to Ann Arbor, courting a speeding ticket, so anxious were we to be free of our vehicular incarceration. The new car smell had gotten stale.

Sniff Test

Yes, there have been a lot of studies of indoor air quality, and the reason, in this couch-potato age, is likely obvious: the average resident of an industrialized country spends more than 90 percent of his or her life in enclosed spaces. To be even more precise, Americans have been found to spend almost 87 percent of their time indoors and an incredible 5.5 percent of their lives in an enclosed vehicle. For those of you who aren't fans of math, this leaves only about 8 percent of our lives for skiing, raking leaves in the autumn, sunbathing on docks, walking kids to school, golfing, enjoying picnics and all other outdoor pursuits combined (see figure 16).

Figure 16. Where Americans spend their lives.[4]

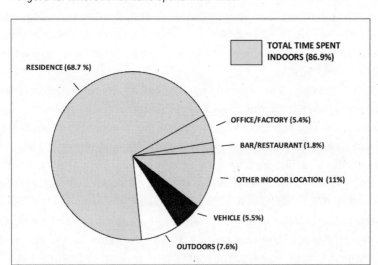

Scientists have increasingly turned their attention to indoor air pollution because, quite simply, this is where much of the world is spending their lives.

Indoor air pollutants are an incredibly varied lot, and virtually all Americans (and, it would be reasonable to assume, residents of other industrialized nations) have measurable levels of VOCs and other pollutants in their bodies.[5] Not surprisingly, the presence or absence of tobacco smoke is a huge determinant of indoor air quality. So is your home's attached garage, if it has one (because of the inevitable and smelly assortment of jerry cans, lawn mowers, broken-down cars and sundry abandoned painting supplies). And if you've recently been exposed to fossil fuel combustion (for example, if you've been sitting in traffic) or have worked with glues and solvents (doing home renovations, for instance), your body levels of VOCs will be through the roof.

Sometimes, though, it's the innocuous activities that contribute to our toxic chemical load, like simply sitting in a car. Researchers have found that we are exposed to over 275 pollutants floating around inside the average automobile. More of these chemicals seem to be released from car interiors in the warmth of summer. Cars less than three years old and luxury automobiles (maybe because if you've paid a lot for a car, you want as much "new car smell" as possible) have above-average smelliness. Studies have underlined the fact that in many vehicles the interior air quality is significantly worse than is considered safe in indoor environments. However, it hasn't been at all clear that these ambient levels result in measurable increases in the human body.[6]

Of all the chemicals we could have looked for, we zeroed in on those known to pose health concerns.[7] We looked for the metabolites, or breakdown products, of hexane (2,5-hexanedione), heptane (2,5-heptanedione), benzene (phenyl mercapturic acid), toluene (benzyl mercapturic acid), and xylenes (methylbenzyl mercapturic acid). Hexane is one of the most common VOCs in many glues, and prolonged exposure to it can lead to neurological damage. Heptane is common in some paints and coatings and certain kinds of rubber cement. Benzene is a well-known human carcinogen, and exposure to toluene and xylene can cause changes in the central nervous system and other damaging neurological effects.

The results of our experiment were astonishing (see figure 17). For all the chemicals in question (including benzene and xylenes, not shown here), both Jeff and I saw significant increases in our bodies after eight hours of breathing the off-gassing. Look at the trends: in all cases our VOC levels rose—sometimes quadrupling. The implications of this are significant, since the average citizen in an industrialized country spends 5 percent of his or her *life*(!) in an enclosed vehicle. The Canadian government tells me that I, as an average Canadian guy, can expect to live until about eighty years of age: that's four entire years of my life spent in a car. And for some of my fellow Torontonians who spend three hours a day commuting to and from work, I guarantee this number will be much higher. Granted, not every car will have the air-quality issues of a new Chevy Tahoe. But many will.

Figure 17. VOC increases in Jeff and Rick after eight hours in a warm, new car (all units mg/L).

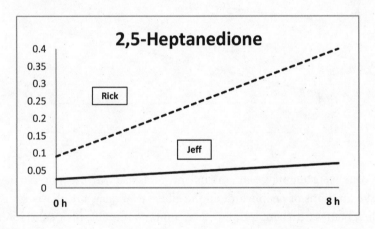

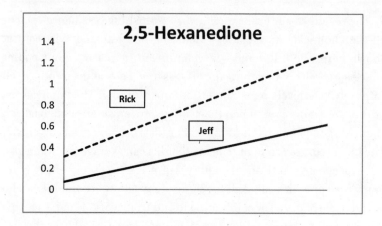

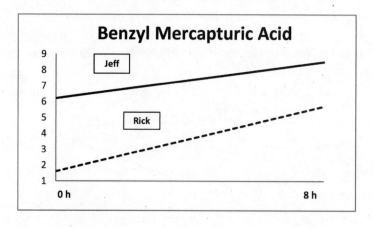

Our experimental result, in a nutshell, was that with every breath they take, millions of people around the globe, every day, are slowly filling their bodies with benzene and other, unpronounceable toxic substances as they take a trip to the grocery store, pack the kids into the car to take them to soccer or head off for a summer vacation. We've included some specific conclusions regarding what to do about this in the last chapter of the book. Suffice it to say for the moment, if you have a new car, rolling the windows down and letting it air out is a good place to start!

"Toxic Soup"

One way to deduce how these sorts of pollutants impact us is to examine their effects on people who work with the stuff every day.

Though occupational exposure to chemicals and resulting health outcomes are poorly understood, one scientific study in particular is noteworthy for its connection to automobiles. A team of researchers led by University of Windsor professor Dr. Jim Brophy, through the support of the Canadian Breast Cancer Foundation (CBCF), decided to investigate whether certain types of work posed occupational risks for increased rates of breast cancer.[8]

Brophy and his team conducted a case-control study of over 2,000 women in Essex and Kent Counties in southwestern Ontario—an industrial expanse known for its flat landscape, automotive parts plants and plastic-manufacturing facilities. The case group of 1,005 women with breast cancer and the control group of 1,146 randomly selected members of the same communities were asked to provide detailed information about their occupational and reproductive histories. Here's the simple but powerful result: industries characterized by high levels of occupational chemical exposure showed an increased risk for breast cancer.

The results of Brophy's study are especially worrisome for women who work in automotive plastics plants. The plastics industry is characterized by a very high concentration of female workers; in Canada, for example, 37 percent of the plastics workforce is female—a higher proportion than any other industry in the manufacturing sector.[9] In Brophy's geographic study area, Windsor–Essex County, where the majority of plastics products are produced for the automobile industry, women make up over half the plastics workforce.[10] Similar proportions occur in plastics-related industries in the United States.

The plastic-manufacturing work done by the women in Brophy's study involved mostly injection moulding, which can be described as follows. After a product is designed—any product really, but in the automotive case, let's say a dashboard or the console between the seats with those handily designed cup holders—a mould is made to form the features of the plastic part. The injecting material for the part is fed into a heated cylinder, mixed around and forced into the mould cavity, where it cools and hardens.[11]

What does this mean in terms of the female workers' exposure to chemicals? The molten mixtures that become the final product are made up of resins, multiple additives and sometimes lamination films. The heating process emits vapours and mists into the plant that can include plasticizers, UV protectors, pigments, dyes, flame retardants and unreacted resin components, among other things.[12] Many plastics release estrogenic chemicals, and additives like phthalates and flame retardants in the molten mixture are known endocrine-disrupting chemicals. Furthermore, some of the ingredients present in the manufacturing of polymers (such as BPA and vinyl chloride) are carcinogenic.[13] So it's no surprise that Brophy and his team discovered that women in the plastics industry had double the risk of developing breast cancer as compared to the control group.

When I interviewed Brophy about the study, I was curious to know how these chemicals actually get into workers' bodies. Are they inhaled, absorbed through the skin or what? "These people are getting exposed in just about every way imaginable," he responded. "It's very important to emphasize that they're not just getting exposed to one toxic substance. They're getting exposed to the most unbelievable mixture of substances, all of which are known to potentially pose a threat to their health. And we know that when you get exposed to these mixtures, it's even more potent than if you get exposed to just one thing on its own." He told me that, during interviews, his team repeatedly heard complaints of improper ventilation, and one of the women working with automotive plastics likened being in her workplace to being "in a toxic soup."

Studies like Brophy's show that the people who deal with high levels of these chemicals every day are at *significant* risk of truly terrible health outcomes. They are "canaries in the coal mine," warning of possible effects on the rest of us even at much lower exposures. Their stories and their illnesses should also make us reflect on the tangible impact that our society's consumption patterns have on the workers who sustain them—in southwestern Ontario and anywhere else where workers are exposed to toxic chemicals.

Strange Symptoms

In this chapter we've focused on VOCs, but other chemicals cause big problems when it comes to indoor air pollution—the ones that can enter our bodies in ways other than inhalation. Flame retardants, common in a wide range of household products, building materials, electronics, furnishing, cars, airplanes, and upholstered products illustrate this very well.

Our friend Miriam Diamond, a super-dynamic professor and researcher in the University of Toronto's Department of Chemistry, has done some impressive research on flame retardants in everyday environments. In 2004 she and her colleagues collected the grime from interior and exterior household windows throughout Toronto and surrounding areas to measure their relative levels of PBDEs. The results showed significantly higher levels of PBDEs on the interior films—especially in more urban environments.[14] This finding prompted further investigation, after which Miriam and her team published a groundbreaking study: the first exposure assessment of PBDEs indicating that house dust was likely the main route of exposure for individuals with high levels of the chemical in their bodies.[15] Miriam's research earned her the Scientist of the Year award from *Canadian Geographic* as well as the honorific "Dust Doctor" from her students. I phoned up the good doctor to ask her a few further questions about flame retardants, dust and indoor air quality.

"If flame retardants are ingredients in seemingly inert items like the foam in seat cushions," I asked, "how do they get into our bodies? Is it as straightforward as the fabrics and foams containing flame retardants breaking down over time and becoming dust that we inhale?" While this could be true of some older, ripped pieces of furniture, Miriam explained that it's actually more complicated. She thinks there are two main ways flame retardants get into dust. She likened the first way to taking a hot shower and watching the water vaporize and condense on the cold window. "A product—like your computer or TV—heats up when you use it. As a result of heating, the flame retardants de-gas, or move from the plastic into the air. But flame retardants don't want to stay in the air, because of the low vapour pressure and also because the air is colder than the electronic product. So then they partition into stuff, stuff like the greasy film on walls and floor and plant surfaces."

Another avenue for flame retardants entering household dust involves humans. Recent research by Miriam's colleagues showed higher concentrations of flame retardants on the bottom of the hand versus the top, indicating that the chemicals are getting onto our palms when we touch them. "We know that bits of chemicals come off the surface of objects that contain them," Miriam explained. "And we know that because all you have to do is touch something containing a flame retardant, like a computer, and you're going to get it on your hand. A little bit of the plastic or fabric seems to come off just by microabrasion." She went on, "Here's another scenario: You've got dust on your couch, and when you sit down, some dust floats up and is resuspended in the air. While the dust was settled on the couch, it had the opportunity to pick up the flame retardant from the couch, and when it's resuspended, it moves into the room."

A study published in the spring of 2013 reminds us that it's not only dust in the home that we should be worried about. Researchers at Duke University looked at a new-to-the-market flame retardant known as V6 and its concentrations in foam baby products and household and automobile dust.[16] With the slow phase-out of PBDEs, V6 has been developed as an alternative, so it's no surprise that the newer flame retardant was found in high concentrations in the baby products and dust that were examined. What's more, the study found that concentrations of V6 were significantly higher in car dust than in house dust.[17]

When I think of dust, I tend to think of dust bunnies. But it seems that toxic dust, in your home or car is actually more likely to be distributed in places that you wouldn't normally expect. "Dust bunnies are what we call the reservoir dust," Miriam said. "It's *active* dust, the stuff in the centre of the room that gets resuspended in the air, that's the concern." Think of dust bunnies as dust carcasses: dead creatures mouldering away on the ground that won't bother anyone ever again. In contrast, the living dust, the really small and sneaky particles that we inhale and often eat (the motes visible in the sunlight as it streams through your kitchen window), actively move around.

In the same way that biologists track animals with radio receivers, Miriam Diamond tracks dust—and with equal zeal. Her work has revealed much about how these chemicals start out residing in the seat cushion under your butt and then go on to be an invasive pollutant in your bloodstream. And once flame retardants are in us, bad things start to happen. Miriam referred to a recent epidemiological study examining the effects of prenatal PBDE exposure on indicators of neurodevelopment in children one to six years of age.[18] The study recruited 210 women in Manhattan who were pregnant during the 9/11 attacks and subsequently delivered at one of three downtown hospitals. Each baby's umbilical blood was taken at birth and analyzed for the presence of toxic chemicals. At 12, 24, 36 and 72 months of age, various types of developmental tests were administered, and scores were compared to known developmental norms. The research team had hypothesized that prenatal exposure to toxins, particularly PBDEs, emitted from the World Trade Center buildings after the attack would affect neurodevelopment in children. They were right; the cohort study reported lower scores on mental and physical development and lower IQ in infants and toddlers, especially in children whose umbilical blood had the highest concentrations of PBDEs.

"It's weird," Miriam said. "As a mom, when I read the adverse effects, it just felt uncomfortably close to my circumstance. I thought of all those years working in front of a computer prior to and during pregnancy." She has always sent her children outside to play, and thinks that maybe we should all play outside more.

Allergic Generation

Indoor air–quality researchers have also focused on another family of chemicals: our old friends the phthalates.

Not content to enter our bodies only through the personal-care products they infuse, phthalates also comprise a significant chunk of the dust in our homes. A particularly convincing series of studies has linked phthalate exposure to asthma and, perhaps surprisingly, the development of allergies.[19] One of the key researchers in this area, Carl-Gustaf Bornehag, of Karlstad University in Sweden, told me that when he started his pioneering research, he didn't have phthalates in mind at all. "In the 1990s in Sweden, we were collecting scientific data on environmental issues related to asthma and allergies, and we were focusing on moisture-related problems in buildings." Bornehag had noticed that something was happening in damp buildings—resulting in higher rates of asthma and allergies in children—and he wanted to know why.

So he started one of the world's biggest studies, called "Dampness in Buildings and Health." It includes forty thousand kids and has tracked their lives and their health status in five-year increments since 2000. As Bornehag and his colleagues started to put together their mountain of data, they encountered a problem: no matter how hard they sifted, they couldn't find a relationship between moisture-related exposures and asthma and allergies. For a while they were stumped. Clearly they were measuring the wrong things, so they kept analyzing and reanalyzing their air and dust samples, looking for some new trends. Finally, in 2004, they found the common thread: it was phthalates. The more phthalates in household dust, the higher the rates of asthma and eczema in kids. Given that a great deal of flooring in Sweden contains polyvinyl chloride (PVC), which is very rich in phthalates, the concentration of the chemical in household dust in many cases was through the roof. "We looked for something," said Bornehag. "We couldn't find it, but we did find something else."

Bornehag expanded his study to another eight countries around the world and a whopping hundred thousand children. It's slow going, but similar results linking phthalates to respiratory and skin problems as well as allergic reactions in children are popping up with growing frequency.[20]

Bornehag ended our conversation with an intriguing observation: "There's no question that there has been a significant increase in allergies in people during the last five or six decades. And if you take not only phthalates but a number of these endocrine-disrupting chemicals, they have all been introduced during exactly the same time period." One attempt to get at this casual connection occurred at the Boston Children's Hospital.

Doctors there realized they were seeing an unusually high number of asthma patients from certain low-income neighbourhoods.[21] They knew that asthma attacks can be set off by things like dust, mould, polluted air and other environmental aggravations common in low-income neighbourhoods, and they wondered if they could do something about it. The Community Asthma Initiative was born.

The programme identifies children who make frequent visits to the hospital's emergency ward suffering from asthma attacks. Willing parents of these kids are then visited by a community health worker, who helps identify and educate the families about problem conditions and products in the indoor environment that can trigger attacks.[22] Visits from the community health worker mean going through a checklist of asthma triggers and indicators of problem environments—things like mould, cockroaches and mice.

The programme has been a success. A report noted "a 56 percent reduction in patients with any emergency room visits, and an 80 percent reduction in patients with any hospitalizations."[23] All this has been done through simple and low-cost changes such as dusting and vacuuming more often, avoiding chemical-heavy cleaners and minimizing the use of fragranced products like room fresheners, which can all aggravate asthma. Who knew that a simple spring cleaning could have such tangible detox benefits?

Good News, Bad News

I had ploughed my way through a tonne of papers on hundreds of different indoor air pollutants, and my head was hurting. I needed someone to give me the bottom line. For an overview of what's been getting better and what's been getting worse when it comes to indoor air quality, I turned to one of Bornehag's occasional co-authors: Dr. Charles Weschler, a researcher at the Rutgers Environmental and Occupational Health Sciences Institute. Weschler had penned a refreshingly clear "everything you wanted to know but were afraid to ask" treatise titled "Changes in Indoor Pollutants Since the 1950s."[24]

"In terms of many known or suspected carcinogens, at least in the U.S. and Canada, things have improved significantly," Weschler explained. For benzene, formaldehyde, asbestos and radon, the levels in typical homes and offices today are much lower than they were in the 1960s and '70s. He cited two large surveys of VOCs in the indoor air of U.S. homes, one conducted between 1981 and 1984 and another between 1999 and 2001. "The average level of benzene went down from about 14 micrograms per cubic metre to about 2 micrograms per cubic metre. And we saw similar declines for other aromatic solvents: toluene, xylenes and ethylbenzene. So that's good news."

Weschler's assessment of "classic toxic gases" like carbon monoxide (CO), sulphur dioxide (SO_2) and nitrogen oxides (NOx) is similarly upbeat. "Fewer people are dying of carbon monoxide poisoning today, per capita, than were dying forty or fifty years ago," he said. "We have CO detectors in homes, but more importantly, CO emissions from a lot of combustion appliances are just much lower than they used to be." He adds cars as another household item whose CO emissions have been vastly reduced. Similarly, levels of sulphur dioxide are down because of reduced use of sulphur-containing fuel and coal. And nitrogen oxides indoors are way down, a result of the most innocuous of changes. "Do gas ranges in Canada still have pilot lights?" he asked. Not many, I told him. "Right!" he continued. "So pilot lights were this continuous source of nitrogen oxide that could actually reach elevated levels in a tightly sealed home. No more."

Heavy metals are another good story. "Lead, mercury, cadmium—they're all much lower in homes today. You collect dust samples today and compare the levels to what you would have found twenty or thirty years ago and again you see orders-of-magnitude reduction. Lead and mercury used to be used in paints to prevent mould and mildew—same with cadmium. And as you know, that's no longer permitted for indoor paints. So that's good news." The last rosy update Weschler underlined was the change in pesticides and the fact that many of the most toxic ones have been curtailed. "You no longer see DDT or chlordane or chlorpyrifos or Mirex used indoors."

Weschler is also interested in focusing specifically on the extent to which our bodies' chemical burden is a result of the indoor environment and exposure through the dermal pathway (that is, our skin). In his 2012 journal article "SVOC Exposure Indoors: Fresh Look at Dermal Pathways," Weschler examined the concentration of several semi-volatile organic compounds (SVOCs)—a category that includes common chemicals like BPA, phthalates, pesticides and flame retardants—in indoor air and on indoor surfaces. Using these levels, he then developed equations to estimate the levels of SVOCs that got through the skin of experiment participants.[25] What he found was that air-to-skin transdermal uptake can be comparable to, or larger than, inhalation intake for many SVOCs of current or potential interest indoors.[26] His results indicate that exposure to these indoor chemicals through the skin has previously been underestimated and that this pathway should be given more weight by exposure scientists and health officials when examining exposure to indoor SVOCs.

Why is this particular type of transmission of SVOCs such a concern? Because the nature of the dermal pathway means that the dose of chemical entering the body is potentially much higher than for a comparable amount of chemical that is inhaled or ingested. Whereas inhaled or ingested SVOCs have to pass through various systems (respiratory and digestive) where their appearance can trigger defence mechanisms, SVOCs passing through the skin can go *directly* to the blood and organ tissue. So it's no wonder that human exposure to these chemicals indoors is a serious concern. Weschler makes the case for improved biomonitoring for these indoor pollutants—that is, ongoing measurement of levels of these chemicals in the human body. This will certainly help illustrate the dimensions of the off-gassing problem, but as always, we also need to make our homes and other indoor environments healthier through our own efforts.

Industry Responds

I can still remember what my hard-bitten Newfoundland grandmother used to say about latex paint. "Pah!" (dismissive wave of the hand). "That stuff never lasts, b'y. Oil is what you need!" But what she might have thought in the 1980s isn't the case today. In fact, as Carl Minchew, director of environment, health and safety at Benjamin Moore Paints, told me, you'll be hard pressed to find anything other than latex paints now. And this is a good thing.

Those older oil paints, Minchew said, were really solvent paints: 50 percent of the volume of the paint in the can was a solvent mixture that evaporated as the paint dried. Given that latex paints dry more quickly, don't make your eyes burn and can be cleaned off your hands with soap and water rather than paint thinner, it's no surprise that latex has enjoyed a rapidly increasing market share. The difference between VOC levels in my grandmother's standby oil paint and modern zero-VOC paints like Benjamin Moore's Natura brand "is almost infinite," according to Minchew. The early latex paints contained about 10 percent of the VOCs contained in oil paints, and with improving paint technology, this proportion is now down to virtually zero. Natura, according to Minchew, is simply "a better-performing paint. It goes on better, dries better, hides better and is more durable under use." And it doesn't fill your house with noxious pollutants. What's not to like?

The market's transition from oil to latex paints is just one example of the ongoing revolution in the way that building materials are made. Whether your house paint is smelly or not is a fairly tangible and obvious thing, but many recent advances are far subtler, though no less important.

In North America the introduction of the LEED (Leadership in Energy and Environmental Design) certification system marked the turn toward better building materials. LEED is a third-party certification programme for the design, construction and operation of high-performance green buildings.[27] It provides building owners and operators with a specific framework that allows them to identify and meet practical and measurable green building design, construction, operations and maintenance solutions that will help contribute to a healthier overall environment.

I spoke to Thomas Mueller, president of the Canada Green Building Council, the group dedicated to promoting LEED in Canada, about the extent to which LEED is now paying attention to indoor air quality. He explained to me that within the LEED system, there are five main credit categories, and one of these is called Indoor Environmental Quality. The core of this category is related specifically to the products that are being used in a building. "These are usually what we call finishing materials," Mueller told me, meaning things like paints, varnishes and sealants, "and they tend to off-gas harmful pollutants during their life in the building."

Mueller said it was the 2000 version of LEED (the second version in the United States, the first in Canada) that really broke into the marketplace and became popular. "The 2000 version focused on and addressed in a more consistent way the idea that some of these products and chemicals needed to be avoided, to enhance the health of building occupants," he explained. Mueller noted the impact LEED has had by way of the paint example. "When paint first came up in LEED, there was a certain threshold for VOCs in paint. If you want these points [the Indoor Environmental Quality points] in LEED, you cannot use paints that have a threshold above so many milligrams of VOCs per litre of paint." These LEED standards introduced the idea of low-VOC paint to the wider marketplace for the first time, and since then low-VOC paints have increased in quality and availability in the building sector. Now carpeting can also be rated according to Indoor Environmental Quality points, and Mueller explained that this point system is being extended to other product categories as well.

Mueller was quick to point out that improvements in building materials can't all be attributed to LEED but noted that the power of the rating system allowed it to become a market mechanism. "The interesting thing is that these products—paint, carpet—are marketed commercially, and they're sold at a price point to be competitive in the marketplace with other products. All the paint manufacturers, all the carpet tile manufacturers, they all have to have these low-VOC products. And that gets rid of the premium. People just say, 'I'm not using this old stuff anymore,' and they don't buy it."

Since its inception in 1998 and relaunch in 2002, LEED's impact has grown exponentially. According to the U.S. Green Building Council, the total floor area of LEED-certified buildings now expands by over 2.2 million square feet a day.[28] Moreover, roughly 92,000 new projects adopt the LEED rating system on a daily basis in over 165 countries and territories around the world.[29] In the United States alone, LEED-certified and -registered projects now represent over 10.5 billion square feet of total building space.[30] The LEED certification program for existing buildings has also experienced explosive growth since its launch in 2004. Indeed, in 2011 the square footage of LEED-certified existing buildings surpassed that of new construction by 15 million square feet.[31] Through such initiatives, we now have the chance to right some of our previous wrongs and ensure that future buildings are safer and more environmentally sustainable than ever before.

At its inception, LEED was considered to be "aspirational" in terms of greening the building industry, but today it's considered to be a reasonable benchmark. A newer certification system, the Living Building Challenge (LBC), is looking to further transform the building industry with the idea of "nutrition labels" for building materials and increased transparency around what's in the products we use. I spoke to Jason McLennan, the author of the Living Building Challenge codification system and CEO of the International Living Future Institute (ILFI), a non-governmental organization that focuses on creating a world that is socially just, culturally rich and ecologically restorative.[32]

Jason is considered one of the most influential figures in the green building movement today, and he was the recipient in 2012 of the prestigious Buckminster Fuller Prize. But his humble beginnings in Sudbury—an Ontario mining city known for both its toxic and its regreening experiences—are what really started him on his path. "I was inspired by my community and its environmental legacy," he told me, "and also its legacy of trying to heal the landscape and regenerate what we had so degraded. I was a participant as a young child in the regreening process and was connected to the environmental changes that

occurred. When I went into architecture, I went into it explicitly wanting to make this my focus."

The philosophy of the Living Building Challenge arose out of Jason's
graduate research and his work with "green" architects throughout the
United States and Europe in the 1990s, but the actual LBC rating system
wasn't launched until 2006. Much like LEED, it is a certification programme that addresses development at all scales. It consists of seven
"performance areas": site, water, energy, health, materials, equity and
beauty. These are subdivided into a total of twenty "imperatives," each of
which focuses on a specific goal.[33] An important aspect of the LBC is the
idea of transparency and toxicity prevention within the building industry. Through the LBC, Jason and his colleagues have developed a "Red
List" of materials and chemicals forbidden to use in any project seeking
Living Building Challenge certification. The Red List also itemizes materials that should be phased out of production because of health concerns
and known toxicity issues.

The Living Building Challenge is still in its infancy in terms of its
scale and impact on manufacturers, but Jason believes the building
industry is starting to take notice. In May 2011, Google announced that
it would abide by the Challenge's Red List and drop any and all of the
cited suppliers. Considering that the company is expanding into
roughly 40,000 square feet of office space a week (and that a recent
acquisition was over 300,000 square feet[34]), Google's decision is a
powerful market signal.[35] Other organizations have committed themselves as "communities" to the LBC. The prestigious Williams College
in Massachusetts, for instance, obtained LBC status for its environmental centre in 2016 and has since then committed to acquiring similar designations for as many campus buildings as possible.[36]

When I asked Jason to describe his preferred green building uni-
verse, he wasn't shy about suggesting that the system he's developed is
where we need to go. "All buildings should be Living Buildings: net
zero energy, net zero waste, net zero water, carbon neutral and free of
toxins. We have to have a completely renewable energy–powered world
without pumping more carbon." Jason's basic point is that we shouldn't
have to think so hard about these things. It should be easy to do good,
rather than easy to do bad. "Everything I've said sounds crazy," he
acknowledged. "But it's all doable now. The only reason it sounds crazy

is because we live in a paradigm that thinks the way we design and build now is 'normal.' And it's not."

Money-Pit Musings

Much of this chapter was written while I was sitting on my living-room couch, listening to the banging and drilling of renovations beneath my feet. Our house in east-end Toronto is one hundred years old, and our basement was showing its age: mould appearing on the 1970s faux-wood wall panelling, water bubbling up through the concrete pad. The *Toronto Star* newspaper we found in the wall was dated November 29, 1941 (with the headline "Sink Nazis in Arctic").

As I was writing about indoor air quality, we were making related choices about new windows, carpeting, paint and furniture. Most of our decisions involved trade-offs of one sort or another. In order to secure windows with fibreglass rather than vinyl framing, we delayed construction an extra month. Instead of going with bare floors, as recommended by the dust-averse Miriam Diamond, we decided to carpet the cold (now waterproof) concrete pad. We did, however, use Interface Flor carpet tiles made from recycled materials and free of VOCs, as well as natural wool carpeting on the stairs. We were careful to use low-VOC paint and carpet underlay, and despite some recent traces of problematic things in IKEA sofas, I chose to believe their renewed corporate commitment to ban any harmful flame retardants from their products.[37] (According to a 2017 online statement, IKEA strives to "totally refrain" from use of "chemical flame retardants" except where required by law.[38]) The Månstad sofa bed in a lovely Gobo blue grey fits in just fine.

In the real world, such trade-offs are the rule. But as a result of the "new car smell" experiment that Jeff and I undertook, I will never again take for granted the quality of the air in the places where I spend 90 percent of my life. In the summer, when the slush and sleet disappear from Toronto's streets, we plan to have the basement windows and the new energy-efficient back door open as much as possible.

Bruce likes to say that detox isn't a one-shot deal but a philosophy and a lifestyle—a statement that is entirely apt when it comes to managing the quality of the air itself.

TWELVE: CLEAN, GREEN ECONOMIC MACHINE

[BRUCE REIMAGINES ECONOMY]

Water, air and cleanliness are the chief articles in my pharmacopoeia.

—NAPOLEON I[1]

ONE LINE OF QUESTIONING Rick and I often hear had me stumped: "What should I do with my old Teflon frying pan, and what happens to the toxic coating when I throw it in the garbage?"

I had to admit I had no idea.

We are so often told by our readers that we "made" them throw away their Teflon pans, BPA plastic containers, triclosan-filled personal-care products and countless other toxic items that I felt obligated to figure out what happens to all this stuff after it's discarded.

We've talked in previous chapters about why it's important to avoid exposure to toxic chemicals in the first place and about what can be done to help our bodies expel these chemicals once they're in us. In this chapter I'll be focusing on the importance of discarding synthetic toxins responsibly—though, of course, the best approach would be to stop producing these chemicals in the first place.

Why subject you to this chapter on garbage and manufacturing policy? Because of the tight connection between waste, toxic chemicals and you (check out figure 18 for a simple explanation of this cycle). The waste we create winds up in landfills, and chemicals from those discards (such as BPA, triclosan and flame retardants) then leach into the surrounding environment.[2] Pharmaceuticals and personal-care products tossed down the drain or flushed away can end up in biosolids and effluents from wastewater treatment plants.[3] They also make their way into the source water that finds its way through our taps and back into our bodies.[4] Population pressures, water shortages and increasing evidence of pharmaceuticals and other chemicals in drinking water have pushed this issue to the forefront of global public health concerns.[5] In the Great Lakes, for instance, the drinking-water source for forty million people, concentrations of some flame retardants have doubled in the past five years.[6]

Figure 18. The toxic chemical cycle.

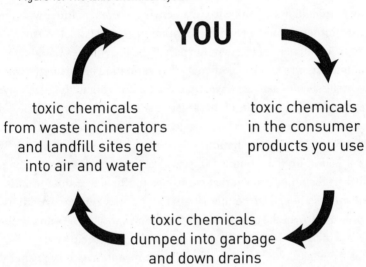

So when we detox our waste, we're detoxing ourselves.

The global economy is based on the manufacture of goods that release harmful chemicals when discarded, and it needs a detox diet—a really big one. Greening the economy requires drastically rethinking what we produce and what we consume, right down to the chemical makeup of those items. It means taking a serious look at where our toxic trash ends up and how we manage to produce so much garbage in the first place, with so little thought about where it all goes. If we are to make any significant progress in reducing the volume of toxic chemicals being released into the environment every day, we'll have to answer the question of where those old Teflon pans go to die.

Trash of the Stars

I was standing on top of the Puente Hills Landfill, the largest landfill in the United States, a mountain of garbage over two hundred metres high and covering nearly two square kilometres of land. It seems fitting that my environmental investigative work had taken me back to California, where conspicuous consumption collides head-on with North America's leading environmental standards and the world headquarters for personal trainers, health nuts and detox fad diets.

My tour guide was Sam Pedroza, an environmental planner with the joint administration office of the Sanitation Districts of Los Angeles County (an independent agency, not part of the Los Angeles County government, Sam was quick to point out). The sanitation departments were first established to manage waste water in the LA basin in the 1920s and have since evolved into one of the largest waste management agencies in the world. Back in the 1920s Los Angeles was the tenth-largest city in the United States, with a population of just over half a million people. By 1930 it had more than doubled in size as oil and the American dream fuelled tremendous growth that continues to this day. Sanitation districts were established to better manage the privately run garbage dumps popping up all over the county. Most of the dumps were in LA's numerous valleys, which also happened to be sources of local drinking water.

Los Angeles's response to garbage is representative of the general history of trash throughout the industrialized world. A hundred years ago people didn't produce much garbage. They grew their own vegetables and raised animals or bought their food from local farmers, and they didn't have electronic toys and devices that broke or became obsolete after a year. Burning waste wasn't a bad thing, because farmers and ranchers in the 1920s weren't burning plastic, mercury-filled batteries or Teflon-coated pans.

During the Industrial Revolution people started moving into cities and creating refuse at a rapid rate. They tossed rubbish into rivers, down wells or into the streets, creating a serious public health issue. Over the course of the twentieth century, waste generation increased tenfold, from an equivalent of 42 kilograms per individual to 565 kilograms per person per year.[7]

It wasn't until the 1950s, when we first faced a "garbage problem," that we started to pay attention to waste disposal, Sam explained.

Backyard incinerators were producing as much smog as cars, and water pollution from hundreds of little unregulated dumps in the valleys of SoCal was increasing. But, as Sam told me, in the 1970s the "garbage problem" hit LA especially hard, reflecting what was happening in most of the world. I attribute this problem to the plasticization of the economy. Within the two decades from about 1950 to 1970, paper bags, wooden toys, wooden furniture and cotton or wool fabrics were replaced by plastics and other synthetics. With the onset of plasticization came the disposable society: many plastic products broke easily and could not be repaired, while other items (plastic packaging, for example) were designed simply to be used once and thrown away. Sam identifies the mindset of "people just tossing out whatever they want" that led to overflowing garbage dumps and the need to create more and bigger landfill sites. Almost fifty years later, with all our composting programmes and recycling efforts, surely things must be getting better, right? Wrong. The amount of personal garbage produced by city dwellers today is almost double what it was *just fifteen years ago*—from 0.64 kilograms of solid waste per person per day in 2002 to 1.2 kilograms per person per day in 2012 and still rising.[8] The global trends of urbanization and plasticization are making it difficult for us to manage our colossal garbage systems failure.

In 2004, China surpassed the United States as the world's largest waste producer, and it is forecast to generate twice as much trash as the United States by 2030.[9] Most of us in Canada are convinced that with our world-leading recycling programmes we are producing less garbage and more useful recycled goods. I'm afraid not. Plastic takeout plates, water bottles, food wrapping and plastic bags can be recycled, but most aren't. What's worse, much of that plastic doesn't even make it into the garbage, or if it does, it manages to escape, blowing off garbage barges or simply tossed into ditches.

Plastics are bad news. And the news keeps getting worse—8.3 billion tonnes of plastics produced since 1950, half of that in the past thirteen years, and only 9 percent of it recycled.[10] It's safe to say that a couple of billion tonnes of plastic has entered the world since we wrote *Slow Death*. And some of it is floating in the Pacific Ocean amongst an island of trash called the Great Pacific Garbage Patch. It's hundreds of kilometres across and contains more garbage than any landfill site on

Earth. Ninety percent of this swirling mess is plastic. Marine debris is threatening not just oceans and lakes but our supplies of food and water as well.[11] In 2012 a group of scientists collecting water samples from the Great Lakes found up to 600,000 plastic pieces per square kilometre, almost twice as many as the highest count ever made in the Great Pacific Garbage Patch. Plastics are out of control. Governments really need to start banning plastic, or we may end up like ocean turtles, birds and fish, choking ourselves to death on bits of toxic plastic.

Japanese researchers discovered a further problem with all this debris: seaborne plastic pellets attract and concentrate harmful chemicals like PCBs; DDE, or 1,1-dichloro-2,2-bis(p-chlorophenyl) ethylene, a breakdown product of DDT; and nonylphenols (breakdown products from detergents) that don't dissolve in water.[12] So in addition to the problem of plastics leaching, they also act as magnets for highly toxic pollutants, and these infused plastic particles are then ingested by marine animals.

Scientists at the University of British Columbia's Department of Zoology examined sixty-seven northern fulmars (foraging seabirds) on B.C.'s northwest coast and found that 93 percent of the birds had plastic in their stomachs, including twine, candy wrappers and polystyrene foam.[13] One of the birds had ingested 454 pieces of plastic.

Gulls *love* garbage. This was all too apparent when Sam drove me to the working face of the landfill, where massive bulldozers push the garbage and spread it out as it is dumped from truck after truck. Hundreds of gulls circled the freshly spread waste. In the fifteen minutes I spent mesmerized by the operation, there must have been forty huge trucks that pulled in, dumped their loads and left.

It all looked so easy. Dump the garbage, push it around, compact it by driving over it in machines with huge studded steel wheels, scrape some topsoil onto it and *voilà*: a budding recreation area! I remarked on the lush vegetation that had clearly been planted on the steep-angled slopes—no doubt well fed by the organic nutrients in the waste stream. Sam was pleased that I'd noticed.

I asked Sam to isolate the biggest waste problems Los Angeles faces today. "The changing face of garbage," he replied, explaining to me that plastic packaging is a much larger percentage of the waste now than the easy and more valuable recyclables such as glass, garden waste, paper, cardboard and aluminum, which are separated at the source for recycling. Just as I suspected. This was obvious, seeing the plastic bags and packaging being dumped truckload after truckload. Sam mentioned the 3R waste management mantra, "reduce, reuse, recycle," but admitted that we were not really making much progress on the first "R."

As we were writing this tenth-anniversary edition of *Slow Death by Rubber Duck*, the issue of plastics pollution was finally starting to enjoy the focus it deserves. The 2018 G7 meeting of global leaders in Charlevoix, Quebec, included a commitment to dramatically scale back plastics use over the next few decades. Slow progress, but progress nonetheless. And with the most recent science showing the presence of plastic microparticles in many different kinds of food and drinking water all over the world (it's only a matter of time before they're found in human bodies), we don't have a moment to waste.[14]

e-Trash

Sam and I walked past a pile of old television sets and computer monitors in the multi-material recycling facility, which is largely a depository for electronic waste. "E-waste," Sam said, "is a major challenge."

When it comes to the conspicuous consumption spelling bee, A is for Apple. Apple's ubiquitous i-devices are the epitome of trendiness and style. Every time the company introduces a new device, sales grow faster than those of the gadget it replaces. Within two years of its launch, the iPad exceeded 55 million units sold worldwide. Apple's CEO, Tim Cook, sums up the trend: "This 55 [million] is something no one would have guessed. Including us. To put it in context, it took us 22 years to sell 55 million Macs. It took us about 5 years to sell 22 million iPods, and it took us about 3 years to sell that many iPhones. . . . And so, this thing is . . . on a trajectory that's off the charts."[15]

That's not the only trajectory that's off the charts. Developing countries are facing a tidal wave of e-waste as we seek cheap ways to dispose of defunct electronics that still contain valuable metals to be recycled. For instance, about 70 percent of the world's 500 million tonnes of yearly e-waste ends up in China.[16] The discarded TVs Sam showed me were next to bales of plastic bottles. Sam tells school kids that these recycled plastic bottles "will be your new toys from China." Plastic, paper, aluminum, steel and e-waste—even unsorted garbage from some cities—are destined for China, where cheap and abundant labour makes hand sorting feasible.

A smartphone is replaced, on average, every eighteen months,[17] and in 2017 alone, over 1.5 billion smartphones were sold worldwide.[18] And they don't just sell themselves. In 2012 Samsung and Apple spent over three-quarters of a billion dollars on advertising campaigns trying to convince us to buy new ones. How much do they spend dealing with the e-waste from the phones they encourage people to toss out? We still don't know. We do know that in 2016 global e-waste hit 45 million tonnes, a new record.

Planned obsolescence—the practice of deliberately limiting a product's useful life—is one of the chief culprits of overconsumption. A home telephone used to last about twenty years. My parents still own a functioning fridge that was built in 1952 (an ecological coup, energy inefficiency aside). But now we tend to expect products to either malfunction or become technologically obsolete within years, or even months, of purchasing them. Many printers are designed with a built-in "kill switch," effectively "timing out" once a predetermined number of pages is reached—not when the ink runs out.

Although I didn't see any discarded smartphones, iPads or plasma TVs at the landfill site, Sam assured me they were there and that we'd find some if we wanted to dig for them. We weren't too far from some of the wealthiest addresses in the world, along the coastline of Newport Beach and Laguna Beach. I imagined some local conversations along the following lines: "It's only an iPad 2, for heaven's sake. Throw it out," or "Are you kidding me? A 42-inch plasma TV? I wouldn't be caught dead with that thing in my house!"

China Syndrome

The region of Guiyu, China, has been in the media spotlight since the mid-2000s as the e-waste dump of the world. The area has been dubbed "the Chernobyl of electronic waste." In Guiyu an estimated 5,000 small businesses and 150,000 workers, many of them women and children, comb through our electronic refuse, separating components.[19] According to studies prepared by nearby Shantou University, women living there have an elevated incidence of miscarriages, children's bodies contain deadly amounts of lead and the soil contains the world's highest level of cancer-causing dioxins. Shantou professor Huo Xia has been measuring lead levels in the blood of local children since 2004. The 2010 test results showed the highest levels ever recorded, with 88 percent of children[20] exceeding the threshold for lead poisoning established by the Centers for Disease Control in the U.S. Recent studies show that the poisoning continues as e-waste numbers skyrocket.[21] The future for Guiyu will improve, eventually, with China's 2018 ban on imports of e-waste, but the toxic legacy will continue for decades.

Cindy Coutts is president of Sims Recycling Solutions Canada, a top-notch e-waste recycling company that has the capacity to extract and sort leaded glass, metal and plastic from e-waste, maximizing recycling and minimizing the need to incinerate the leftovers or send them to landfill. With over fifty facilities worldwide, they are also one of the largest providers of this service.

Cindy described the ever-growing and ever-changing mix of e-waste and what it contains: brominated flame retardants and heavy metals like mercury, leaded glass, cadmium, lithium, cobalt and radioactive materials—not to mention hundreds of different plastic compounds. As with most e-waste, her company was shipping it to China—before the new Chinese waste-import ban came into effect. Twice a year she travelled there for a first-hand inspection of plastics recycling facilities across the country. She described the scene in early 2013 of enormous black-and-white-speckled mounds lining the roads and paths in village after village—like snowbanks—going right up to people's doorways. "Plastic is everywhere. It's part of the landscape," she said. In one town Cindy asked about their waste management practices and was told that (incredibly) they had none. On her way out of town she could see evidence of this: a bulldozer was pushing plastic garbage from the land straight into a river.

At another site, where chemicals were used to help sort plastics, Cindy asked to see the wastewater treatment system. Officials pointed to a series of cement basins full of thick, dark water with bits of plastic floating around in them. It all evaporates, she was told, but finding this hard to believe, Cindy inspected the basins further and discovered a small hose at the bottom of each one. She followed the hoses down to the river, where she saw untreated chemicals draining out.

Arriving at a recycling facility in yet another town, Cindy was welcomed by the workers, who were all dressed up to greet their special Canadian guest. She observed carefully their process of manually sorting plastics. One worker, in this case a young man, held a flame to a piece of plastic to see if it would burn. The plastics that didn't burn were tossed into a pile labelled "brominated flame retardants." For any that did burn, he waited a few seconds, blew the flame out and held the smoking plastic under his nose. He identified the type of plastic based on the scent of the toxic fumes and then sorted it accordingly.

Cindy wasn't in China to expose poor recycling practices or toxic waste dumping. She just wanted to find e-waste recycling companies that she could trust. Of the seventy recycling facilities she visited, she approved eight as eligible to receive Sims' plastic e-waste. How is it that most manufacturers don't take responsibility for how or where their products are manufactured or disposed of, let alone for the toxic materials they use? Changes are happening in this area as manufacturers start subscribing to extended producer responsibility (EPR) programmes. But how is this new waste mantra working out?

Exaggerated Producer Responsibility

Sam Pedroza told me that he sees extended producer responsibility as the future of waste management. But others are not so sure. For instance, my close colleague and global EPR expert Clarissa Morawski. "It's a great idea in theory. It basically makes companies responsible for their products at the end of life. Governments really like EPR too," Clarissa noted, "because along with shedding the responsibility of collecting and managing waste go the costs of running EPR programmes. But this is where they tend to fall apart. The vast majority of EPR programmes are run by industry consortia that work collectively to implement the cheapest recycling option under the law." A 2017 report found that EPR programmes in Canada were achieving modest success; however, without landfill bans, disposal charges or other supporting policies, they are unlikely to achieve their potential.

Battery manufacturers are a case in point. Batteries can contain a slew of heavy metals such as cadmium, cobalt, lead, lithium and mercury, and their use is growing exponentially, even while the vast majority are thrown away and eventually end up in municipal landfills or incinerators.

A voluntary battery collection programme that ran in Quebec for many years saw 85 percent recycling rates for the batteries, which were sent to a mechanical recycling facility in Ontario. Following the Quebec government's 2012 decision to regulate battery collection, the manufacturers organized themselves[22] and now send all the batteries they collect to a smelting facility in Pennsylvania, where only 25 percent of the materials are recovered; the rest are converted to a rock-like by-product called slag and used in road construction. It is a far cheaper option than the mechanical recycling, but with three-quarters of the material going to slag, it hardly qualifies as successful recycling.

I spoke with Sam's colleague Mario Iacoboni, supervising engineer for the Los Angeles County Sanitation Districts, to find out more about the water and air quality at Puente Hills. I was curious to know whether anybody there ever measured (or even considered) what happened to BPA plastics, phthalates in discarded vinyl and, of course, perfluorinated compounds (PFCs), the chemicals used to make Teflon pans and stain-resistant carpets. Mario stated that they follow government regulations and none of those substances are regulated, so they don't test for them—a simple lesson in why it's crucial to regulate toxic chemicals.

The Minnesota Pollution Control Agency found perfluorinated compounds in the leachate (the liquid that seeps out of landfills) and in the gas emitted into the atmosphere at every Minnesota landfill site they tested.[23] PFCs are among the most persistent chemicals ever invented, meaning they do not break down easily in the environment and can build up in our bodies. The medical researchers examining the health effects of the PFC-contaminated drinking water in Parkersburg, West Virginia (described in chapter 2) have since found that PFCs in drinking water are linked to various cancers, high blood pressure in pregnant women, bowel disease, thyroid problems and childhood obesity.[24]

The Teflon pan question was still bothering me, so I asked some waste chemists what should be done with discarded Teflon wares. These chemists work at an experimental synthetic gas facility in Canada, where garbage is converted directly into inert slag and useable gas by zapping it at extreme temperatures. They use plasma technology, which (in simple terms) allows for a process that's like blasting garbage into oblivion with lightning. They gave my question some serious thought before getting back to me with an answer. Landfill, they said, was probably the best option, presenting the lowest likelihood of the non-stick PFC chemicals breaking down into more toxic by-products and getting into the environment. Incineration, as I suspected, was the worst option for PFCs, and one that should be absolutely avoided because of the temperature of incinerator fires and the highly toxic gases emitted from the burning Teflon. Plasma technology should be safe, they figured, because the plasma torches break down the molecular structure of the chemicals into simpler forms that are non-toxic. So—

Step 1: Don't buy non-stick pans, because of the associated health hazards.

Step 2: Hope that your town doesn't incinerate garbage. If it does, drive to the closest town that landfills municipal waste, make sure it's garbage day and sneak your old pans into somebody's garbage can when they aren't looking.

I left the joint administration office of the Sanitation Districts of Los Angeles County with mixed feelings. I was genuinely impressed with the remarkable engineering feat I had witnessed at Puente Hills. But what about the non-stick pans, all that e-waste, the plastic being sent to China, and the Great Pacific Garbage Patch? Or the fact that even the most advanced extended producer responsibility programmes are at best performing poorly and at worst creating a false impression of environmental progress while industry consortia opt for the cheapest recycling methods? Digging into waste, so to speak, gave me that "Houston, we have a problem" feeling. There was little evidence that we'd be able to keep our air and water safe by relying only on the waste end of the detox economy.

Detox Cleanse or Greenwash?

I strolled into the spiffy lobby of a Washington, D.C., hotel looking for signs that would point me to the 16th Annual Green Chemistry and Engineering Conference. I had come to Washington to understand whether we were on the verge of a green chemistry revolution or whether this detox cleanse for the economy was mostly a greenwash. Hanging above an escalator to the second floor was a banner with a large red diamond and the name Dow in it.

There were sessions on "recombinant cellulolytic bacillus subtilis," "methacrylated lignin model compounds as monomers" and "synthesis of bioactive 4-methyl-6-[(1-alkyl-1H-1,2,3,-triazol-4-yl) methoxy]-2H-chromen-2-one." I approached the information desk. "Is there a session called 'Green Chemistry for Dummies?'" I inquired hopefully. A pleasant woman smiled and handed me a conference agenda and a pocket card with the Twelve Principles of Green Chemistry printed on it (more on those below). Reviewing the schedule in greater detail, I was pleased to see some familiar names among the presenters: my close colleague Pete Myers, an environmental scientist and among America's leading environmental health advocates, and Terry Collins, one of the world's green chemistry gurus.

Terry Collins is the Teresa Heinz Professor of Green Chemistry and Director of the Institute for Green Chemistry at Carnegie Mellon University. After seeing the destruction and health problems caused by pesticides and pulp mills in his native New Zealand, Terry devised an oxygen-based catalyst to replace chlorine in pulp and paper manufacturing. His quiet voice, soft New Zealand twang and friendly smile belie his stature as one of the world's most sought-after chemists and as the first professor of green chemistry. We met for dinner and I had Terry to myself for two hours.

Over the course of the conference I would ask a few people, including Terry, whether green chemistry was the "real deal" or whether it was thinly disguise to corporate greenwashing. They all had the same response: "It depends."

Terry believes the philosophical underpinnings of green chemistry are very real. But he cautioned that there's a huge risk of its being co-opted by the conventional chemical industry. "Take Dow [the sponsor of the conference], for example. They are expanding chlorine use and therefore producing more PVC and building up dioxins," he said. "Or consider ethane from methane in fracking gas, used to make PVC. People miss the ethane-to-ethylene-to-PVC plastics connection." He is referring to the environmentally contentious technique called hydraulic fracturing (fracking), which is used to extract methane (natural gas) from shale, from which ethane is derived, followed by ethylene—a primary feedstock in the manufacture of PVC.

This is the classic environmental conundrum. The only way we are going to succeed in cleaning up chemistry is if the big companies change, yet it is often in their best interest to maintain the status quo and slow the pace of change. The Dows of the world need to be advancing green chemistry and should be sponsoring these conferences, as long as their intentions are legitimate.

The Twelve Principles of Green Chemistry

I started to get the gist of green chemistry the next day after attending several sessions. In each one the Twelve Principles of Green Chemistry moulded the discussion. Here are the Twelve Principles:

1. *Prevention.* Preventing waste is better than treating or cleaning up waste after it is created.
2. *Atom economy.* Synthetic methods should try to maximize the incorporation of all materials used in the process into the final product.
3. *Less hazardous chemical syntheses.* Synthetic methods should avoid using or generating substances toxic to humans and/or the environment.
4. *Designing safer chemicals.* Chemical products should be designed to achieve their desired function while being as non-toxic as possible.
5. *Safer solvents and auxiliaries.* Auxiliary substances should be avoided wherever possible, and as non-hazardous as possible when they must be used.
6. *Design for energy efficiency.* Energy requirements should be minimized, and processes should be conducted at ambient temperature and pressure whenever possible.
7. *Use of renewable feedstocks.* Whenever it is practical to do so, renewable feedstocks or raw materials are preferable to non-renewable ones.
8. *Reduce derivatives.* Unnecessary generation of derivatives— such as the use of protecting groups—should be minimized or avoided if possible; such steps require additional reagents and may generate additional waste.
9. *Catalysis.* Catalytic reagents that can be used in small quantities to repeat a reaction are superior to stoichiometric reagents (ones that are consumed in a reaction).
10. *Design for degradation.* Chemical products should be designed so that they do not pollute the environment;

when their function is complete, they should break down into non-harmful products.

11. *Real-time analysis for pollution prevention.* Analytical methodologies need to be further developed to permit real-time, in-process monitoring and control before hazardous substances form.

12. *Inherently safer chemistry for accident prevention.* Whenever possible, the substances in a process, and the forms of those substances, should be chosen to minimize risks such as explosions, fires, and accidental releases.[25]

As one speaker put it, "Green chemistry needs to become an attitude, not a slogan."

Cleaning Up the Chemistry Act

John Warner's name was all over the green chemistry conference. He is, after all, the co-author of the green chemistry "bible" (titled, not surprisingly, *Green Chemistry: Theory and Practice*), where the Twelve Principles of Green Chemistry first appeared.[26] Warner has a PhD in chemistry from Princeton, ten years' experience working as a chemist for Polaroid, ten years in academia and 250 patents and research papers, and he now heads his own private research institute.

I was struck by how John's credentials dwarf those of the chemists who make careers out of dismissing the pollution concerns of environmental and health advocates and who defend the use of toxic chemicals. So I asked him why some chemists ignore the health hazards posed by low levels of synthetic chemicals and seem to dismiss green chemistry. "For the past forty years universities have not taught chemistry students anything about toxicity—not until Terry Collins started at Carnegie Mellon," he said.

During his own chemistry studies at top universities, John never once had a class in toxicology and was never required to learn what makes a molecule toxic. That is why, he claims, so many conventional chemists—who are completely unregulated—don't understand toxicity. "Anyone can make a molecule that has never existed in the world before. Even if it's the most potent carcinogen in history, nowhere in their education are they ever required to have any knowledge of how to look at a molecule and say: 'Gee whiz, this might be a carcinogen. I might not want to make it.'" Changing the curriculum for chemistry students seemed crucial to John, so he created the "Green Chemistry Commitment" to accelerate learning. His goal is to have all six hundred universities in the United States that have chemistry departments commit to teaching toxicology and green chemistry through Beyond Benign, the organization he co-founded. The group works with kindergarten to grade 12 teachers, too, and has developed two hundred lesson plans to help teach green chemistry.

John narrowed down the Twelve Principles of Green Chemistry to five underlying principles that need to be followed for green chemistry to succeed:

1.   Standardize toxic testing protocols.
2.   Test products, not molecules.
3.   Label products, not ingredients.
4.   Establish timelines for companies to phase out toxic products.
5.   Create a network of toxicology testing centres and train a workforce of testing technicians.

Priority number 1, John said, is to focus on tests used to determine toxicity, not on tests of individual chemicals. Manufacturers of chemicals and consumer products pass all the safety tests before a product goes to market, but different organizations use different safety tests and reach different conclusions. The tests need to be consistent across the industry. Priority number 2: we need to move from testing molecules to testing products, and that might mean grinding up a smartphone, for example, and having it tested. In that way we can label the smartphone—not just a molecule—as containing a carcinogen or an endocrine disruptor. Priority 3 is labelling. Companies hide behind trade secrets as a way to avoid labelling ingredients, but if they are required to label products, that concern disappears (recall the hidden chemicals in hair products). By indicating that *something* in the product is a carcinogen, the label gives consumers the choice to buy it or not. Priority 4 gives companies a set window of time to find non-toxic alternatives for toxic ingredients they are currently using in their products. And priority number 5 is to create a toxicology-testing infrastructure. The European

Environmental Agency estimates that toxicology data exist for only 25 percent of industry chemicals used around the world.[27] Coupled with training and workforce development, this could become a politically attractive programme that focuses on skills development in the biotech sector, including improving the skills of community college students and displaced workers. Not only would workers be trained for entry (or re-entry) into the workforce, they would also have an immediate and useful function to play in supporting a stable, greener economy.

John's standards are obviously high. But he's also pragmatic. "We need to be working *with* Dow, 3M and DuPont," he told me, "not *against* them. We've got to allow them molecular redemption and let them find a path forward that doesn't vilify them."

John was frustrated that too many people want to focus only on the problems. "I can find infinite amounts of money to scare pregnant women, inject bunnies and publicize the dangers of some toxic chemical. But try finding money to invent a safe alternative and the same people say, 'That's not what we do.'" He lumps certain environmental groups and foundations together as having "romantic" ideas, with little hope of succeeding. "We need workable solutions to people dying and getting sick from toxic chemicals, not people trying to take down capitalism."

Copying Nature

John and Terry are two parts of a green chemistry triad. The third is Janine Benyus, founder of the Biomimicry Institute and author of *Biomimicry: Innovation Inspired by Nature*.[28]

Biomimicry, much as it sounds, is the emerging field of modelling chemical and industrial design after the designs found in nature. Janine described it more poetically: "We are asking nature for inspiration." We are the students; nature is the teacher. And here are some examples of biomimicry in action: the aerodynamic nose of a high-speed train mimicking the bill of a kingfisher, the super-slippery fabric of an Olympic swimsuit modelled after sharkskin, and water collection nets (capable of extracting water from fog) designed to imitate the shell of a desert beetle.

When I asked her to explain green chemistry from the perspective of biomimicry, Janine used nature's medium for chemical experimentation to explain. "Life chose water, not solvents," she said. In the natural world chemistry is based on water, but industrial chemistry relies on high temperature, high pressure and petroleum-based toxic ingredients. "Nature, for example, does not add sulphuric acid to things," said Janine. The Holy Grail for green chemists is shifting from petroleum-based to water-based chemicals in manufacturing.

Janine explained that in nature, atoms line up and self-assemble into molecules. The process is somewhat like shaking a box of Lego pieces, pouring them out onto the floor and having the contents self-assemble into a castle. Nature makes sure that the "pieces" (the atoms) find each other in some medium (while they're swirling around in a pool of tepid water, for instance). Nature's chemistry relies on negatively and positively charged atoms being attracted to each other to produce stable chemicals and also on shapes being drawn to each other, Janine explains. Modern synthetic chemistry is much more about *forcing* atoms. There's a concept called "atom efficiency" in nature, which means that atoms are not wasted, and it's this phenomenon that's described as "atom economy" in the second of the Twelve Principles of Green Chemistry. Most industrial chemistry requires the addition of many more chemicals than will end up in the final product. And this leads to vast amounts of wasted chemicals that may be discarded or discharged in waste water. In nature, however, there is no waste. The ingredients that go into creating a naturally occurring chemical stay in that chemical. Nothing comes out, so there are no by-products and therefore no toxic by-products. In addition, nature does not add solvents, catalysts or other chemical agents. In following nature's lead, biomimicry helps avoid the use of toxins in manufacturing.

Life Chose Water

What could be a simpler way of framing our future priorities as a species than basing them on the principle that Janine described: life chose water. Because life chose water, we need to choose and protect water in order to safeguard our lives and the lives of our children and their children. Consuming adequate quantities of water is one of the most important things we can do to detox our bodies—but that's true only if we have access to clean, fresh water. Air, of course, is just as important to life as water, and if we can't maintain clean air and pure water, we have no hope of staying healthy—regardless of the detox protocols we follow. People often ask me whether I use a water filter at home. I do—even though I know that Toronto's drinking water is among the best municipal water in the world. Toronto Water's accredited laboratory, for example, performs over fifteen thousand bacteriological tests each year on my drinking water, and it monitors over three hundred potential chemical contaminants[29]—hazardous metals such as aluminum and zinc, and dozens of poisonous organic compounds from ammonia to xylenes, among many others. But there's one exception: endocrine-disrupting (that is, hormone-disrupting) synthetic chemicals (EDCs), which are rarely included in drinking water protocols. This is mostly because of the high costs of testing and the lack of analytical technologies and infrastructure needed to detect a wide range of endocrine-disrupting chemicals and their many metabolites. Therefore, most of the data on EDCs in drinking water come from targeted research projects, so we don't know the true levels of these chemicals in our water.

I take the quality of my tap water for granted. But so did the people of Milwaukee, Wisconsin, in 1993 and the residents of Walkerton, Ontario, in 2000. Milwaukee is a mid-size American city on the coast of Lake Michigan about 160 kilometres north of Chicago. Walkerton is a small Canadian farming town near Lake Huron about 160 kilometres northwest of Toronto. The two are about 500 kilometres apart as the crow flies, over two Great Lakes. Milwaukee is home to the largest single water-contamination event in recorded American history, when more than 400,000 people fell ill and over a hundred people died from *Cryptosporidium* contamination.[30]

Cryptosporidium is a nasty parasite that lives in the gastrointestinal tracts of many animals, including cows and humans.[31] It still isn't clear how it ended up in Milwaukee's drinking water—possibly through human sewage or possibly because of cows getting into a local river. Runoff from cattle manure was *definitely* part of the problem in Walkerton, which caused one of the most deadly drinking water incidents in Canadian history. In May 2000 the town's water supply was contaminated by a highly infectious strain of *E. coli* from farm runoff. About 2,500 residents became ill and seven people died as a direct result; many more have permanent kidney damage. An investigation into the tragedy, known as the Walkerton Inquiry, laid most of the blame on improper operating practices and negligent behaviour of the Walkerton Public Utilities Commission. However, the Ontario provincial government was also faulted for cutting back on environmental monitoring, poor water-quality regulation and failing to enforce the existing water-quality guidelines.[32] The inquiry's report resulted in sweeping reforms of Ontario's water-testing standards.

These tragic events have also contributed to surging interest in home water filters. Sales of water-filtration systems in Canada shot up after 2000, as did sales of bottled water. In 1999, bottled water consumption in Canada was about twenty-four litres per person; by 2005 that number had jumped to sixty litres per person, with bottled water sales exceeding C$650 million.[33] By 2017 annual sales in bottled water in Canada topped an unbelievable $2.5 billion.[34] The Milwaukee and Walkerton events awakened North American families to the quality of their drinking water, and for many others they raised concerns about the adequate protection of water systems.

Consider the very basics of the hydrological cycle. Oceans, lakes and rivers store water. The water evaporates and condenses, forming clouds, and falls to the earth as precipitation. The process of evaporation and condensation, together with movement through rivers, soil and rock formations, cleanses and purifies water. Unless the process is interrupted. Human activities are serious interruptors of this natural water cycle: we spray pesticides and herbicides and we run factories, manufacturing facilities, coal-fired electricity stations, garbage incinerators and wastewater treatment plants. In North America the governance of water quality and safety is a shared duty, with states and provinces responsible for drinking water guidelines and municipalities that oversee water treatment facilities doing the day-to-day management and monitoring.[35] Governments issue water-quality limits, standards and/or permits, but many of those limits were established decades ago when populations were smaller, competition for water was not so fierce and the chemicals we used were not nearly as complex as they are today.

Despite all the reassuring work done by my city, by late summer my tap water, which comes from Lake Ontario, smells a little swampy. This is the main reason why I have my water filter. It gets rid of odour and it helps remove other contaminants that may be present. Water-quality guidelines, however, are designed to make sure that people do not actually become *sick*, and the threshold of safety for heavy metals, pesticides, pharmaceuticals and sundry other things is debatable.

Let's look at trace pharmaceuticals as one example of the contaminants people ingest from their tap water. A 2012 World Health Organization report noted that the previous decade had seen a significant increase in the number of studies investigating pharmaceuticals in drinking water, and concerns have been increasing about the potential risks to human health related to low-level exposure.[36] Early studies in the United States in the 1970s first reported the presence of active ingredients from heart medications, pain relievers and birth control pills in waste water. Since then, peer-reviewed research has found between fifteen and twenty-five different pharmaceuticals in treated drinking water worldwide.[37] And synthetic endocrine-disrupting chemicals like BPA and phthalates from landfill leachate and municipal sewage effluent may end up in tap water as well.[38] These chemicals are additives in plastics and are released from products as they degrade over their life in landfills. BPA and phthalates get into the leachate and, especially in landfills with no leachate treatment facilities, they're discharged into the surrounding rivers and groundwater, which can be sources of drinking water.

Some people don't use water-filtration systems but still distrust tap water, so they look to other sources of pure, clean water—including bottled water. But few people stop to ask whether bottled water is, in fact, the safer choice.

Bad Bottle

With images of snow-peaked mountains on the labels, we imagine bottled water gushing from a brook in the Swiss Alps into a little plastic container that somehow makes its way onto our grocery store shelf. However, much bottled water is "purified water"—nothing more than packaged municipal drinking water—the same water that would come out of your tap, put through a filtering system and sold to you at a high price. In Canada bottled water is actually regulated as a food product.[39] It's subject to monitoring for microbiological content, but limited details of these analyses are provided.[40] Manufacturers are not required to test for trace toxic contaminants such as those tested for by municipalities in tap water, nor are they required to report any testing analyses to any authority.

In 2011, Americans bought over nine billion gallons of bottled water, outlays valued at US$22 billion.[41] The manufacture of the plastic bottles alone used up seventeen million barrels of crude oil.[42] In 2016, bottled water overtook soda as the most sold drink in the U.S.[43] Only 30 percent of these plastic bottles are recycled and, of that 30 percent, only a fifth is repurposed for the food and beverage industry.[44] These bottles take centuries to decompose, and if they are incinerated, they emit toxic by-products into the atmosphere. Finally, for a city with one million people, tap water costs approximately 80 cents per 1,000 litres, while bottled water costs, on average, US$527 per 1,000 litres, not including the enormous environmental costs.[45]

If there is one simple thing that every human can do to improve environmental conditions, it is to *stop buying bottled water*.

Filtering Out the Negatives

Removing unwanted contaminants from your drinking water is one of the simplest ways to detox your personal environment. Household water filters generally fall into two categories: point-of-entry units and point-of-use units. Point-of-entry units treat water before it is distributed through the house, while point-of-use units, which include countertop filters, faucet filters and under-sink units, are self-contained and generally portable.[46] But can you be guaranteed that either type is doing its job?

Many filters use more than one kind of filtration technology within their systems. NSF International is a widely recognized independent not-for-profit organization that provides standards development and certification for the world's food, water, health and consumer products,[47] and as a general rule, filters labelled as meeting NSF Standard 53 are certified to remove contaminants of concern in your tap water. Standard 53 addresses point-of-use and point-of-entry systems designed to reduce specific health-related contaminants, such as *Cryptosporidium*, *Giardia*, lead, VOCs and MTBE (methyl tertiary-butyl ether), which may be present in public or private drinking water.[48] Generally, filters that meet NSF Standard 53 are geared toward treating water for health and not just aesthetic qualities. The NSF certification programme is not flawless—and certainly doesn't cover all products—but it does provide assurance that at least some manufacturers' claims have been independently tested and verified.

You can see the results for specific types of filters in table 8, and the

NSF International website provides a useful product database that can help you choose a filter that meets your needs.[49]

Table 8. Types of filters and their uses and mechanisms of elimination.[50]

Type of Filter	How It Works	Use	Elimination
Activated carbon filter	Positively charged and absorbent carbon in the filter attracts and traps impurities.	Countertop, faucet filters and under-the-sink units	•tastes and odours •heavy metals such as copper, lead and mercury •disinfection by-products •parasites such as *Giardia* and *Cryptosporidium* •pesticides •radon •VOCs like dichlorobenzene and trichloroethylene (TCE)
Cation exchange softener	"Softens" hard water by trading minerals with a strong positive charge for one with a lesser charge.	Household point-of-entry units	•calcium and magnesium •barium and other, similar ions hazardous to health
Distiller	Boils water and recondenses the purified steam.	Countertop or whole-house, point-of-entry units	•heavy metals like cadmium, chromium, copper, lead and mercury •arsenic, barium, fluoride, selenium and sodium

Type of Filter	How It Works	Use	Elimination
Reverse osmosis	A semipermeable membrane separates impurities from water (process wastes significant amount of water).	Under-the-sink units	•parasites like *Cryptosporidium* and *Giardia* •heavy metals like cadmium, copper, lead and mercury •arsenic, barium, perchlorate, nitrate/nitrite and selenium
UV disinfection	Ultraviolet light kills bacteria and other microorganisms.	Under-the-sink units (with a carbon filter)	•bacteria and parasites •class A systems protect against harmful bacteria and viruses •class B systems designed to make non-disease-causing bacteria inactive

The Wrong Rules

Back to Los Angeles County and the Puente Hills landfill. In many ways, our modern waste-disposal system is a marvel. In the morning at home you toss out a few tin cans, that old radio and lots of plastic packaging, and within a matter of hours it has been collected, trucked here, dumped, spread, packed and buried in an almost seamless, odourless marvel of engineering and logistics. But what about toxic leachate and gas emissions? We don't have a very good handle on how much of this garbage (or garbage in any landfill) is polluting our air and water. And did anyone ever stop to ask how and why we produce all this refuse?

Yes, in fact, someone has, and her name is Annie Leonard, executive director of Greenpeace USA and the creator of a project called "The Story of Stuff." Not only has she thought a great deal about this issue, she has also turned it into her life work. It started off as a way for Annie to show the world how dumb it is to waste as much as we do. She was giving many presentations on the topic before realizing it didn't really make sense for her to fly around America wasting fuel. So she turned her presentation into a wonderful animated video. It took off like wildfire on YouTube and has been viewed more than five million times to date! Imagine how much jet fuel Annie has saved by not flying to various destinations and presenting in person. From that simple idea, the Story of Stuff evolved into a movement of people asking "Why did we let this happen?" *This* being the creation of the most wasteful society in history.

Annie has landed on the idea that if we describe ourselves as "consumers," then we're part of the problem—we're self-defining as, in my words, "those who buy stuff." Citizens have a right to work, live and become politically active in a particular country, while consumers are politically detached global buyers of goods. Why, Annie was asking, would we ever want to define ourselves as consumers? I did push back a little and suggested that we can't just ignore consumers. Garbage is a colossal problem, and it's getting worse. We've seen where all that stuff goes. It becomes garbage containing thousands of toxic chemicals—unknown, untested, untracked and unhealthy. We need to be working on all fronts to stem wasteful production and consumption. And consumers are part of the equation. I agreed with her that at the end of the day, the big issue isn't simply what kinds of stuff we should buy; it's the fact that we need to buy way less stuff, period. Furthermore, that stuff—whether it's a car, a soft drink or a smartphone—needs to be regulated by governments, not by companies who have no interest apart from endless growth in sales. These regulations need to cover what the products contain and how they are disposed of. Moreover, the costs for proper recycling and disposal need to be built into the products so that scarce natural resources don't end up being buried or burned.

Of course, it's not as though economists and environmentalists haven't been warning us against the folly of disposable products since at least the original Earth Day, more than forty-five years ago. In fact, some of the very first Earth Day placards read "Clean Air, Pure Water." We just can't seem to get our collective heads around the challenges of that simple message because, as much as anything, the rules our society is playing by are the wrong ones. The rules of the game we're playing now are best defined by the Malcolm Forbes maxim "He who dies with the most toys wins." We need a different game, with different rules—perhaps "Those who use the least stuff win." And our economic and regulatory systems need to reinforce that motto with another one—such as this: The more you use, waste, pollute and discard, the more you'll lose financially.

Greening the Economy

Pollution is a broad economic and societal problem, not merely an ecological challenge. Though humans seem to have an inkling that we can't survive without air, water and food, there appears to be less consciousness of the fact that these needs will exist in the future. We're acutely aware of the need for food and water on a daily or weekly basis, but we don't pay as much attention to long-term requirements. Therefore, without deliberate economic instruments designed to capture the long-term environmental damage caused by our consumption (such as fees, tolls, taxes and pollution-trading schemes), we won't succeed in stemming the growth of toxic waste and pollution. This is why we need to "green the economy." Working to ban a chemical that is known to increase the risk of cancer is rewarding and can sometimes be relatively straightforward. But this type of action is not nearly enough. Making the shift to a green economy—one where hazardous chemicals are not manufactured or put in infants' toys in the first place—is more daunting but far more effective. Will we soon see a greener world where our chemistry is green too? Can we overcome the failure of our economy to properly address the health and environmental costs associated with unfettered economic expansion? I'm afraid the jury is still out on those questions. Green chemistry is an exciting concept, but I'm not convinced it will take hold unless we create broader social, cultural and economic demand for what it is attempting to accomplish.

I returned to my Teflon pan question, which John Warner said was an excellent example of the complicated challenges facing green chemistry. He has invented a replacement technology for non-stick coatings that is stain resistant, water resistant and free from toxic perfluorinated compounds. It's in the early stages of development, but he requires some of the scarce pre-commercialization research dollars that our economic system cannot seem to cough up. For now, old-fashioned cast iron, enamel-coated cast iron and stainless steel remain the best options for green-minded cooks.

Without economic incentives or penalties, companies will continue to manufacture toxic products, consumers will buy them thinking they are safe, garbage dumps and incinerators will accept them along with other throwaways containing persistent pollutants, our drinking water will become contaminated and people will get sick. The safer alternatives will never be produced. And so my quest to find out what happens to a Teflon pan led me to discover the failure of global waste systems, plans to retool chemistry education and the need for economic reform. As of 2018, there are no non-stick pan recycling programs to be found.

We need a truly green economy, one that goes far beyond the modest efforts of current corporate social responsibility (CSR) efforts espoused by multinational corporations. The only real answer to getting rid of toxic chemicals is to move from a linear economic model of one-time material extraction, throughput and dumping to a circular economy that mimics nature by creating closed-loop systems, where resources and nutrients are fed back into the process and the concept of waste is eliminated (see figure 19).[51] What's more, rather than finding out after the fact that chemicals in our food and cosmetics cause harm, testing protocols need to be followed to ensure that cancer-causing and endocrine-disrupting chemicals are not manufactured in the first place. One such protocol now exists. Developed by a scientific panel of chemical and health experts, including Terry Collins and John Warner, it is called the "tiered protocol for endocrine disruption" (TiPED), and it's an example of the new collaborative thinking that may just move us to healthier, greener chemistry.[52] TiPED is a design tool to detect whether or not a chemical will cause endocrine disruption. It consists of five testing tiers, each designed to "broadly interrogate" a chemical's potential effect on the endocrine system of different species.[53]

Figure 19. Linear vs. circular economies.

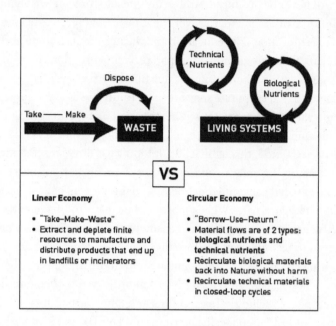

There are other hints of a new economy on the horizon. Companies are producing a wide array of green products, including cosmetics and cleaning products, as we've described in earlier chapters of this book. And exciting green chemistry breakthroughs are taking place in research labs throughout the globe. At present, German scientists seem to be leading the way—manufacturing biodegradable plastic polymer from milk, using algae or straw to make chemical feedstocks at an economically workable scale and designing colourful pigments based on iron oxide, a.k.a. rust.[55] Even the famous little blue pill, Viagra, has benefited from green chemistry. Chemists at Pfizer, the manufacturer of Viagra, have designed a chemical reaction process that requires dramatically fewer toxic solvents, eliminates the use of tin chloride (an environmental pollutant) and allows for production to happen with only a fraction of the waste involved in the original manufacturing process.[56]

Renewable power and electric cars are the global green trends that have blown past everyone's predictions from ten years ago. Electric car sales in the third quarter of 2017 increased 63 percent over the same quarter one year earlier. In the original edition of *Toxin Toxout*, we cited estimates of global electric car sales hitting 670,000 by 2020. We weren't optimistic enough. In 2017 over 1.2 million electric and plug-in hybrid electric cars were sold worldwide. And the story behind that increase has to do with more than just media darling Tesla and the U.S. market. China is where the rapid growth in electric cars is happening.

The same kind of sharp trajectory is happening for renewable power. Solar power now outcompetes new conventional power facilities in Germany and the U.S., and will outperform coal in China and India by 2021.[57] Global renewable electricity capacity added in 2016 is sufficient to power nearly all of Western Europe.[58] Energy efficiency is going gang-busters too. Every dollar invested in energy efficiency saves two dollars in generation and distribution costs.[59] Countries around the world are starting to make energy efficiency the first choice in the energy resource mix. In other words, the news was good in 2012 and the news today is even better. The transformation we predicted is in full flight.

But not so much on waste. Monster-sized hills of garbage are still piling up all over the world, and there's a mountain of work to do if we're going to detox our economic systems before we do irreparable damage to our environment and ourselves.

THIRTEEN: THE SLOW DEATH BY
RUBBER DUCK TOP TEN

Be careful about reading health books. You may die of a misprint.

—MARK TWAIN

DIET BOOKS ARE DIFFERENT from detox books in one very important respect: following the advice of the former yields obvious results, whereas doing so for the latter may not. If you try a diet and you don't see the pounds coming off, chances are you won't continue. But there's no such built-in quality control with the welter of detox articles and books out there, which provide often conflicting prescriptions for potions and pills and odd foods, often claiming to be "100% GUARANTEED!" to eliminate toxins from your body. Who's to know whether or not these recommendations will really work? It would be nice if you could buy a "Tox-o-Meter" from your local pharmacy, put it under your tongue and get a simple read out of the various poisons in your body. Alas, this is not possible.

That's where this book comes in. Through much trial and error, pricey self-testing and numerous uncomfortable situations, we have done your homework for you. You can't paralyze yourself into inaction worrying about all the 80,000 or so chemicals that are in circulation today. So we've tried to focus on the ones that exhibit the following two characteristics: (1) The best scientific evidence points to them as harmful to human health and (2) Recent science, and our self-tests, shows that you can measurably reduce their levels in your body if you do certain things.

We've summarized our various experimental results in table 9 in this chapter. As you can see, if you do a few ordinary, daily things a little differently, you can dramatically reduce levels of certain pollutants in your body—sometimes very quickly.

This final chapter provides what we hope is a useful summary of the ways you can reduce those toxins. We've boiled down the voluminous amounts of information in this book to create an easy-to-read list that you can tear out and stick on your refrigerator. It's the Slow Death by Rubber Duck Top Ten list on page 292 of this book.

Read it, follow its advice . . . and you'll get a whole lot of toxins out of your body in no time flat.

Table 9: Magnitude of toxic changes we achieved through experimentation.

Experiment	Changes in Chemical Levels
Introduction Levels of BPA and BPS after handling cash register receipts (Rick, Bruce, Sarah and Muhannad)	BPA levels up by 42 times (see Figure 2) BPS levels up by 115 times (see Figure 2)
Chapter 1 Levels of phthalates after using common personal-care products (Rick)	MEP levels up by 22 times (see Figure 3)
Levels of phthalates and para-bens after using green and not-so-green personal-care products (Jessa and Ray)	MEP levels down by 10 times on average* when using conventional products (see Figure 4) Methyl paraben levels down by 77 times on average* when using conventional products (see Figure 4)
Chapter 4 Levels of mercury after eating tuna (Bruce)	Mercury levels up by 2.5 times (see Figure 6)
Chapter 5 Levels of triclosan after using common personal-care products (Rick)	Triclosan levels up by 2,907 times (see Figure 7)

Experiment	Changes in Chemical Levels
Chapter 7 *Levels of BPA after using BPA-containing containers and food (Rick)*	BPA levels up by 7 times (see Figure 8)
Chapter 8 *Levels of organophosphate pesticides after eating organic food (nine children)*	Levels down by 3 times on average (see Figure 10)
Chapter 9 *Levels of heavy metals during chelation (Bruce)*	Levels of removal from body up between 4 and 23 times (see Figure 11)
Chapter 10 *Levels of BPA and phthalates (MEP and MBP) during use of sauna (Bruce)*	BPA released in sweat in all 5 weeks (see Figure 13) MEP and MBP released in sweat in all 5 weeks (see Figures 14 and 15)
Chapter 11 *Levels of VOCs after sitting in new car (Rick)*	Levels up between 1.2 and 5 times (see Figure 17)
NBC experiment** *Levels of BPA and triclosan after ceasing the use of common personal-care products (Andrea Canning)*	BPA levels down by 88 times Triclosan levels down by 99 times

* Increases and decreases were calculated by dividing the peak level by the trough level. The numbers documented here are the average of Ray's and Jessa's respective changes in chemical levels

** In late 2012, during the writing of *Toxin Toxout*, we did an experiment with reporter Andrea Canning for NBC's *Dateline* that looked at BPA, triclosan and phthalate levels. The experiment, similar to our experiment with Jessa and Ray in chapter 1 of this book, consisted of three phases: a washout, then heavy use of conventional products, followed by another washout where products containing those chemicals were avoided. The results above are from the BPA and triclosan experimentation. The segment aired on *Dateline* March 24, 2013.

The Most Important "To Do" List of Your Life

Managing what we absorb, breathe, eat and drink is the first line of defence against toxins like phthalates, parabens, pesticides and volatile organic compounds. Once chemicals are in our body, Bruce has some clear ideas on the detox methods that work and those that are modern-day snake oil. Ultimately, of course, we need to get synthetic toxins out of our economy and our world, but in the meantime, these ten simple steps (summarized in the Slow Death by Rubber Duck Top Ten list) will lead to a healthier life for all.

1. **Use natural personal-care products that don't contain chemicals such as phthalates or parabens.**
   In a study published in 2012, Shanna Swan investigated associations between women's reported use of various personal-care products and phthalate metabolite levels in their urine, tested within twenty-four hours of the women's interviews (see chapter 1).[1] Swan found that concentrations of MEP (the primary metabolite of diethyl phthalate) in women increased with the number of products used. Swan also found, more generally, that women's more frequent use of these products, particularly perfumes and fragranced products, was associated with higher urinary concentrations of multiple phthalate metabolites.

   Here are some important tips and tools—and actions to carry out—to reduce toxic chemicals in your personal-care products:
   - Less is less. Limit your use of personal-care products whenever possible.
   - Use natural and/or organic cosmetics and personal-care products.
   - Check out the Environmental Working Group's (EWG's) Skin Deep database for information and safety scores of your products (it includes the scores of natural and organic products).
   - Whenever possible, avoid personal-care products with complicated chemical names on the labels

(especially products with "fragrance" or "parfum" in the ingredients list).

- Avoid problem products such as chemical hair straighteners.
- Avoid antibacterial products, especially the ones that list triclosan on their labels. Instead, wash your hands regularly and vigorously.

2. **Eat more organic food to avoid pesticides.**

We really are what we eat. In chapter 8 Rick saw how effective an organic diet is in lowering the levels of pesticides in the bodies of young children. And why should we all avoid those pesticides in the first place? Pesticide exposure has been linked to some very serious negative health effects. Here are just some of them: general developmental problems and cognitive deficits in children, endocrine disruption, non-Hodgkin's lymphoma, low birth weight, reproductive problems, asthma, risk of obesity and diabetes and infertility.[2] And a 2017 study in the prestigious *Journal of the American Medical Association* showed that women seeking to get pregnant could significantly improve their chances by eating conventional produce with fewer pesticide residues or, better yet, eating organic.[3] In simple terms, an organic diet can lower your body pesticide levels. Here's what you can do to reduce the pesticides in your life:

- Eat seasonal local and organic produce whenever you can.
- Choose conventional produce that are lowest in pesticides (usually those with thick skins, such as onions, corn, pineapple and avocados).
- Wash your produce well before eating it.
- Be proud of your chemical-free lawn, yard and neighbourhood.

3. **Drink the water from your tap! And lots of it!**

We can lower our toxic burden by controlling what we eat, but what about the real "staff of life"—the water that we drink? On average, we are made up of two-thirds water by weight. Add to that the critical role that water plays in our bodily detox mechanisms, and we'd better be sure that we safeguard our drinking water. Water is vital to detoxification—personal and ecological.

Public health officials and municipal governments everywhere work together to rigorously test our tap water supplies for hundreds of potential chemical contaminants. And they do it every day. If that doesn't give you enough assurance, you can install an affordable and effective filter in your home. Plenty of them are available. Revisit that handy table 8 in chapter 12, comparing some common in-house filters. For many of the chemicals we're concerned about, activated carbon filters are the best bet, and they're affordable. It's a lot easier to install a point-of-use tap filter or to refill that countertop filter than to keep lugging flats of individual-sized water bottles from the grocery store, and it's a whole lot better for the environment and you. So drink up and detox: six glasses of liquid a day for women and nine glasses a day for men (that includes all liquids).

4. **Use natural fibres and green products like low-VOC paints in your homes and avoid products that might off-gas.** With so many of us spending so much time indoors and with so many smelly, off-gassing products surrounding us, indoor air quality has become an area of growing environmental and human health concern. As mentioned in chapter 11, the average person in an industrialized country now spends over 90 percent of their life indoors, including about 5 percent in enclosed vehicles.[4] With that in mind, air quality inside is more important than it is outside.

In terms of reducing your exposure to off-gassing chemicals in road vehicles, toxic chemicals like benzene, phthalates and flame retardants are an issue, as Rick discovered. But manufacturers are starting to get rid of them. Ask the car company you're dealing with what they're doing to reduce the "new car smell."

As in the case of cars, there's some bad news about the buildings people spend so much time in, and some good news. First the bad: chemicals like flame retardants and phthalates are getting into the dust that gathers in our homes and offices, and they've been linked to some serious health outcomes like asthma and increased allergenicity.[5] On the upside: you can take preventive steps to reduce your exposure:

- Open your windows and get outside!
- Incorporate furniture and textiles made from natural fibres into your life, avoid furniture made from polyurethane foam, and reupholster your old furniture whenever it begins to rip.
- Clean and dust interior surfaces frequently (especially those that come in contact with food) and use a vacuum cleaner with a HEPA filter (a type of high-efficiency air filter, usually made from randomly arranged fibreglass—they're designed to capture ultra-fine particles).
- Look for furniture and electronics retailers who carry products that are free of toxic flame retardants.
- Avoid vinyl products.
- Use green building materials, like low-VOC paint, when possible.
- When buying or renting a home or office, choose LEED-certified premises when possible.

5. **Eat more vegetables and less meat to avoid toxin-grabbing animal fat.**

Toxic chemicals are like a bad rash—they keep coming back, and they appear where you least expect or want them. This is the case for toxins like DDT and PCBs, chemicals that were banned as many as forty years ago. Some of the newer toxic chemicals on the market today—flame retardants and commonly used pesticides—also bioaccumulate. These toxins, transported by air and water, are lipophilic (fat-loving), so they find their way into the fat cells of wildlife like fish and move up the food chain into humans.

What's the solution to avoiding these persistently pesky chemicals in the food chain? Well, it's not all that different from what doctors and nutritionists (and many mothers) already recommend: eat your veggies and stay away from fatty foods!

6. **Sweat more—toxic chemicals like BPA and phthalates leave your body through your sweat.**

   When researching his chapters, Bruce learned first-hand about the sheer volume of resources (useful or otherwise) that exist on the topic of diet- and exercise-based detox routines. Do check out some of the resources we recommend at the end of the book. Saunas have been used for spiritual and therapeutic reasons alike, across cultures, for hundreds and hundreds of years. The sauna detox experiment Bruce undertook was a novel design. And though it wasn't possible to show before-and-after body concentrations, the experiment demonstrated unmistakably that synthetic chemicals like BPA are removed through sweating—one of our body's most basic natural detox methods.

7. **Exercise!**

   Though the science of detox is in its infancy, some methods do clearly work—as evidenced by the research of Stephen Genuis.[6] But some methods don't work. The effectiveness of a given detox method often depends on the toxic chemical in question. Some of the common ones that we've mentioned in this book (phthalates and parabens, for instance) are metabolized and excreted quickly through the body's natural mechanisms, whereas others find their way into fat cells and therefore bioaccumulate. To help get rid of these lipophilic chemicals, do plenty of exercise. This breaks down the fat cells, releasing the stored toxins and allowing them to be excreted via lung exhalation and sweat.[7]

   In one recent example, a study carried out at the University of Montreal evaluated the impact of physical exertion on human exposure to the volatile organic compounds (VOCs) toluene and n-hexane. The researchers subjected the test subjects to toluene and n-hexane in

equal amounts and found that breathing from physical
exercise, higher concentrations of toluene and n-hexane
levels were being exhaled from the lungs.[8]

8. **Avoid wacky quick-fix detoxes and optimize your body's
    natural detox mechanisms by adopting a detox lifestyle.**
    Since we know that chemicals are entering our bodies on a
    daily basis, shouldn't we make sure that they're leaving
    our bodies on a daily basis? And shouldn't we train our
    bodies to be in the best possible condition to do this?
    Ridding your body of pollutants you can't actively avoid
    requires a certain lifestyle approach that, frankly, may
    take a bit of effort. Recall that myth-busting table 7 from
    chapter 9 about the effectiveness of various detox treat-
    ments? As Bruce explored the depths of the detox indus-
    try, he debunked some of the phony detox techniques that
    are being peddled on the market today. He also learned
    that to succeed in eliminating toxic chemicals, we have to
    overthrow the notion of quick-fix, fad-based diets and
    cleanses. Focus instead on our healthy detox lifestyle rec-
    ommendations.

9. **Buy less and buy green.**
    As consumers we need to protect ourselves and our fami-
    lies by making informed choices—since it appears that
    many corporations have little concern for our health.
    Fortunately, however, there's also a growing trend among
    small and big businesses to do better by us. Johnson &
    Johnson has voluntarily phased out the use of formaldehyde-
    releasing preservatives in their baby shampoo sold in
    Canada, the U.S., China, Australia and Indonesia. In
    September 2013, Procter & Gamble announced that
    phthalates and triclosan would be eliminated from its
    products by 2014 and Walmart U.S. said in 2016 that it
    would "push" suppliers to "remove or restrict" the use
    of eight hazardous chemicals in household cleaning,
    personal-care and beauty items.[9] All this was a direct
    response to calls for action from consumers (many of
    them readers of the first edition of *Slow Death by Rubber*

Duck) and groups like the Campaign for Safe Cosmetics and Environmental Defence Canada.

Things have changed. While doing some research for a media story in New York, we popped into a local grocery store to purchase some BPA microwaveable food containers. Much to our amazement (and dismay, in terms of the experiment we were preparing), we couldn't find any. All the brand-name plastic containers were now BPA-free. This is a clear signal that, despite the whining from chemical companies, the days are numbered for many synthetic toxins, thanks to active and vocal consumers like you.

These may appear to be small steps, but they are a big reminder that consumers have the power to demand healthier products and win.

As we, individually, become more adept at the Slow Death by Rubber Duck Top Ten list, we must also recognize that these same steps need to be applied to society as a whole: we have to get our collective act together to create a greener, less toxic economy.

In our role as consumers, we're doing a pretty good job of just that—consuming, and creating more waste per day than ever before. Garbage, in itself, is not a problem, but too much of it is toxic, and we make and consume way too much. We need more—way more—initiatives like IKEA's recent announcement that it's looking to replace all its polystyrene packaging with material made from mushroom waste. People like Terry Collins, John Warner and Janine Benyus are leaders in green chemistry, and they're working to make materials and designs available for the stuff we already create. Software programmes are being developed to better predict the toxicity of chemicals so we can avoid using any that will harm human health, and chemists are looking into shifting away from petroleum-based chemical manufacturing. But does this mean that we're just learning to make more stuff in a less harmful way? Green chemistry may be gaining ground, but it solves only part of the problem.

10. **Support politicians who believe in a greener economy and organizations that work for a cleaner environment.** Consumers have power, and when we make different choices, we can encourage change in the products that are available. But it's only by mobilizing our power as consumers *and also as citizens* that we can create a modern green economy. If we think of ourselves only as consumers, we'll end up as part of the problem. We don't need more consumers; we need active citizens, as Annie Leonard reminded us.

   To meet the challenges of detoxing our economy, citizens will need to be informed and engaged. We also need governments that will put public health ahead of corporate profits. Governments decide which chemicals can be sold, where our garbage ends up and what levels of toxins will be allowed in our food, water and air. That's why we need to elect politicians who understand the importance of keeping toxic chemicals out of our lives. We all respond to economic signals, and we need governments to develop effective pricing policies that capture the full cost of pollution, including the pollution of our bodies by toxic chemicals.

Start Somewhere

Is all of the above a perfect recipe for being toxin-free? Of course not. But by following these guidelines, you'll make a huge difference in creating a cleaner, healthier lifestyle. It's the most reliable, evidence-based prescription that we know of to get chemicals out of your environment and your body. Scientists have observed that some of us are more susceptible to the effects of toxic chemicals than others. But how do we know? Well, this issue is similar to the smoking debate.

Rick's beloved grandmother Marjorie Braive could have been a poster girl for the tobacco industry. She smoked at least a pack a day of Du Maurier Regulars dating back to the 1930s. In the early 1970s she had a mastectomy but then carried on, undeterred, to the ripe old age of eighty-five. One of Rick's enduring childhood memories is of her swimming off the dock of their Adirondack cottage, a floppy-brimmed straw sunhat on her head and a cigarette hanging out of her mouth. Her family sprinkled a few cigarettes on top of her coffin to carry her through to the afterlife.

On the other hand, how many of us know of people whose lives were clearly cut short by the effects of smoking? Rick's grandfather on his father's side, a heavy smoker, dropped dead of a massive heart attack in his mid-forties.

The effects of pollution are similar. Some of us remain relatively unaffected by toxic synthetic chemicals. Others can be damaged even by apparently minor exposure. All of us benefit when exposure to cigarette smoke is reduced, and the same is true of exposure to synthetic chemicals.

The key is to start. Start somewhere.

Now rip out page 292, stick it on your refrigerator and get going!

THE SLOW DEATH BY RUBBER DUCK TOP TEN

1. Use natural personal-care products that don't contain chemicals such as phthalates or parabens.
2. Eat more organic food to avoid pesticides.
3. Drink the water from your tap! And lots of it!
4. Use natural fibres and green products like low-VOC paints in your home and avoid products that might off-gas.
5. Eat more vegetables and less meat to avoid toxin-grabbing animal fat.
6. Sweat more—toxic chemicals like BPA and phthalates leave your body through your sweat.
7. Exercise!
8. Avoid wacky quick-fix detoxes and optimize your body's natural detox mechanisms by adopting a detox lifestyle.
9. Buy less and buy green.
10. Support politicians who believe in a greener economy and organizations that work for a cleaner environment.

www.slowdeathbyrubberduck.org

NOTES

Introduction

[1] E. Zander, "Human Exposure to Preventable Environmental Chemicals Is Resulting in Health Costs of 10% of Global GDP," *Health and Environment Alliance*, December 5, 2017 (www.env-health.org/resources/press-releases /article/human-exposure-to-preventable; accessed April 18, 2018).

[2] More recent studies have also found the presence of toxic chemicals in umbilical cord blood. See A. Dursun, K. Yurdakok, S. S. Yalcin, G. Tekinalp, O. Aykut, G. Orhan and G. K. Morgil, "Maternal Risk Factors Associated with Lead, Mercury and Cadmium Levels in Umbilical Cord Blood, Breast Milk and Newborn Hair," *Journal of Maternal-Fetal and Neonatal Medicine*: 954–61. doi: 10.3109/14767058.2015.1026255.

[3] M. Warhurst, "It's a No Brainer! Action Needed to Stop Children Being Exposed to Chemicals That Harm Their Brain Development!" *ChemTrust*, March 7, 2017 (www.chemtrust.org/brain/; accessed April 18, 2018).

[4] L. Glodman and N. Tran, "Toxics and Poverty: The Impact of Toxic Substances on the Poor in Developing Countries," *World Bank*, August 2002 (http://documents.worldbank.org/curated/en/689811468315541722/pdf /445580WP0BOX0327404B01PUBLIC1.pdf; accessed March 29, 2018).

[5] A. Westervelt, "Phthalates Are Everywhere and the Health Risks Are Worrying. How Bad Are They Really?" *The Guardian*, February 10, 2015 (https://www.theguardian.com/lifeandstyle/2015/feb/10/phthalates -plastics-chemicals-research-analysis; accessed March 30, 2018).

[6] R. J. Bertelsen, M. P. Longnecker, M. Løvik, A. M. Calafat, K.-H. Carlsen, S. J. London and K. C. Lødrup Carlsen, "Triclosan Exposure and Allergic

Sensitization in Norwegian Children," *Allergy*, no. 1 (January 2013) 68: 84–91 (https://www.ncbi.nlm.nih.gov/pmc/articles/PMC3515701/; accessed March 29, 2018).

[7] K. M. Rice, E. M. Walker Jr., M. Wu, C. Gillette and E. R. Blough, "Environmental Mercury and Its Toxic Effects," *Journal of Preventive Medicine and Public Health*, no. 2 (March 2014) 47: 74–83 (https://www.ncbi.nlm.nih.gov /pmc/articles/PMC3988285/; accessed March 29, 2018).

[8] See I. Andersen, O. Voie, F. Fonnum and E. Mariussen, "Effects of Methyl Mercury in Combination with Polychlorinated Biphenyls and Brominated Flame Retardants on the Uptake of Glutamate in Rat Brain Synaptosomes: A Mathematical Approach for the Study of Mixtures," *Toxicological Sciences* 112 (2009): 175–84.

[9] H. Willer and J. Lernoud, "The World of Organic Agriculture: Statistics and Emerging Trends 2017," Research Institute of Organic Agriculture and International Federation of Organic Agriculture Movements, February 2017 (https://shop.fibl.org/CHen/mwdownloads/download/link/id/785/?ref=1; accessed March 30, 2018).

[10] Agriculture and Agri-Food Canada, "Market Trends: Organics," Market Analysis Report, 2010 (http://publications.gc.ca/collections/collection _2015/aac-aafc/A74-2-2010-11-eng.pdf; accessed March 29, 2018).

[11] T. Granger, "McDonald's to Stop Using Foam Packaging by End of Year," *Earth 911*, January 12, 2018 (https://earth911.com/business-policy/mcdonalds -foam/; accessed April 1, 2018).

[12] "Sustainability Nears a Tipping Point," *MIT Sloan Management Review* 53 (Winter 2012): 69–74.

[13] Ibid.

[14] L. Tan, N. Neilsen, D. Young and Z. Trizna, "Use of Antimicrobial Agents in Consumer Products," *Archives of Dermatology* 138 (2002): 1082–86; Environmental Defence Canada, *The Trouble with Triclosan* (Toronto, November 2012); Health Canada, "Canada Concludes Preliminary Assessment of Triclosan," press release, March 30, 2012 (https://www. canada.ca/en/news/archive/2012/03/canada-concludes-preliminary- assessment-triclosan.html; accessed March 29, 2018).

[15] S. Lunder, "Washington Is First State to Ban Fluorinated Chemicals in Food

Packaging," *Environmental Working Group*, March 22, 2018 (https://www.ewg.org /news-and-analysis/2018/03/washington-first-state-ban-fluorinated -chemicals-food-packaging#.WsDHodPwbOR; accessed April 1, 2018).

[16] M. L. Wind, "Response to Petition HP 99-1: Request to Ban PVC in Toys and Other Products Intended for Children Five Years of Age and Under," August 2002, quoted in *Trouble in Toyland*, NYPIRG 2002 Toy Safety Report (https://slidex.tips/download/trouble-in-toyland-table-of-contents; accessed March 21, 2018).

[17] I. Colón, D. Caro, C. J. Bourdony and O. Rosario, "Identification of Phthalate Esters in the Serum of Young Puerto Rican Girls with Premature Breast Development," *Environmental Health Perspectives* 108 (2000): 895– 900; R. Moral, R. Wang, I. H. Russo, D. A. Mailo, C. A. Lamartinière and J. Russo, "The Plasticizer Butyl Benzyl Phthalate Induces Genomic Changes in Rat Mammary Gland after Neonatal/Prepubertal Exposure," *BMC Genomics* 8 (2007): 453.

[18] D. Smith, "Worldwide Trends in DDT Levels in Human Milk," *International Journal of Epidemiology* 28 (1999): 184; P. Pinsky and M. Lorber, "A Model to Evaluate Past Exposure to 2,3,7,8-TCDD," *Journal of Exposure Analysis and Environmental Epidemiology* 8 (1998): 325; Health Canada, *Risk Management Strategy for Lead*, February 2013, 25 (http://www.hc-sc.gc.ca/ewh-semt /pubs/contaminants/prms_lead-psgr_plomb/index-eng.php; accessed April 1, 2018).

[19] Ami R. Zota, Antonia M. Calafat, and Tracey J. Woodruff, "Temporal Trends in Phthalate Exposures: Findings from the National Health and Nutrition Examination Survey, 2001–2010" *Environmental Health Perspectives*, doi: 10.1289/ehp.1306681.

[20] Modified from Ami R. Zota, Antonia M. Calafat and Tracey J. Woodruff, "Temporal Trends in Phthalate Exposures: Findings from the National Health and Nutrition Examination Survey, 2001–2010," *Environmental Health Perspectives*, doi:10.1289/ehp.1306681.

[21] RICK AND BRUCE'S TEST SCHEDULE

Saturday, March 1, 2008

Rick limits exposure to products that contain phthalates, bisphenol A and triclosan.

Sunday, March 2, 2008 (Day 1)

Rick continues to limit exposure to products containing phthalates, bisphenol A and triclosan.

Rick begins the 1st 24-hour urine collection.

1 p.m. Rick and Bruce meet to have first blood samples taken.

2 p.m. Bruce has two tuna sandwiches for lunch.

Monday, March 3, 2008 (Day 2)

9 a.m. Rick and Bruce arrive at the condo.

9:45 a.m. Bruce drinks Earl Grey tea.

10:15 a.m. Carpet cleaning company arrives to protect/Stainmaster the test-room carpet and couch.

11 a.m. Rick drinks first coffee, brewed in polycarbonate French press. Rick gets ready for the day (showers, shaves, brushes teeth, etc.).

11:30 a.m. Rick and Bruce settle into the test room.

12:15 p.m. Rick washes hands with antibacterial hand soap.

1 p.m. Bruce has tuna sandwich and tea for lunch.

1:30 p.m. Rick has chicken noodle soup and canned spaghetti for lunch, both microwaved in Rubbermaid microwavable containers. Rick also brews a fresh pot of coffee.

2 p.m. Rick begins second 24-hour urine collection and takes a urine spot sample.

2:30 p.m. Rick does dishes and washes up, then uses lotion, brushes teeth and washes hands.

3 p.m. Bruce has a tuna sandwich and tea for a mid-afternoon snack.

3:15 p.m. Rick drinks two small (275 mL) cans of Coke.

4:30 p.m. Rick brews fresh coffee and then drinks it.

5:15 p.m. Rick and Bruce have second blood samples taken.

5:45 p.m. Bruce has a trayful of tuna sushi and sashimi.

6:45 p.m. Rick has tuna casserole for dinner.

7 p.m. Bruce eats a trayful of tuna sashimi, sushi roll and nigiri sushi for dinner, along with a beer or two.

7:15 p.m. Rick washes dishes, washes hands and brushes teeth.

8:15 p.m. Rick moisturizes hands.

9:00 p.m. Rick takes second urine spot sample.

9:30 p.m. Rick and Bruce leave the condo for the night.

Tuesday, March 4, 2008 (Day 3)

10 a.m. Rick arrives at the condo and makes first cup of coffee of the day. He settles into the room.

11 a.m. Rick brews fresh pot of coffee and plugs in room air freshener.

11 a.m. Bruce arrives at the condo and settles into the room.

11:15 a.m. Rick showers.

11:45 a.m. Rick has canned pineapple for a snack.

1 p.m. Rick unplugs air freshener, removes it from the room and then makes lunch.

1 p.m. Bruce has tuna sandwich for lunch.

3 p.m. Rick takes third urine spot sample.

7 p.m. Bruce has seared tuna steak for dinner.

9 p.m. Rick and Bruce leave the condo for the night.

Wednesday, March 5, 2008 (Day 4)

9:30 a.m. Rick and Bruce have final blood samples taken. Rick has additional samples of blood drawn to analyze his PBDE levels.

12 noon All blood and urine samples shipped to AXYS Analytical Services.

Thursday, March 6, 2008

10 a.m. Blood and urine samples arrive at AXYS.

[22] S. Ndaw, A. Remy, D. Jargot and A. Robert, "Occupational Exposure of Cashiers to Bisphenol A via Thermal Paper: Urinary Biomonitoring Study," *International Archives on Occupational and Environmental Health* 89, no. 6: (August 2016) 935–46 (https://www.ncbi.nlm.nih.gov/pubmed/27126703; accessed March 29, 2018).

[23] In fact, Fred vom Saal, the grandfather of BPA research, has found exactly this. See A. M. Hormann, F. S. vom Saal, S. C. Nagel, R. W. Stahlhut, C. L.

Moyer, M. R. Ellersieck, W. V. Welshons et al., "Holding Thermal Receipt Paper and Eating Food after Using Hand Sanitizer Results in High Serum Bioactive and Urine Total Levels of Bisphenol A (BPA)," *PLoS One*, 9, no. 10 (October 2014): e110509; doi: 10.1371/journal.pone.0110509, eCollection 2014 (https://www.ncbi.nlm.nih.gov/pubmed/25337790; accessed March 29, 2018).

[24] S. LaMotte, "BPA-Free Plastic Alternatives May Not Be As Safe As You Think," CNN, February 1, 2016 (https://www.cnn.com/2016/02/01/health/bpa-free-alternatives-may-not-be-safe/index.html; accessed March 29, 2018).

[25] See Hormann et al., "Holding Thermal Receipt Paper."

[26] "Global Bisphenol A (BPA) Market by Application (Appliances, Automotive, Consumer, Construction, Electrical & Electronics) Expected to Reach USD 20.03 Billion by 2020," Grand View Research, June 2015 (https://www.grandviewresearch.com/press-release/global-bisphenol-a-bpa-market; accessed March 29, 2018).

One: Wellness Revolution

[1] R. Raphael, "What's Driving the Billion-Dollar Natural Beauty Movement?" *Fast Company*, May 28, 2017 (https://www.fastcompany.com/3068710/whats-driving-the-billion-dollar-natural-beauty-movement; accessed April 10, 2018).

[2] "EcoFocus Trend Survey 2010–2012," EcoFocus Worldwide (https://ecofocusworldwide.com/new-global-trend-survey/; accessed March 13, 2018). More recent research, commissioned by Unilever, has found that roughly a "third of consumers [now choose] to buy from brands they believe are doing social or environmental good." (See "Report Shows a Third of Consumers Prefer Sustainable Brands," Unilever, May 1, 2017 (https://www.unilever.com/news/Press-releases/2017/report-shows-a-third-of-consumers-prefer-sustainable-brands.html; accessed March 13, 2017).

[3] McGinley, L. "FDA Bans Common Ingredients in Antibacterial Soaps and Body Washes," *Washington Post*, September 2, 2016 (https://www.washingtonpost.com/news/to-your-health/wp/2016/09/02/fda-bans-some-antibacterial-soaps-and-body-washes/?noredirect=on&utm_term=.bb983614fb95; accessed May 31, 2018).

4 U.S. Food & Drug Administration, "What Are Parabens and Why Are They Used In Cosmetics?," February 22, 2018 (https://www.fda.gov/Cosmetics/ProductsIngredients/Ingredients/ucm128042.htm#what_are_parabens; accessed May 31, 2018).

5 See: Government of Canada, "Registration Decision RD2014-03, Sodium Lauryl Sulfate,"March 19, 2014 (https://www.canada.ca/en/health-canada/services/consumer-product-safety/reports-publications/pesticides-pest-management/decisions-updates/registration-decision/2014/sodium-lau-ryl-sulfate-rd2014-03.html) and American Cleaning Institute, "Sodium Lauryl Sulfate (SLS),"2018 (https://www.cleaninginstitute.org/policy/sls.aspx; both accessed May 31, 2018).

6 IBISWorld, a Los Angeles–based business intelligence company, estimated the total value of the global cosmetic market in 2017 at $301.7 billion. See "Global Cosmetics Manufacturing—Global Market Research Report," IBISWorld, June 2017 (https://www.ibisworld.com/industry-trends/global-industry-reports/manufacturing/cosmetics-manufacturing.html; accessed March 27, 2018).

7 Estée Lauder official website (https://www.esteelauder.com/; accessed July 30, 2012).

8 "Weleda: 4.2% Increase in Sales Worldwide," *Organic Market Info*, March 15, 2018 (http://www.organic-market.info/news-in-brief-and-reports-article/weleda-4-2-increase-in-sales-worldwide.html; accessed April 18, 2018).

9 "Ecocert Greenlife & Cosmos," Ecocert, March 30, 2016 (www.ecocert.com/en/ecocert-greenlife-cosmos; accessed April 18, 2018).

10 J. Saunders, "Making Sense of 'Organic' Labels for Non-food Products," Organic Council of Ontario, October 26, 2017 (www.organiccouncil.ca/news/making-sense-of-organic-labels-for-non-food-products; accessed April 10, 2018).

11 United States Department of Labor, Occupational Safety and Health Administration, "Hazard Alert Update: Hair Smoothing Products That Could Release Formaldehyde" (http://www.osha.gov/SLTC/formaldehyde/hazard_alert.html; accessed August 1, 2012).

12 State of California Department of Justice, Office of the Attorney General, "Attorney General Kamala D. Harris Announces Settlement Requiring Honest Advertising over Brazilian Blowout Products," press release, January 30, 2012

(http://oag.ca.gov/news/press-releases/attorney-general-kamala-d-harris-announces-settlement-requiring-honest; accessed August 1, 2012).

[13] Health Canada, "Media Advisory and Product Safety Recall: Brazilian Blowout Solution Contains Formaldehyde," October 26, 2010, http://www.healthycanadians.gc.ca/recall-alert-rappel-avis/hc-sc/2010/13437a-eng.php (accessed August 2, 2012).

[14] Environmental Defence Canada, *Not So Sexy: The Health Risks of Secret Chemicals in Fragrance* (Toronto: Environmental Defence, 2010). In 2013, *CTV News* reported on a University of Guelph study that found that "nearly 60 percent of [herbal supplements] contained DNA from at least one plant species that wasn't listed on the product label." (See "Do You Take Herbal Supplements? Find Out What's Really in That Bottle," *CTV News*, October 11, 2013 (https://www.ctvnews.ca/health/do-you-take-herbal-supplements-find-out-what-s-really-in-that-bottle-1.1493311; accessed March 27, 2018).

[15] The term "girlcott" was first coined in 2005 by a group of high school girls who were protesting sexist T-shirt slogans by Abercrombie & Fitch. In her book *Not Just a Pretty Face* (Gabriola Island, BC: New Society Publishers, 2007), Stacy Malkan discusses synthetic chemicals and quotes Dr. Devra Davis as saying: "Boycotts mean saying no. Girlcotts mean yes. Women are the main purchasers of products and take responsibility for what goes into the home. We can organize to change market forces by saying we don't want cancer-causing products and we do want safer products. When enough women get together, we can make things happen." Since 2007, the term has continued to be applied to girl-led protests against a variety of companies and organizations, including Starbucks, Abercrombie & Fitch (again) and the National Rifle Association.

[16] C. Martina, B. Weiss and S. Swan, "Lifestyle Behaviours Associated with Exposures to Endocrine Disruptors," *Neurotoxicology* 6 (2012): 1247–1433, http://dx.doi.org/10.1016/j.neuro.2012.05.016.

[17] O. Geiss, S. Tirendi, J. Barrero-Moreno and D. Kotzias, "Investigation of Volatile Organic Compounds and Phthalates Present in the Cabin Air of Used Private Cars," *Environment International* 35 (2009): 1188–95.

[18] R. Rudel, J. Gray, C. Engel, T. Rawsthorne, R. Dodson, J. Ackerman, J. Rizzo et al., "Food Packaging and Bisphenol A and Bis(2-ethyhexyl) Phthalate Exposure: Findings from a Dietary Intervention," *Environmental Health Perspectives* 119 (2011): 914–20.

[19] P. Greenfield, "Eating Out Increases Levels of Phthalates in the Body, Study Finds," *The Guardian*, March 29, 2018 (https://www.theguardian.com /society/2018/mar/29/eating-out-increases-levels-of-phthalates-in-the -body-study-finds?CMP=share_btn_tw; accessed April 18, 2018).

[20] R. Kwapniewski, S. Kozaczka, R. Hauser, M. Silva, A. Calafat and D. Duty, "Occupational Exposure to Dibutyl Phthalate among Manicurists," *Journal of Occupational and Environmental Medicine* 50 (2008): 705–11.

[21] L. Parlett, A. Calafat and S. Swan, "Women's Exposure to Phthalates in Relation to Use of Personal Care Products," *Journal of Exposure Science and Environmental Epidemiology*, November 21, 2012, doi: 10.1038/jes.2012.105.

[22] J. Meeker, S. Sathyanarayana and S. Swan, "Phthalates and Other Additives in Plastics: Human Exposure and Associated Health Outcomes," *Philosophical Transactions of the Royal Society of London B: Biological Sciences* 364 (2009): 2097–113.

[23] S. Swan, K. Main, F. Liu, S. Stewart, R. Kruse, A. Calafat, C. Mao et al., "Decrease in Anogenital Distance among Male Infants with Prenatal Phthalate Exposure," *Environmental Health Perspectives* 113 (2005): 1056–61.

[24] S. Swan, F. Liu, M. Hines, R. Kruse, C. Wang, J. Redmon, A. Sparks et al., "Prenatal Phthalate Exposure and Reduced Masculine Play in Boys," *International Journal of Andrology* 33 (2010): 259–69.

[25] "Phthalate Levels in Expectant Fathers Influence Sperm Epigenetics, Study Suggests," *Medical Life Sciences*, September 12, 2017 (https://www.news -medical.net/news/20170912/Phthalate-levels-in-expectant-fathers-influence -sperm-epigenetics-study-suggests.aspx; accessed April 18, 2018).

[26] A. Calafat, X. Ye, L. Wong, A. Bishop and L. Needham, "Urinary Concentrations of Four Parabens in the U.S. Population: NHANES 2005– 2006," *Environmental Health Perspectives* 118 (2010): 679–85.

[27] P. Darbre, A. Aljarrah, W. Miller, N. Coldham, M. Sauer and G. Pope, "Concentrations of Parabens in Human Breast Tumours," *Journal of Applied Toxicology* 24 (2004): 5–13.

[28] N. Janjua, G. Mortensen, A. Andersson, B. Kongshoj, N. Skakkebaek and H. Wulf, "Systemic Uptake of Diethyl Phthalate, Dibutyl Phthalate and Butyl Paraben Following Whole-Body Topical Application and Reproductive and Thyroid Hormone Levels in Humans," *Environmental Science and Technology* 41 (2007): 5564–70.

[29] L. Barr, G. Metaxas, C. Harbach, L. Savoy and P. Darbre, "Measurement of Paraben Concentrations in Human Breast Tissue at Serial Locations across the Breast from Axilla to Sternum," *Journal of Applied Toxicology* 3 (2012): 219–32.

[30] P. Darbre, D. Pugazhendhi and F. Mannello, "Aluminium and Human Breast Diseases," *Journal of Inorganic Biochemistry* 105 (2011): 1484–88.

[31] U.S. Food and Drug Administration, "Does FDA Regulate the Use of Preservatives in Cosmetics?" February 22, 2018, https://www.fda.gov /Cosmetics/ProductsIngredients/Ingredients/ucm128042.htm#regulations (accessed May 31, 2018).

[32] Since 2012, Dabre has continued her important research and advocacy. In 2015 she contributed a chapter to *Endocrine Disruption and Human Health*, arguing that "personal care products" contain endocrine-disrupting chemicals absorbed through the skin, potentially generating a range of harmful side effects. See P. D. Dabre and P. W. Harvey, "Regulatory Considerations for Dermal Application of Endocrine Disrupters in Personal Care Products," chapter 19 of *Endocrine Disruption and Human Health* (Cambridge, MA: Academic Press, 2015); https://www.sciencedirect.com/science/article/pii /B9780128011393000193. She has also authored two reports since then on applied toxicology and breast tissue, as well as an astute but depressing research overview on endocrine disruptors and obesity. See P.D. Darbe, "Endocrine Disruptors and Obesity," *Current Obesity Reports* no. 1 (March 2017) 6: 18–27 (https://link.springer.com/article/10.1007/s13679-017-0240-4).

[33] S. Khanna and P. Darbre, "Parabens Enable Suspension Growth of MCF-10A Immortalized, Non-transformed Human Breast Epithelial Cells," *Journal of Applied Toxicology*, June 29, 2012, (https://www.ncbi.nlm.nih.gov /pubmed/22744862; accessed March 13, 2018).

[34] P. Darbre and A. Charles, "Environmental Oestrogens and Breast Cancer: Evidence for Combined Involvement of Dietary, Household and Cosmetic Xenoestrogens," *Anticancer Research* 30 (2010): 815–28.

[35] My phthalate shopping list included the following:

Hair

Pantene Pro-V Sheer Volume shampoo and conditioner; Pantene Body Builder mousse; TRESemmé European Freeze Hold hairspray

Shaving

Gillette Deep Cleansing shave gel

Other Toiletries

Calvin Klein Eternity for Men; Right Guard Sport regular deodorant; Jergens original scent lotion

Kitchen

Dawn Ultra Concentrated liquid/antibacterial hand soap (apple blossom scent)

Test Room

Glade Plug-in Scented Oil, Morning Walk scent (plugged in for 2 hours on Tuesday)

[36] Ibid.

[37] One study concluded that consumer products and different indoor sources dominate the exposure to dimethyl, diethyl, benzyl butyl, diisononyl and diisodecyl phthalates, whereas food has a major influence on the exposure to diisobutyl, dibutyl and di(2-ethylhexyl) phthalates. See M. Wormuth, M. Scheringer, M. Vollenweider and K. Hungerbühler, "What Are the Sources of Exposure to Eight Frequently Used Phthalic Acid Esters in Europeans?" *Risk Analysis* 26, no. 3 [2006]). Another, more recent study found, somewhat hopefully, that both "legislative activity and advocacy campaigns" may have played a beneficial role in limiting Americans' exposure to phthalates. See: A. R. Zota, A. M. Calafat and T. J. Woodruff, "Temporal Trends in Phthalate Exposures: Findings from the National Health and Nutrition Examination Survey, 2001–2010," *Environmental Health Perspectives* 122, no. 3 (March 2014): 235–41.

[38] In the orioginal version of *Slow Death by Rubber Duck,* we conducted a much simpler experiment comparing phthalate levels during and after wearing conventional personal-care products. In this experiment, we wanted to design something that would be more useful for consumers: a comparison of synthetic chemical levels from conventional and natural cosmetics, since virtually nobody will go cosmetics-free. As far as we know, the paraben experiment and comparison of levels resulting from conventional and natural cosmetics is a "first."

[39] The following are the products they used:

Jessa Blades—Conventional Products

Neutrogena Pore Refining Cleanser; Neutrogena Alcohol-Free Toner; Estée Lauder DayWear Plus Multi Protection Anti-Oxidant Crème; Pantene Pro-V Moisture Renewal 2-in-1 shampoo; Pantene Pro-V Moisture Renewal conditioner; Herbal Essences Set Me Up mousse; Herbal Essences Set Me Up Extra Hold styling gel; John Frieda Luxurious Volume Extra Hold hairspray; Olay Body Ultra Moisture Body Wash with Shea Butter; Irish Spring Original deodorant soap; Lady Speed Stick 24/7 antiperspirant deodorant in Cool Breeze; Vaseline Intensive Care Total Moisture Dry Skin lotion; Alfred Sung Forever perfume; Dial Complete Antibacterial Foaming Hand Wash; Covergirl TruBlend pressed powder; Physicians Formula Summer Eclipse Radiant Bronzing Powder; Revlon ColorStay Mineral Blush; L'Oréal Neutrals eyeshadow; Covergirl Professional Super Thick Lash mascara; Revlon ColorStay Overtime Lipcolor; Sally Hansen Insta-Dri nail color

Jessa Blades—Green Products

Aubrey Organics shampoo; Aubrey Organics conditioner; Dr. Hauschka eyeshadow; Zosimos Botanicals eyeliner; Couleur Caramel mascara; Organic Pharmacy Honey and Jasmine Mask; Earth Tu Face Body Butter; TMS Beauty concealer; Jane Iredale PurePressed powder; Nine Naturals body wash; Sprout lip balm; Organic Pharmacy blush

Ray Civello—Conventional Products

Gillette Fusion shaving gel Neutrogena Men Post Shave lotion; Neutrogena Pore Refining cleanser; Nivea for Men moisturizer; Pantene Pro-V Always Smooth shampoo; Pantene Pro-V Sheer Volume conditioner; Bed Head for Men Matte Separation Workable Wax; Dove Men+Care Deep Clean bodywash; Irish Spring Original deodorant soap; Old Spice deodorant; Vaseline Men Fast Absorbing lotion; Axe body spray; Dial Complete Antibacterial Foaming Hand Wash

Ray Civello—Green Products

Aveda Caribbean Therapy Body Crème; Aveda Calming body cleanser; Aveda Rosemary Mint Hand and Body Wash; Aveda Hand Relief; Aveda Foot Relief; Aveda Tourmaline Charged Hydrating Crème; Aveda Men Pure-Formance shampoo; Aveda Men Pure-Formance conditioner; Aveda Men Pure-Formance Grooming Clay; Aveda Men Pure-Formance shave cream; Aveda Men Pure-Formance Dual Action aftershave

Though it's impossible to nail down with complete precision which amounts of phthalates and parabens came from which specific products, the selection—according to a variety of sources—both likely contained the chemicals in question and replicated the typical product selection of countless consumers.

[40] R. Dodson, M. Nishioka, L. Standley, L. Perovich, J. Brody and R. Rudel, "Endocrine Disruptors and Asthma-Associated Chemicals in Consumer Products," *Environmental Health Perspectives* 20 (2012): 935–43.

[41] Environmental Working Group, Skin Deep Cosmetics Database (http://www.ewg.org/skindeep/; accessed September 20, 2012).

[42] The lab in British Columbia analyzed the urine samples for the following phthalates and parabens: monoethyl phthalate (MEP), mono(2-ethylhexyl) phthalate (MEHP), mono(2-ethyl-5-hydroxyhexyl) phthalate (MEHHP), mono(2-ethyl-5-oxohexyl) phthalate (MEOHP), monobenzyl phthalate (MBzP), mono(3-carboxypropyl) phthalate (MCPP), monomethyl phthalate (MMP), mono-isobutyl phthalate (MiBP), mono-n-butyl phthalate (MnBP) and methyl, ethyl, n-propyl, butyl and benzyl parabens.

[43] N. Janjua, H. Frederiksen, N. Skakkebaek, H. Wulf and A. Andersson, "Urinary Excretion of Phthalates and Parabens after Repeated Whole-Body Application in Humans," *International Journal of Andrology* 3 (2008): 118–30.

[44] T. Chen, "The Impact of the Shea Nut Industry on Women's Empowerment in Burkina Faso: A Multi-dimensional Study Focusing on the Central, Central-West and Hauts-Bassins Regions," *United Nations Food and Agriculture Organization*, 2017 (http://www.fao.org/3/a-i8062e.pdf; accessed April 12, 2018).

[45] Tonnages of shea nuts: J. Funt, managing director, Global Shea Alliance, personal correspondence with author, July 18, 2012.

[46] "Shea Nut Production Provides Jobs and Empowerment for West African Women,"*Africa Dispatch* (https://journalism.nyu.edu/publishing/africadispatch /2013/06/28/shea-nut-production-provides-jobs-and-empowerment-for -west-african-women/; accessed April 12, 2018).

[47] "Loblaw Companies Limited," George Weston Limited, 2011 (http://www.weston.ca/en/Loblaw-Companies-Ltd.aspx; accessed April 1, 2018).

Two: The World's Slipperiest Substance

¹ U.S. Centers for Disease Control and Prevention, PFOA Factsheet
(https://www.cdc.gov/biomonitoring/PFOA_FactSheet.html; accessed
December 8, 2008).

² Ibid.

³ Environmental Protection Agency, "Phaseout of PFOS," correspondence
from Charles Auer, May 16, 2000 (http://www.chemicalindustryarchives.org/
dirtysecrets/scotchgard/pdfs/226-0629.pdf; accessed December 5, 2008).

⁴ T. Lougheed, "Environmental Stain Fading Fast," *Environmental Health
Perspectives* 115, no. 1 (January 2007): A20.

⁵ Danish Environmental Protection Agency, Survey of Chemical Substances in
Consumer Products, no. 99, "Survey and Environmental/Health Assessment of
Fluorinated Substances in Impregnated Consumer Products and Impregnating
Agents," October 2008 (http://chm.pops.int/Portals/0/download.aspx?d=UNEP
-POPS-NIP-GUID-ArticlePaperPFOSInv-4.En.pdf; accessed December 15, 2008).

⁶ J. Eilperin, "Compound in Teflon a 'Likely Carcinogen,'" *Washington Post*,
June 29, 2005. In 2005, the EPA moved the rating for PFOA up from "possible carcinogen" to "likely human carcinogen," based on its review of the evidence. At the time, DuPont actively disputed this categorization. As of March
2018, the EPA has established a "health advisory" for PFOA based on its
assessment of the "latest peer-reviewed science." See Environmental
Protection Agency, "Drinking Water Health Advisories for PFOA and PFOS"
(https://www.epa.gov/ground-water-and-drinking-water/drinking-water
-health-advisories-pfoa-and-pfos; accessed March 8, 2018).

⁷ A. Kärrman, B. van Bavel, U. Järnberg, L. Hardell and G. Lindström,
"Perfluorinated Chemicals in Relation to Other Persistent Organic
Pollutants in Human Blood," *Chemosphere* 64, no. 9 (August 2006): 1582–91.

⁸ "Scientists Find Rising PFC Levels in Polar Bears," "Pesticide and Toxic
Chemical News," Chemical Business News Base, March 31, 2008.

⁹ W. Vetter, V. Gall and K. Skírnisson, "Polyhalogenated Compounds (PCBs,
Chlordanes, HCB and BFRs) in Four Polar Bears (*Ursus maritimus*) That
Swam Malnourished from East Greenland to Iceland," *Science of the Total
Environment*, November 2015, 533: 290–6 (https://www.ncbi.nlm.nih.gov
/pubmed/26172596; accessed April 4, 2018).

[10] J. W. Martin, M. M. Smithwick, B. M. Braune, P. F. Hoekstra, D. C. G. Muir and S. A. Mabury, "Identification of Long Chain Perfluorinated Acids in Biota from the Canadian Arctic," *Environmental Science and Technology* 38 (2004a): 373–80.

[11] C. Lyons, *Stain-Resistant, Nonstick, Waterproof and Lethal: The Hidden Dangers of C8* (Westport, CT: Praeger, 2007).

[12] "DuPont in Sticky Situation over Teflon Chemical" (including interview with Della Tennant), *Living on Earth*, National Public Radio, broadcast January 6, 2006.

[13] Amended Class Action Complaint, Civil Action no. 01-C-2518, Circuit Court of Kanawha County, West Virginia, 17, https://www.hpcbd.com /dupont/Amended-Complaint.PDF (accessed March 21, 2018).

[14] Environmental Protection Agency, "EPA Settles PFOA Case Against DuPont for Largest Environmental Administrative Penalty in Agency History," news release, December 14, 2005, http://yosemite.epa.gov/opa /admpress.nsf/68b5f2d54f3eefd2852570150051τfbf/fdcb2f665cac66bb8525 70d7005d6665!OpenDocument (accessed March 21, 2018).

[15] K. Cook, "EWG TSCA 8(e) Petition to U. S. EPA," correspondence from Ken Cook to Christine Todd Whitman, Administrator, EPA, April 11, 2003, https://www.ewg.org/news/testimony-official-correspondence/ewg-tsca -8e-petition-us-epa#.Wp8KrJPwbOQ (accessed December 5, 2008).

[16] "3M and Scotchgard: 'Heroes of Chemistry' or a 20-Year Coverup?" *Chemical Industry Archives*, http://www.chemicalindustryarchives.org /dirtysecrets/scotchgard/1.asp (accessed August 10, 2008).

[17] Ibid.

[18] Dupont, "DuPont Participation in Voluntary EPA PFOA Stewardship Program," January 27, 2006, http://www2.dupont.com/Media_Center/en _US/news_releases/2006/article20060127c.html (accessed December 8, 2008).

[19] Environmental Working Group, "PFCs: Global Contaminants: DuPont's Spin about PFOA," research report, April 3, 2003. The EWG report describes an unpublished report in which 3M discovered these birth defects while conducting studies on rats in 1983. DuPont made the results available as part of the class action suit.

[20] Law Firm of Hill, Peterson, Carper, Bee & Deitzler, "C-8 Class Action Settlement," https://www.hpcbd.com/Personal-Injury/DuPont-C8/C8 -Class-Action-Settlement.shtml (accessed December 5, 2008).

[21] H. Brubaker, "DuPont Settles Pollution Lawsuit: The Firm Will Pay $108 Million to Resolve Allegations That Discharge from a W. Va. Plant Contaminated Water Supplies," *Philadelphia Inquirer*, September 9, 2004.

[22] "DuPont Position Statement on PFOA,"DuPont, 2018, www.dupont.com /corporate-functions/our-company/insights/articles/position-statements /articles/pfoa.html (accessed April 4, 2018).

[23] DuPont, 2007 Annual Review, http://library.corporate-ir.net/library/73 /733/73320/items/283770/DD_2007_AR_v2.pdf (accessed November 8, 2008).

[24] R. E. Wells, "Fatal Toxicosis in Pet Birds Caused by Overheated Cooking Pan Lined with Polytetrafluoroethylene," *Journal of the American Veterinary Medical Association* 182 (1983): 1248–50.

[25] Dupont, "Learn More about DuPont™ Teflon®."

[26] J. Houlihan, K. Thayer and J. Klein, "Canaries in the Kitchen: Teflon Toxicosis," research report, May 15, 2003.

[27] Ibid.

[28] Ibid.

[29] R. F. Brown and P. Rice, "Electron Microscopy of Rat Lung Following a Single Acute Exposure to Perfluoroisobutylene (PFIB): A Sequential Study of the First 24 Hours Following Exposure," *International Journal of Experimental Pathology* 72 (1991): 437–50.

[30] M. Son, E. Maruyama, Y. Shindo, N. Suganuma, S. Sato and M. Ogawa, "A Case of Polymer Fume Fever with Interstitial Pneumonia Caused by Inhalation of Polytetrafluoroethylene (Teflon)," *Japanese Journal of Toxicology* 19, no. 3 (2006): 279–82.

[31] A. M. Calafat, L.-Y. Wong, Z. Kuklenyik, J. A. Reidy and L. L. Needham, "Polyfluoroalkyl Chemicals in the U.S. Population: Data from the National Health and Nutrition Examination Survey (NHANES) 2003–2004 and Comparisons with NHANES 1999–2000," *Environmental Health Perspectives* 115, no. 11 (November 2007): 1596–1602.

[32] M. J. A. Dinglasan-Panlilio and S. A. Mabury, "Significant Residual

Fluorinated Alcohols Present in Various Fluorinated Materials,"
Environmental Science and Technology 40 (2007): 1447–53.

[33] 1. Total condo room volume was roughly 26.6 m³.

2. Total surface area of protected material was roughly 19 m² (drapes = 1
   m², couch = 3 m² and carpet = 15 m²).

3. Teflon Advanced recommends an application rate of 200 ft² per gallon of
   diluted product (one part pure product, four parts water). In metric
   measurement this equates to roughly 19 m² per 4 L (litres) of "diluted
   product." So, considering the recommended application rate, 4 L of
   diluted product, which is equal to 800 mL of pure product, would need
   to be applied (since the coverage area was about 19 m²).

4. In 800 mL of pure product, there would be about 0.15 g of fluorotelomer
   alcohols (FTOHs), the precursors to PFOA. Assuming this was all
   released (which is unlikely), the result would be an air concentration of
   2.5 µg/m³. This is on the high side of what has been calculated for indoor
   air, Butt told us, but not absurdly high.

5. The conversion of expected indoor air concentration to a response in the
   blood levels is where things got tricky. Over the twenty-four hours of
   exposure (two days, twelve hours per day), Butt assumed that Rick would
   breathe about 9 m³ of air, which, at a rate of 2.5 µg/m³, would result in
   exposure to 22.5 µg of FTOH. If we assume that all of the FTOH is taken up
   across the lungs (a worst-case scenario) and that all of it is converted to
   PFOA and other perfluorinated acids (again, at a conversion efficiency far
   greater than what would be expected in reality), Rick would accumulate
   22.5 µg of FTOH in his blood. Based on average human blood volumes,
   Butt assumed that Rick (who, at six foot six, is taller than most) had about
   8 L of blood. So if all the perfluorinated acids accumulated in his blood
   (which again is unlikely, as they would presumably also accumulate in the
   liver and kidneys), the concentration would increase to roughly 3 ng/mL,
   similar to Rick's existing PFOA value.

Three: The New PCBs

[1] A. R. Horrocks and D. Price, *Fire Retardant Materials* (Cambridge:
Woodhead, 2001).

[2] Chlorinated flame-retardants work in a very similar manner and present similar environmental concerns. There is a great deal of concern over the use of chlorinated tris-BP (2, 3-dibromopropyl phosphate) as a flame retardant.

[3] M. Alaee, P. Arias, A. Sjödin and Å. Bergman, "An Overview of Commercially Used Brominated Flame Retardants, Their Applications, Their Use Patterns in Different Countries/Regions and Possible Modes of Release," *Environment International* 29, no. 6 (September 2008): 683–89.

[4] L. Charlton, "Intentions Gone Astray: The Facts about Tris Don't Leave Much Choice," *New York Times*, July 3, 1997, 97.

[5] N. Brozan, "Flame Retardant Sleepwear: Is There a Risk of Cancer?" *New York Times*, April 10, 1976, 38.

[6] Ibid.

[7] "Ban Asked on Children's Wear with Flame Retardant," *New York Times*, February 9, 1977, 21.

[8] A. Blum, M. D. Gold, B. N. Ames, C. Kenyon, F. R. Jones, E. A. Hett, R. C. Dougherty et al., "Children Absorb Tris-BP Flame Retardant from Sleepwear: Urine Contains the Mutagenic Metabolite, 2,3-Dibromopropanol," *Science* 201, no. 4360 (September 15, 1978): 1020–23.

[9] M. Hosenball, "Karl Marx and the Pajama Game," *Mother Jones*, November/ December 1979.

[10] Ibid.

[11] L. J. Carter, "Michigan's PBB Incident: Chemical Mix-Up Leads to Disaster," *Science* 92, no. 4236 (April 16, 1976): 240–43.

[12] M. R. Reich, "Environmental Politics and Science: The Case of PBB Contamination in Michigan," *American Journal of Public Health* 73, no. 3 (March 1983): 301–13.

[13] Michigan Department of Community Health, "PBBs (Polybrominated Biphenyls) in Michigan Frequently Asked Questions – 2011 Update," www.michigan.gov/documents/mdch_PBB_FAQ_92051_7.pdf (accessed March 7, 2018).

[14] Reich, "Environmental Politics and Science."

[15] J. Brody, "Perils in a Chemical World: PBB Incident in Michigan Is Viewed

as Latest Evidence of Need for New Investigative System," *New York Times*, November 11, 1976, 61.

[16] J. Lowy, "Safety of a New Flame Retardant Questioned," Scripps Howard News Service, October 11, 2004.

[17] T. Yoshimura, "Yusho in Japan," *Industrial Health* 41, no. 3 (2003): 139–48.

[18] K. Hooper and T. A. McDonald, "The PBDEs: An Emerging Environmental Challenge and Another Reason for Breast Milk Monitoring Programs," *Environmental Health Perspectives* 108, no. 5 (May 2000): 387–92.

[19] Ibid.

[20] The ability of PCBs and PBDEs to act as endocrine disruptors has received more public scrutiny than their neurotoxicity during development. The *yu-cheng* children were mentally handicapped, and several high-quality epidemiological studies have documented adverse effects of PCBs on IQ and other behaviours at environmental levels. The effects of PCBs and PBDEs on behaviour in animals are pretty much the same. Moreover, the biochemical effects in brain tissue are the same for both kinds of chemicals. So, although the epidemiological studies on PBDEs have not been done, it is highly likely that PDBEs are developmental neurotoxicants in humans. Although the mechanisms are largely independent of endocrine disruption, the endocrine system may produce some behavioural effects.

[21] A. Blum and B. N. Ames, "Flame Retardant Additives as Possible Cancer Hazards," *Science* 195, no. 4273 (January 7, 1997): 17–23.

[22] A. Sjodin, L.-Y. Wong, R. S. Jones, A. Park, Y. Zhang, C. Hodge, E. Depietro et al., "Serum Concentrations of Polybrominated Diphenyl Ethers (PBDEs) and Polybrominated Biphenyl (PBB) in the United States Population: 2003–2004," *Environmental Science and Technology* 42, no. 4 (February 15, 2004): 1377–84.

[23] Note that the "P" in PBDE stands for "poly" and refers to a number of individual BDEs.

[24] "Methyl Bromide Bill Riles 'Greens,'" *Chemical Marketing Reporter* 248, no. 1 (July 3, 1995), 4.

[25] "Global Flame Retardant Market Projected to Reach US$11.96 Billion by 2025,"*Additives for Polymers*, 2017, no. 1 (January 2017): 10–11

(https://www.sciencedirect.com/science/article/pii/S0306374717300143; accessed June 14, 2018).

[26] According to the U. S. Environmental Protection Agency, PBDEs remain widely used in "textiles, plastics, wire insulation and automobiles" and often "serve as flame retardants for electrical equipment, electronic devices, furniture, textiles and other household products." See "Polybrominated Diphenyl Ethers (PBDEs)," Environmental Protection Agency, January 19, 2017, https://www.epa.gov/assessing-and-managing-chemicals-under-tsca /polybrominated-diphenyl-ethers-pbdes (accessed April 3, 2018) and "Technical Fact Sheet – Polybrominated Diphenyl Ethers (PBDEs)" Environmental Protection Agency, November 2017, https://www.epa.gov /sites/production/files/2014-03/documents/ffrrofactsheet_contaminant _perchlorate_january2014_final_0.pdf (accessed April 4, 2018).

[27] Bromine Science and Environmental Forum, "An Introduction to Brominated Flame Retardants," October 19, 2000. According to the BSEF, "Brominated flame retardants have saved thousands of lives . . . In the last 10 years, a 20% reduction in fire deaths is a result of the use of flame retardants."

[28] Monsanto Company, "PCB Environmental Pollution Abatement Plan," 1969, https://www.documentcloud.org/documents/3032105-Monsanto-PCB-Pollution-Abatement-Plan.html (accessed July 5, 2008).

[29] D. Rosenbaum, "Monsanto Plans to Curb Chemical," *New York Times*, July 15, 1970, 27.

[30] "Phase Out Is Set of PCBs Chemical: Monsanto Acts after Years of Public Health Hazard," *New York Times*, January 27, 1976, 54.

[31] World Health Organization, "Fact Sheet on Reduced Ignition Propensity

[32] World Health Organization, "Fact Sheet on Reduced Ignition Propensity (RIP) Cigarettes," November 2014 (www.who.int/tobacco/industry/product_regulation/factsheetreducedignitionpropensitycigarettes/en/; accessed June 14, 2018).

[33] http://media.apps.chicagotribune.com/flames/index.html (accessed September 10, 2018).

[34] W. Guo, A. Holden, S. Crispo Smith, R. Gephart, M. Petreas, J.-S. Park, "PBDE Levels in Breast Milk Are Decreasing in California" Chemosphere 150, (2016): 505-13.

[35] E. Leamy, "How to Find Flame-Resistant Pajamas for Kids, Without Toxic Chemicals," *Washington Post*, November 16, 2017 (https://www.washingtonpost.com/lifestyle/on-parenting/how-to-find-flame-resistant -pajamas-for-kids-without-toxic-chemicals/2017/11/08/fe587216-c32d -11e7-afe9-4f60b5a6c4a0_story.html?utm_term=.c51ab2b30bff; accessed April 2, 2018).

Four: Quicksilver, Slow Death

[1] L. B. Wright, "Actress Describes Mercury Poisoning Ordeal: Daphne Zuniga Was Eating a High Seafood Diet," *ABC News*, October 21, 2005.

[2] Ibid.

[3] U.S. Centers for Disease Control and Prevention, "Biomonitoring Summary: Mercury," CAS No. 7439-97-6 (https://www.cdc.gov/biomonitoring /Mercury_BiomonitoringSummary.html; accessed April 10, 2018).

[4] R. Canuel, S. Boucher de Grosbois, M. Lucotte, L. Atikessé, C. Larose and I. Rheault, "New Evidence on the Effects of Tea on Mercury Metabolism in Humans," *Archives of Environmental and Occupational Health* 61, no. 5 (2006): 232–38.

[5] S.-M. Shim, M. G. Ferruzzi, Y.-C. Kim, E. M. Janle and C. R. Santerre, "Impact of Phytochemical-Rich Foods on Bioaccessibility of Mercury from Fish," *Food Chemistry* 112, no. 1 (January 2009): 46–50

[6] Environmental Protection Agency, "National Listing of Fish Advisories General Fact Sheet 2011" (https://www.epa.gov/fish-tech/national-listing-Fish-advisories-general-fact-sheet-2011; accessed March 7, 2018).

[7] Oceana, "Mercury Health Effects" (http://oceana.org/our-work/stop-ocean-pollution/mercury/learn-act/mercurys-health-effects; accessed November 30, 2008).

[8] U.S. Food and Drug Administration, "An Important Message for Pregnant Women and Women of Childbearing Age Who May Become Pregnant about the Risks of Mercury in Fish," consumer advisory (https://www.fda.gov/ OHRMS/DOCKETS/ac/02/briefing/3872_Advisory%201.pdf; accessed August 5, 2008).

[9] C. Johnson, "Elemental Mercury Use in Religious and Ethnic Practices in Latin American and Caribbean Communities in New York City," *Population and Environment* 20, no. 5 (May 1999): 443–53.

[10] There are only a few examples of mercury being used for murder, as slow death and the telltale signs that mark its use make it less desirable than arsenic as a poison.

[11] K. L. Rasmussen, J. L. Boldsen, H. K. Kristensen, L. Skytte, K. L. Hansen, L. Molholm, P. M. Grootes, "Mercury Levels in Danish Medieval Human Bones," *Journal of Archaeological Science* 35, no. 8 (August 2008): 2295–96.

[12] "Mercury Was Once Seen as a Cure-all," *Free Lance–Star*, August 7, 2006.

[13] J. J. Putman, "Quicksilver and Slow Death," *National Geographic*, October 1972, 506–27.

[14] T. Ogura, J. Ramírez-Ortiz, Z. M. Arroyo-Villaseñor, S. Hernández Martínez, J. P. Palafox-Hernández, L. H. García de Alba and Q. Fernando, "Zacatecas (Mexico) Companies Extract Hg from Surface Soil Contaminated by Ancient Mining Industries," *Water, Air, and Soil Pollution* 148, no. 1–4 (September 2003): 167–177 (https://link.springer.com/article/10.1023 /A:1025497726115; accessed March 22, 2018).

[15] Pollution Probe, *Mercury in the Environment: A Primer* (Toronto: Pollution Probe, 2003).

[16] T. Clarkson, L. Magos and G. J. Myers, "The Toxicology of Mercury: Current Exposures and Clinical Manifestations," *New England Journal of Medicine* 349, no. 18 (October 30, 2003): 1731–37.

[17] A. C. Rennie, M. McGregor-Schuerman, I. M. Dale, C. Robinson and R. McWilliam, "Mercury Poisoning after Spillage at Home from a Sphygmomano-meter on Loan from Hospital," *British Medical Journal* 319 (August 7, 1999): 366–67.

[18] "Colleagues Vow to Learn from Chemist's Death," *New York Times*, October 3, 1997.

[19] Clarkson et al., "The Toxicology of Mercury."

[20] The World Health Organization is unequivocal on these links, stating on its website that "The primary health effect of methylmercury is impaired neurologi-cal development." See "Mercury and Health," World Health Organization, March 2017 (www.who.int/mediacentre/factsheets/fs361/en/; accessed April 4, 2018).

[21] M. J. Vimy and F. L. Lorscheider, "Dental Amalgam Mercury: Background," a summary of research results on dental amalgam mercury to date, Faculty of Medicine and Medical Physiology, University of Calgary, May 1993.

22 Canadian Council of Ministers of the Environment, *Canada Wide Standard on Mercury for Dental Amalgam Waste*, September 2001.

23 J. A. Martin and J. R. Guernsey, "A Comprehensive Review of the Health Effects of Fungicides," poster presentation, Department of Community Health and Epidemiology, Dalhousie University, Halifax, Nova Scotia, 2008 (http://resources.cpha.ca/CPHA/Conf/Code/PresentationsAbstract.php?r=0&Year=2008&ID=A08-211&l=F&site=am; accessed November 30, 2008).

24 An investigative piece from the *Globe and Mail* in 2007 also looked into links between the use of pesticides on Prince Edward Island and higher-than-average rates of cancer. The article presented several anecdotal accounts of elevated rates of childhood cancer, but noted that the scientific research remained inconclusive. See M. Mittelstaedt, "Pesticides Are What Is Killing Our Kids," *Globe and Mail*, December 6, 2006 (https://www.theglobeandmail.com/news/national/pesticides-are-what-is-killing-our-kids/article18179217/; accessed April 5, 2018).

25 J. Ui, ed., *Industrial Pollution in Japan* (Tokyo: United Nations University Press, 1992).

26 T. Shigeto, *The Political Economy of the Environment: The Case of Japan* (Vancouver: University of British Columbia Press, 2000).

27 A 2017 report from Reuters states that there were "3,000 certified victims of Minamata disease" that "more than 20,000 people have sought to be designated victims." See M. Funakoshi and K. H. Kim, "More than 60 Years On, Japan's Mercury-Poison Victims Fight to Be Heard," Reuters, September 20, 2017 (https://www.reuters.com/article/us-japan-minamata-victims/more-than-60-years-on-japans-mercury-poison-victims-fight-to-be-heard-idUSKCN1BV326; accessed March 27, 2018).

28 National Institute for Minamata Disease (http://www.nimd.go.jp/archives/english/index.html; accessed November 30, 2008).

29 Goldberg. "The Town Where Mercury Still Rises," *New York Times*, April 19, 2017 (https://www.nytimes.com/2017/04/19/opinion/the-town-where-mercury-still-rises.html; accessed November 8, 2017).

30 D. Bruser and J. Poisson, "Ontario Knew about Grassy Narrows Mercury Site for Decades, But Kept It Secret," *Toronto Star*, November 11, 2017

(https://www.thestar.com/news/canada/2017/11/11/ontario-knew-about
-mercury-site-near-grassy-narrows-for-decades-but-kept-it-secret.html;
accessed March 28, 2018).

[31] G. E. McKeown-Eyssen and J. Ruedy, "Methyl Mercury Exposure in
Northern Quebec: 1. Neurologic Findings in Adults," *American Journal of
Epidemiology* 118, no. 4 (1983): 461–69.

[32] B. Wheatley and S. Paradis, "Exposure of Canadian Aboriginal Peoples to
Methylmercury," *Water, Air, and Soil Pollution* 80, no. 1–4 (February 1995):
3–11 (http://www.springerlink.com/content/x317026557217813/fulltext.pdf;
accessed March 22, 2018).

[33] Pollution Probe, *Mercury in the Environment*.

[34] P. Grandjean, P. Weihe, R. White, F. Debas, S. Araki, K. Yokoyama, K. Murata,
et al., "Cognitive Deficit in 7-Year-Old Children with Prenatal Exposure to
Methylmercury," *Neurotoxicology Teratology* 19, no. 6 (1997): 417–28.

[35] Ibid.

[36] R. S. Rasmussen, J. Nettleton and M. T. Morrissey, "A Review of Mercury in
Seafood: Special Focus on Tuna," *Journal of Aquatic Food Product Technology*
14, no. 1 (2005): 1–3.

[37] Various pharmacies in Canada, for instance, have initiated thermometer
"take back" programs. See "Products That Contain Mercury: Thermometers
and Thermostats," Environment Canada, July 9, 2013 (https://www.canada.ca
/en/environment-climate-change/services/pollutants/mercury-environment
/products-that-contain/thermometers-thermostats.html; accessed April 5,
2018).

[38] "Mercury in Fish," Environment Canada, February 3, 2017 (https://www
.canada.ca/en/health-canada/services/food-nutrition/food-safety/chemical
-contaminants/environmental-contaminants/mercury/mercury-fish.html;
accessed April 5, 2018).

Five: Germophobia

[1] Environmental Working Group, "Pesticide in Soap, Toothpaste and Breast
Milk—Is It Kid-Safe?" Washington, D. C., July 17, 2008.

[2] E. Hartmann, "Banned Antimicrobial Chemicals Found in Many Household

Products," CNN, January 25, 2017 (https://www.cnn.com/2017/01/25/health/triclosan-household-items-partner/index.html; accessed April 3, 2018).

[3] Antimicrobial products defend against bacteria, viruses and fungi; antibacterial products defend only against bacteria.

[4] Alliance for the Prudent Use of Antibiotics (www.tufts.edu/med/apua; accessed March 8, 2016).

[5] A. E. Aiello, B. Marshall, S. B. Levy, P. Della-Latta, S. X. Lin and E. Larson, "Antibacterial Cleaning Products and Drug Resistance," *Emerging Infectious Diseases* 11, no. 10 (October 2005): 1565–70.

[6] E. L. Larson, S. X. Lin, C. Gomez-Pichardo and P. Della-Latta, "Effect of Antibacterial Home Cleaning and Handwashing Products: Infectious Disease Symptoms," *Annals of Internal Medicine* 140, no. 5 (2004): 321–29, quoted in A. Glaser, "The Ubiquitous Triclosan: A Common Antibacterial Agent Exposed," *Pesticides and You* 24, no. 3 (2004).

[7] R. Harrington, "Antibacterial Soap Is Not Better, Cleaner, or Safer, and You Probably Should Stop Using It," *Business Insider*, September 25, 2015 (www.businessinsider.com/is-soap-containing-triclosan-better-than-regular-soap-2015-9; accessed April 2, 2018).

[8] Ibid.

[9] M. Allmyr, M. Adolfsson-Erici, M. S. McLachlan and G. Sandborgh-England, "Triclosan in Plasma and Milk from Swedish Nursing Mothers and Their Exposure via Personal Care Products," *Science of the Total Environment* 372, no. 1 (2006): 87–93.

[10] A. M. Calafat, X. Ye, L.-Y. Wong, J. A. Reidy and L. L. Needham, "Urinary Concentrations of Triclosan in the U.S. Population: 2003–2004," *Environmental Health Perspectives* 116, no. 3 (2008): 303–7.

[11] D. W. Kolpin, E. T. Furlong, M. T. Meyer, E. M. Thurman, S. D. Zaugg, L. B. Barber and H. T. Buxton, "Pharmaceuticals, Hormones, and Other Organic Wastewater Contaminants in U.S. Streams, 1999–2000: A National Reconnaissance," *Environmental Science and Technology* 36 (2002): 1202–11.

[12] C. M. Foran, E. R. Bennett and W. H. Benson, "Developmental Evaluation of a Potential Non-steroidal Estrogen: Triclosan," *Marine Environmental Research* 50 (2000): 153–56.

[13] N. Veldhoen, R. C. Skirrow, H. Osachoff, H. Wigmore, D. J. Clapson, M. P. Gunderson, G. Van Aggelen et al., "The Bactericidal Agent Triclosan Modulates Thyroid Hormone-Associated Gene Expression and Disrupts Postembryonic Anuran Development," *Aquatic Toxicology* 80, no. 3 (December 2006): 217–27.

[14] T. L. Miller, D. J. Lorusso, M. L. Walsh and M. L. Deinzer, "The Acute Toxicity of Penta-, Hexa- and Heptachlorohydroxydiphenyl Ethers in Mice," *Journal of Toxicology and Environmental Health* 12, nos. 2–3 (1983): 245–53. The chemical has also been found to affect the onset of puberty in L. M. Zorrilla, E. K. Gibson, S. C. Jeffay, K. M. Crofton, W. R. Setzer, R. L. Cooper and T. E. Stoker, "The Effects of Triclosan on Puberty and Thyroid Hormones in Male Wistar Rats," *Toxicological Sciences* 107, no. 1 (January 2009): 56–64. More recent research on the negative impacts of triclosan includes G. W. Louis, D. R. Hallinger, M. J. Braxton, A. Kamel and T. E. Stoker, "Effects of Chronic Exposure to Triclosan on Reproductive and Thyroid Endpoints in the Adult Wistar Female Rat" *Journal of Toxicology and Environmental Health* 80, no. 4 (2017): 236–49.

[15] L. Tan, N. H. Neilsen, D. C. Young and Z. Trizna, "Use of Antimicrobial Agents in Consumer Products," *Archives of Dermatology* 138, no. 8 (2002): 1082–86.

[16] "Safety and Effectiveness of Health Care Antiseptics: Topical Antimicrobial Drug Products for Over-the-Counter Human Use," *Federal Register*, December 20, 2017 (https://www.federalregister.gov/documents/2017/12/20/2017-27317/safety-and-effectiveness-of-health-care-antiseptics-topical-antimicrobial-drug-products-for; accessed April 5, 2018).

[17] "Fact Sheet: The Top 10 Causes of Death," World Health Organization, January 2017 (www.who.int/mediacentre/factsheets/fs310/en/; accessed April 2, 2018).

[18] "SARS (Severe Acute Respiratory Syndrome)," World Health Organization, 2018 (www.who.int/ith/diseases/sars/en/; accessed April 3, 2018).

[19] K. Ashenburg, *The Dirt on Clean: An Unsanitized History* (Toronto: Knopf Canada, 2007).

[20] G. Sandborgh-Englund, M. Adolfsson-Erici, G. Odham and J. Ekstrand, "Pharmacokinetics of Triclosan Following Oral Ingestion in Humans: Part A," *Journal of Toxicology and Environmental Health* 69 (2006): 1861–73.

[21] R. Sutton, *Pesticide in Soap, Toothpaste and Breast Milk: Is It Kid-Safe?* (Washington, D. C.: Environmental Working Group, 2008).

[22] Calafat et al., "Urinary Concentrations of Triclosan."

[23] C. Shearer, "A Guide to the Nanotechnology Used in the Average Home," The Conversation, July 4, 2016 (http://theconversation.com/a-guide-to-the -nanotechnology-used-in-the-average-home-59312; accessed April 5, 2016).

[24] "Antimicrobial Coatings Market Size by Product," Global Market Insights, August 2016 (https://www.gminsights.com/industry-analysis/antimicrobial -coatings-market-report?utm_source=globenewswire.com&utm_medium =referral&utm_campaign=Paid_Globnewswire; accessed April 8, 2017).

[25] International Center for Technology Assessment, Executive Summary, Legal Petition Challenges EPA's Failure to Regulate Environmental and Health Threats from NanoSilver, May 1, 2008, http://appletonlaw.com/files /2009/PDFs/20_LegalPetition.PDF.

[26] "Silver Nanoparticles May Be Killing Beneficial Bacteria in Wastewater Treatment," Science Daily, April 30, 2008, http://www.sciencedaily.com.

[27] D. McShan, P. C. Ray and H. Yu, "Molecular Toxicity Mechanism of Nanosilver," *Journal of Food and Drug Analysis* 22, no.1 (March 2014) 1: 116–27 (https://www.sciencedirect.com/science/article/pii/S1021949814000118; accessed April 8, 2018).

[28] R. Senjen, "Nanosilver: A Threat to Soil, Water and Human Health?" (Melbourne: Friends of the Earth Australia, 2007).

[29] Ibid.

[30] Ibid.

[31] Ibid.

Six: Risky Business: 2,4-D and the Sound of Science

[1] T. Kiely, D. Donaldson and A. Grube, *Pesticides Industry Sales and Usage: 2000 and 2001 Market Estimates*, EPA-733-R-04-001 (Washington, D.C.: Environmental Protection Agency, 2004).

[2] C. Cox, "2,4-D: Toxicology," *Journal of Pesticide Reform* 19, no. 1 (Spring 1999).

3 W. Mieder, "The Grass Is Always Greener on the Other Side of the Fence: An American Proverb of Discontent," 1995 (www.deproverbio.com; accessed March 8, 2018).

4 E. Russell, *War and Nature: Fighting Humans and Insects with Chemicals from World War I to* Silent Spring (Cambridge: Cambridge University Press, 2001).

5 Ibid.

6 Industry Task Force on 2,4-D Research Data, "Straight Talk about 2,4-D Herbicide," March 17, 2016 (https://www.24d.org/PDF/Backgrounders /Backgrounder-StraightTalk-MythvFact.pdf; accessed March 8, 2018).

7 J. Troyer, "In the Beginning: The Multiple Discovery of the First Hormone Herbicides," *Weed Science* 49, no. 2 (March–April 2001): 290–97.

8 "Taking Stock of DDT," *American Journal of Public Health* 36, no. 6 (June 1946).

9 Russell, *War and Nature*.

10 K. Miller Stacy, "Cancer Risk Lingers for Long-Banned DDT," WebMD, April 29, 2008 (http://men.webmd.com/news/20080428/cancer-risk -lingers-for-long-banned-ddt; accessed March 22, 2018).

11 M. Aubé, C. Larochelle and P. Ayotte, "1,1-dichloro-2,2-bis(pchlorophenyl) ethylene(p,p'-DDE) Disrupts the Estrogen-Androgen Balance Regulating the Growth of Hormone-Dependent Breast Cancer Cells," *Breast Cancer Research* 10, no. 1 (February 2008), quoted in "DDT Compound Speeds Breast Cancer Growth," HealthDay, February 14, 2008 (https://consumer .healthday.com/cancer-information-5/breast-cancer-news-94/ddt-compound -speeds-breast-cancer-growth-612635.html; accessed March 22, 2018).

12 C. Cox, "2,4-D Toxicology: Part 2," *Journal of Pesticide Reform* 19, no. 2 (Summer 1999).

13 J. von Meding, "Agent Orange, Exposed: How U.S. Chemical Warfare in Vietnam Unleashed a Slow-Moving Disaster," The Conversation, October 3, 2017 (http://theconversation.com/agent-orange-exposed-how-u-s-chemical -warfare-in-vietnam-unleashed-a-slow-moving-disaster-84572; accessed April 8, 2018).

14 The testing was conducted by Accu-Chem Laboratories, Richardson, Texas.

15 C. Lu, K. Toepel, R. Irish, R.A. Fenske, D.B. Barr and R. Bravo, "Organic Diets Significantly Lower Children's Dietary Exposure to Organophosphorus

Pesticides," *Environmental Health Perspectives* 114, no. 2 (February 2006): 260–63.

[16] L. L. Needham, V. W. Burse, S. L. Head, M. P. Korver, P. C. McClure, J. S. Andrews Jr., D. L. Rowley, "Adipose Tissue/Serum Partitioning of Chlorinated Hydrocarbon Pesticides in Humans," *Chemosphere* 20 (1990): 975–80.

[17] United Nations Environment Programme, *Central America and the Caribbean: Regional Report*, December 2002.

[18] Centers for Disease Control and Prevention, *Third Report on Human Exposure to Environmental Chemicals* (Atlanta: CDC 2005).

[19] Environmental Working Group, Human Toxome Project (https://www.ewg .org/sites/humantoxome/; accessed March 6, 2018).

[20] Ibid.

[21] A. Pollack, "E.P.A. Denies an Environmental Group's Request to Ban a Widely Used Weed Killer," *New York Times*, April 9, 2012 (https://www.nytimes.com /2012/04/10/business/energy-environment/epa-denies-request-to-ban -24-d-a-popular-weed-killer.html?_r=0; accessed April 8, 2018).

[22] L. Wood, "Global Pesticides Market: Trends and Forecasts," Business Wire, February 24, 2016 (https://www.businesswire.com/news/home /20160224006416/en/Global-Pesticides-Market---Trends-Forecasts-2015 -2020; accessed April 8, 2018).

[23] Environmental Protection Agency, *2,4-D RED Facts*, EPA-738-F-05-00, June 30, 2005 (https://archive.epa.gov/pesticides/reregistration/web/ html/24d_fs.html; accessed March 22, 2018).

[24] C. Atwood and C. Paisley-Jones, "Pesticides Industry Sales and Usage 2008–2012 Market Estimates," Environmental Protection Agency, January 2017 (https://www.epa.gov/sites/production/files/2017-01/documents/pesticides -industry-sales-usage-2016_0.pdf; accessed April 8, 2018).

[25] G. R. Stephenson, K. R. Solomon and L. Ritter, "Environmental Persistence and Human Exposure Studies with 2,4-D and Other Turfgrass Pesticides," Centre for Toxicology, University of Guelph.

[26] D. Boyd, *Unnatural Law: Rethinking Canadian Environmental Law and Policy* (Vancouver: University of British Columbia Press, 2003).

[27] I. Arnold and K. Perrotta, "Cosmetic Pesticides – Provincial Policies and Municipal Bylaws: Lessons Learned and Best Practices," Canadian Association of Physicians for the Environment, August 2016 (https://cape.ca/wp-content/uploads/2016/08/Pesticides-Policy-Report-FINAL.pdf; accessed April 9, 2016).

[28] "Dow Contests Pesticide Ban," *Chemical and Engineering News* 86, no. 44 (November 22, 2008).

[29] K. L. Bassil, C. Vakil, M. Sanborn, D.C. Cole, J. S. Kaur and K. J. Kerr, "Cancer Health Effects of Pesticides: Systematic Review," *Canadian Family Physician* 53, no. 10 (2007): 1704–11.

[30] T. E. Arbuckle, S. M. Schrader, D. Cole, J.C. Hall, C.M. Bancej, L. A. Turner and P. Claman, "2,4-Dichlorophenoxyacetic Acid Residues in Semen of Ontario Farmers," *Reproductive Toxicology* 13 (1999): 421–29.

[31] G. M. Solomon and P. M. Weiss, "Chemical Contaminants in Breast Milk: Time Trends and Regional Variability," *Environmental Health Perspectives* 110, no. 6 (2002): A336–47.

[32] C. Storrs, "Report: Pesticide Exposure Linked to Childhood Cancer and Lower IQ," CNN, September 14, 2015 (https://www.cnn.com/2015/09/14/health/pesticide-exposure-childhood-cancer/index.html; accessed April 9, 2018).

[33] K. L. Bassil, C. Vakil, M. Sanborn, D. C. Cole, J. S. Kaur and K. J. Kerr, "Cancer Health Effects of Pesticides: Systematic Review," *Canadian Family Physician* 53, no. 10 (2007): 1704–11.

[34] M. Sanborn, K. J. Kerr, L. H. Sanin, D. C. Cole, K. L. Bassil and C. Vakil, "Non-cancer Health Effects of Pesticides: Systematic Review and Implications for Family Doctors," *Canadian Family Physician* 53 (October 2007).

[35] Ibid.

[36] Dow AgroSciences, "About Us" (http://www.dowagro.com/about/; accessed December 17, 2008).

[37] M. Chen, C.-H. Chang, L. Tao and C. Lu, "Residential Exposure to Pesticide During Childhood and Childhood Cancers: A Meta-analysis," American Academy of Pediatrics, September 2015 (pediatrics.aappublications.org

/content/early/2015/09/08/peds.2015-0006?sid=b7090daa-bc95-45df-87f5-a64529d4ef3f; accessed April 9, 2018).

[38] T. Colborn, "A Case for Revisiting the Safety of Pesticides: A Closer Look at Neurodevelopment," *Environmental Health Perspectives* 114 (2006): 10–17.

[39] "Pesticides 101," Pesticide Action Network (www.panna.org/pesticides-big-picture/pesticides-101; accessed April 9, 2018).

[40] Dupont, "Comprehensive Scientific Study Confirms Consumer Articles with DuPont Materials Are Safe for Consumer Use: Peer-Reviewed Science Concludes Consumer Use of Articles Are Not a Source of PFOA in People," April 25, 2005 (http://www2.dupont.com/Media_Center/en_US/assets/downloads/pfoa/nr04_20_05a.pdf; accessed March 8, 2016).

[41] S. Sood, "Scientists: EPA 'Under Siege.' Survey of EPA Scientists Finds Rampant Political Interference," *Washington Independent*, April 23, 2008.

[42] The Natural Resources Defense Council (NRDC) has launched a campaign to have Scott Pruitt fired from his post as EPA administrator. See https://www.nrdc.org/case-firing-scott-pruitt (accessed April 14, 2018).

[43] "Global Top 50," *Chemical and Engineering News* 85, no. 30 (July 23, 2007), https://pubs.acs.org/cen/coverstory/85/8530cover.html (accessed March 8, 2018).

[44] Oraclepoll Research, *Survey Report Prepared for Pesticide Free Ontario and the Canadian Association of Physicians for the Environment*, February 2007.

Seven: Mothers Know Best

[1] R. Smith and A. Daifallah, "It's in Tory Genes to Go Green," *Globe and Mail*, February 6, 2006.

[2] T. Corcoran, "Rona Brockovich?" *National Post*, June 3, 2006.

[3] A. M. Calafat, X. Ye, L. Yang, J. A. Reidy and L. Needham, "Exposure of the U.S. Population to Bisphenol A and 4-tertiary-octylphenol: 2003–2004," *Environmental Health Perspectives* 116, no. 1 (January 2008): 39–44.

[4] W. Qiu, M. Yang and N. Wayne, "BPS, a Popular Substitute for BPA in Consumer Products, May Not Be Safer," The Conversation, March 11, 2016 (http://theconversation.com/bps-a-popular-substitute-for-bpa-in-consumer-products-may-not-be-safer-54211; accessed April 9, 2018).

5 Ibid.

6 D. Case, "The Real Story Behind Bisphenol A," Fast Company, February 1, 2009 (https://www.fastcompany.com/1139298/real-story-behind-bisphenol; accessed April 9, 2018).

7 S. Toloken, "SPI Study Disputes Endocrine Disruptor Findings," Plastics News, October 16, 1998.

8 Z. Wang, H. Liu and S. Liu, "Low-Dose Bisphenol A Exposure: A Seemingly Instigating Carcinogenic Effect on Breast Cancer," Advanced Science, November 2016, doi: 10.1002/advs.201600248 (https://www.ncbi.nlm.nih .gov/pubmed/28251049; accessed April 9, 2018).

9 J. T. Wolstenholme, M. Edwards, S. R. J. Shetty, J. D. Gatewood, J. A. Taylor, E. F. Rissman and J. J. Connelly, "Gestational Exposure to Bisphenol A Produces Transgenerational Changes in Behaviors and Gene Expression," Endrocrinology 8, no. 1 (August 2012) 1: 3828–38 (https://academic.oup.com /endo/article/153/8/3828/2424098; accessed April 9, 2018).

10 R. R. Gerona, T. J. Woodruff, C. A. Dickenson, J. Pan, J. M. Schwartz, S. Sen, M. W. Friesen et al., "Bisphenol-A (BPA), BPA Glucuronide and BPA Sulfate in Midgestation Umbilical Cord Serum in a Northern and Central California Population," Environmental Science and Technology 47, no. 21 (2013): 12477–85 (https://www .ncbi.nlm.nih.gov/pubmed/23941471; accessed April 9, 2018).

11 J. R. Rochester, "Bisphenol A and Human Health: A Review of the Literature,"Reproductive Toxicology 42 (December 2013): 132–55 (https://www.ncbi.nlm.nih.gov/pubmed/23994667; accessed April 10, 2018).

12 F. S. vom Saal, B. T. Akingbemi, S. M. Belcher, L. S. Birnbaum, D. A. Crain, M. Eriksen, F. Farabollini, et al., "Chapel Hill Bisphenol A Expert Panel Consensus Statement: Integration of Mechanisms, Effects in Animals and Potential to Impact Human Health at Current Levels of Exposure," Reproductive Toxicology 24, no. 2 (2007): 131–38.

13 "Statement from Stephen Ostroff M.D., Deputy Commissioner for Foods and Veterinary Medicine, on National Toxicology Program Draft Report on Bisphenol A," U. S. Food and Drug Administration, February 23, 2018 (https://www.fda.gov/NewsEvents/Newsroom/PressAnnouncements /ucm598100.htm; accessed April 10, 2018).

[14] A. Yeager, "FDA Report on BPA's Health Effects Raises Concerns," *The Scientist*, February 28, 2018 (https://www.the-scientist.com/?articles.view /articleNo/51931/title/FDA-Report-on-BPA-s-Health-Effects-Raises -Concerns/; accessed April 10, 2018).

[15] A container that, in a recent study, was found to leach bisphenol A. See "Estimates of How Much BPA a Child Could Ingest from Food Products in a Day, Based on Journal Sentinel's Lab Results," *Milwaukee Journal Sentinel* (http://archive.jsonline.com/watchdog/watchdogreports/34532859.html/; accessed March 8, 2018).

[16] "About SafeMama.com," Safe Mama (http://safemama.com/about/; accessed December 28, 2008).

Eight: Organic Tea Party

[1] Complete survey results were as follows. Of the 245 surveys completed:

149 (60.8%) — (A) I am concerned about exposure to toxins in non-organic food.

17 (6.9%)—(B) I believe organic foods taste better.

31 (12.7%)—(C) I think that organic foods have more nutrients than non-organic foods.

19 (7.8%) — (D) I like to support local farmers.

29 (11.8%) — (E) I believe organic food is better for the environment.

[2] 2. S. Lockie, K. Lyons, G. Lawrence and J. Grice, "Choosing Organics: A Path Analysis of Factors Underlying the Selection of Organic Food among Australian Consumers," *Appetite* 43 (2004): 135–46; Maryellen Molyneaux, president, Natural Marketing Institute, "Engaging the Next Wave: An Organic Consumer Study," presentation at Organic Trade Association, "State of the Organic Industry," Baltimore, Maryland, September 2012.

[3] C. Benbrook, "Initial Reflections on the *Annals of Internal Medicine* Paper 'Are Organic Foods Safer and Healthier Than Conventional Alternatives? A Systematic Review,'" 2012 (www.tfrec.wsu.edu/pdfs/P2566.pdf; accessed March 13, 2018).

[4] C. Benbrook, *Simplifying the Pesticide Risk Equation: The Organic Option*, (Boulder, CO: Organic Center, 2008) https://www.organic-center.org

/reportfiles/Organic_Option_Final_Ex_Summary.pdf (accessed March 13, 2018); C. Benbrook, "The Organic Center's 'Dietary Risk Index' – Tracking Relative Pesticide Risks in Food and Beverages," Organic Center, 2011 (https://www.organic-center.org/reportfiles/DRIfinal_09-10-2011.pdf; accessed March 13, 2018).

[5] V. A. Rauh and A. E. Margolis, "Environmental Exposures, Neurodevelopment and Child Mental Health: New Paradigms for the Study of Brain and Behavioral Effects,"*Journal of Child Psychology and Psychiatry*, March 2016 (https://onlinelibrary.wiley.com/doi/full/10.1111/jcpp.12537; accessed April 15, 2018).

[6] C. Lu, K. Toepel, R. Irish, R. Fenske, D. Barr and R. Bravo, "Organic Diets Significantly Lower Children's Dietary Exposure to Organophosphorus Pesticides," *Environmental Health Perspectives* 114 (2006): 260–63.

[7] C. Lu, D. Barr, M. Pearson, L. Walker and R. Bravo, "The Attribution of Urban and Suburban Children's Exposure to Synthetic Pyrethroid Insecticides: A Longitudinal Assessment," *Journal of Exposure Science and Environmental Epidemiology* 19 (2009): 69–78.

[8] C. Lu, K. Warchol and R. Callahan, "In situ Replication of Honey Bee Colony Collapse Disorder," *Bulletin of Insectology* 65 (2012): 99–106.

[9] In 2017, various news outlets reported, however, that there is a growing body of evidence to suggest that neonicotinoids are "harmful to pollinators." As a result, the European Union has declared a temporary moratorium on use of three major neonicotinoids on bee-attractive crops. See S. Wong, "Strongest Evidence Yet That Neonicotinoids Are Killing Bees," *New Scientist*, July 3, 2017 (https://www.newscientist.com/article/2139197-strongest-evidence -yet-that-neonicotinoids-are-killing-bees/; accessed March 27, 2018).

[10] P. Jeschke, R. Nauen, M. Schindler and A. Elbert, "Overview of the Status and Global Strategy for Neonicotinoids," *Journal of Agriculture and Food Chemistry* 59 (2011): 2897–2908.

[11] According to *Newsweek*, the most commonly used agricultural pesticide is now glyphosate. See: D. Mann, "Glyphosate Now the Most-Used Agricultural Chemical Ever," *Newsweek*, February 2, 2016 (www.newsweek.com/glypho-sate-now-most-used-agricultural-chemical-ever-422419; accessed March 27, 2018).

[12] R. Morse and N. Calderone, "The Value of Honey Bees as Pollinators of U.S. Crops in 2000," 2000 (http://citeseerx.ist.psu.edu/viewdoc/download?doi= 10.1.1.472.4894&rep=rep1&type=pdf; accessed March 13, 2018); N. Gallai, J. Salles, J. Settele and B. Vaissière, "Economic Valuation of the Vulnerability of World Agriculture Confronted with Pollinator Decline," *Ecological Economics* 68 (2009): 810–21.

[13] European Commission Animal Health and Welfare, "Bees and Pesticides: Commission Goes Ahead with Plan to Better Protect Bees," May 1, 2013 (https://ec.europa.eu/food/animals/live_animals/bees_en; accessed July 11, 2013).

[14] European Commission, "Neonicotinoids," May 30, 2018 (https://ec.europa.eu /food/plant/pesticides/approval_active_substances/approval_renewal /neonicotinoids_en; accessed June 6, 2018).

[15] United States Department of Agriculture National Honey Bee Health Stakeholder Conference Steering Committee, *Report on the National Stakeholders Conference on Honey Bee Health* (Washington, DC: USDA, 2012).

[16] United States Environmental Protection Agency, "Schedule for Review of Neonicotinoid Pesticides," December 2017 (https://www.epa.gov/pollinator -protection/schedule-review-neonicotinoid-pesticides; accessed June 6, 2018).

[17] K. Harris, and S. Lunn, "New Limits, But No All-Out Ban on Pesticides That Harm Bee Population," CBC, December 19, 2017 (www.cbc.ca/news /politics/bees-environment-pesticides-1.4456011; accessed June 6, 2018).

[18] Government of Ontario, "Neonicotinoid Regulations," January 30, 2017 (https://www.ontario.ca/page/neonicotinoid-regulations; accessed June 6, 2018).

[19] "Quebec Places New Restrictions on Pesticides in Bid to Protect Honeybees," CBC, February 19, 2018 (www.cbc.ca/news/canada/montreal/ quebec-pesticides-honeybees-1.4541996; accessed June 6, 2018).

[20] BC Farms & Food, "Nepnicotinoid Pesticides in Honey," November 23, 2017, https://bcfarmsandfood.com/neonicotinoid-pesticides-in-honey/.

[21] C. Smith-Spangler, M. Brandea, G. Hunter, J. Bavinger, M. Pearson, P. Eschbach, V. Sundaram et al., "Are Organic Foods Safer or Healthier Than Conventional Alternatives? A Systematic Review," *Annals of Internal Medicine* 157 (2012): 348–66.

[22] Benbrook, "Initial Reflections on the *Annals of Internal Medicine* Paper."

[23] K. Brandt, C. Leifert, R. Sanderson and C. Seal, "Agroecosystem Management and Nutritional Quality of Plant Foods: The Case of Organic Fruits and Vegetables," *Critical Reviews in Plant Sciences* 30 (2011): 1–2, 177–97.

[24] A large "meta-analysis" published in the *British Journal of Nutrition* in 2016 found that that there is indeed growing "evidence that organic production can boost key nutrients in foods." Among other things, the analysis found that "organic dairy and meat contain about 50 percent more omega-3 fatty acids." See: A. Aubrey, "Is Organic More Nutritious? New Study Adds to the Evidence," NPR, February 18, 2016 (https://www.npr.org/sections/thesalt /2016/02/18/467136329/is-organic-more-nutritious-new-study-adds-to -the-evidence; accessed March 27, 2018).

[25] As we edited this book, Matt Holmes sent me some highlights from his organization's study of the Canadian organic marketplace. His statistics indicated that the Stanford study couldn't have been as much of a disaster as the media predicted. Canada's organic market had continued to grow in 2012, totalling C$3.7 billion for the year—a tripling in sales from just six years before. Ignoring the naysayers, 58 percent of all Canadians purchased organic products every week. More recent studies from 2017 indicate that the total organic market has now grown to $5.4 billion and that 83 percent of "millennials" purchase organic products every week. See Canada Organic Trade Association, "Canadian Organic Market Report 2017" (https://ota.com /sites/default/files/Canadian%20Organic%20Market%20Report%202017 %20teaser.pdf; accessed March 13, 2016).

[26] G. Gallant, "Promoting the Development of Canada's Organic Sector," news release, Agriculture and Agri-Food Canada, Government of Canada, February 21, 2018 (https://www.canada.ca/en/agriculture-agri-food/news /2018/02/promoting_the_developmentofcanadasorganicsector.html; accessed April 12, 2018).

[27] "Growth and Opportunities in the Food Sector," Export Development Canada, December 8, 2016 (https://www.edc.ca/events/EN/1-BJRZJ2/Pages /overview.aspx; accessed April 12, 2018).

[28] See U.S. Department of Agriculture, "*The Organic Integrity Quarterly: National Organic Program Newsletter*," October 2012 (https://www.ams.usda. gov/sites/default/files/media/2012-Organic-October-Newsletter.pdf;

accessed March 13, 2018); Organic Trade Association, Organic Industry Survey 2018 (https://www.ota.com; accessed September 5, 2018).

[29] S. Ström, "Has 'Organic' Been Oversized?" *New York Times*, July 7, 2012 (http://www.nytimes.com/2012/07/08/business/organic-food-purists -worry-about-big-companies-influence.html?pagewanted=all&_r=0; accessed November 3, 2012).

[30] Cornucopia Institute, *White Paper: The Organic Watergate*, 2012 (https:// www.cornucopia.org/USDA/OrganicWatergateWhitePaper.pdf; accessed March 13, 2018).

[31] "Our Path," Nature's Path Canada (https://www.naturespath.com/en-ca/ our-path/family-owned/; accessed April 12, 2018).

[32] Stonyfield Farm, "History," November 27, 2012 (http://www.stonyfield. com/our-story/history; accessed March 13, 2018).

[33] In 2017, the Latin American Grupo Lala offered to buy Stonyfield for roughly $850 million. See B. Dummett, "Grupo Lala Leads Bids for Danone's Stonyfield Farm," MarketWatch, May 18, 2017 (https://www.marketwatch.com /story/grupo-lala-leads-bids-for-danones-stonyfield-farm-2017-05-18; accessed March 27, 2018).

[34] K. McCormack, "Stonyfield CEO Resigns to Focus on Food Policy," Associated Press, January 12, 2012 (https://www.deseretnews.com/article /700214832/Stonyfield-CEO-resigns-to-focus-on-food-policy.html; accessed March 13, 2018).

[35] B. Kowitt, "Why the Danone Sale Puts Stonyfield at Risk," *Fortune*, March 31, 2017 (http://www.fortune.com/2017/03/31/stonyfield-danone-white- wave-sale/; accessed April 12, 2017).

[36] M. Gunther, "Stonyfield Stirs Up the Yogurt Market," CNN Money Online, January 4, 2008 (http://money.cnn.com/2008/01/03/news/companies /gunther_yogurt.fortune/index.htm; accessed November 27, 2012).

[37] H. Agnew, "Danone Agrees $875m Sale of Stonyfield to Lactalis," *Financial Times*, July 3, 2017 (https://www.ft.com/content/f30e92b0-5ff4-11e7-8814- 0ac7eb84e5f1; accessed April 12, 2018).

[38] "Global Food-Giant Buyouts of Top Organic Brands," CNBC, October 8, 2012 (https://www.cnbc.com/2012/10/08/Global-Food-Giant-Buyouts-of- Top-Organic-Brands.html; accessed March 13, 2018).

[39] A. Bhattarai, "Americans Are Buying More Food at Walmart," *Washington Post*, August 17, 2017 (https://www.washingtonpost.com/news/business /wp/2017/08/17/americans-are-buying-more-food-at-walmart/?noredirect =on&utm_term=.27364277cd22; accessed April 12, 2018).

[40] "Local Produce at Walmart," Walmart, 2018 (https://corporate.walmart. com/_news_/media-library/photos/live-better/local-produce-at-walmart; accessed April 12, 2018).

[41] "About Us," International Federation of Organic Agriculture Movements, 2018 (https://www.ifoam.bio/en/about-us; accessed April 4, 2018).

[42] I know of only one other study in the scientific literature in addition to Lu's that has looked at this question. Cynthia Curl and her colleagues found that mean levels of certain organophosphate pesticides were nine times higher in preschool kids in Seattle who reported a conventional diet versus an organic one. See C. Curl, R. Fenske and K. Elgethun, "Organophosphorus Pesticide Exposure of Urban and Suburban Preschool Children with Organic and Conventional Diets," *Environmental Health Perspectives* 111 [2003]: 377–82). More recent research on the same subject has continued to reveal the dangers of organophosphorus pesticide exposure. See S. M. Engel, A. Bradman, M. S. Wolff, V. A. Rauh, K. G. Harley, J. H. Yang, L. A. Hoepner, "Prenatal Organophosphorus Pesticide Exposure and Child Neurodevelopment at 24 Months: An Analysis of Four Birth Cohorts," *Environmental Health Perspectives* 124 (June 2016): 822–30, doi: 10.1289/ehp.1409474.

[43] Curl et al., "Organophosphorus Pesticide Exposure"; Lu et al., "Organic Diets Significantly Lower Children's Dietary Exposure."

[44] Triple Pundit, "The Shrinking Price-Gap Between Organics and Conventional Food," June 3, 2016, https://www.triplepundit.com/2016/06 /gap-cost-organics-conventional-food-narrowing/.

Nine: Straight Flush

[1] Jay- Z, and A. Winehouse, "Rehab (Remix)" (https://www.youtube.com/ watch?v=oSPvkqqPn9k; accessed March 14, 2018).

[2] B. Dixon, "'Detox': A Mass Delusion," *The Lancet* 5 (2005): 261.

[3] Marketdata Enterprises, a U.S.-based independent market research firm, released a report in 2011 looking at the weight loss and dieting market in the

United States: Marketdata Enterprises Inc., *U.S. Weight Loss and Diet Control Market*, 11th ed. (Tampa, FL: Marketdata Enterprises, 2011). According to their research, the sales of diet and detox pills alone total over US$2.5 billion a year in the United States. Another market intelligence firm, Euromonitor International, looked at the sales of top antioxidant ingredients (e.g., green tea, super-fruit juice, dietary supplements, etc.) and used those figures to estimate the combined global sales in this category: US$34 billion in 2010. See Euromonitor International, *Health and Wellness: Global Briefing Series* (London: Euromonitor International, 2011). Amazingly, these massive figures don't include many of the products and techniques we're about to examine.

[4] For a detailed description of the science of chelation, see B. Halstead, *The Scientific Basis of EDTA Chelation Therapy* (Colton, CA: Golden Quill, 1979).

[5] Weilll Cornell Medicine, "Fecal Microbiota Transplant Is Safe and Effective for Patients with Ulcerative Colitis," April 26, 2017, https://news.weill .cornell.edu/news/2017/04/fecal-microbiota-transplant-is-safe-and -effective-for-patients-with-ulcerative-colitis (accessed April 10, 2018).

[6] E. Ernst, "Colonic Irrigation and the Theory of Autointoxication: A Triumph of Ignorance over Science," *Journal of Clinical Gastroenterology* 24, no. 4 (1997): 196–98.

[7] "UN: Six Billion Mobile Phone Subscriptions in the World," *BBC News*, October 12, 2012 (http://www.bbc.com/news/technology-19925506; accessed March 14, 2018). The World Bank reports that, as of 2016, the global number of cellphone subscriptions per 100 people reached 101.55. See: "Mobile Cellular Subscriptions (Per 100 People)," *World Bank* (https://data .worldbank.org/indicator/IT.CEL.SETS.P2; accessed March 14, 2018).

[8] S. Kemp, "Digital in 2017: Global Overview," WeAreSocial, January 24, 2017, (https://wearesocial.com/special-reports/digital-in-2017-global-overview; accessed April 12, 2017).

[9] "How to Reduce Exposure to Radiofrequency Energy from Cell Phones," California Department of Public Health, 2017 (https://www.cdph.ca.gov /Programs/CCDPHP/DEODC/EHIB/CDPH%20Document%20Library /Cell-Phone-Guidance.pdf; accessed April 13, 2018).

[10] Adapted from S. Genuis, "Elimination of Persistent Toxicants from the

Human Body," *Human and Experimental Toxicology* 30 (2011): 3–18, with added language to simplify the detox effectiveness column.

[11] R. Jandacek, N. Anderson, M. Liu, S. Zheng, Q. Yang and P. Tso, "Effects of Yo-Yo Diet, Caloric Restriction and Olestra on Tissue Distribution of Hexachlorobenzene," *American Journal of Physiology and Gastrointestinal Liver Physiology* 288 (2005): G292-G299; M. Imamura and T. Tung, "A Trial of Fasting Cure for PCB-Poisoned Patients in Taiwan," *American Journal of Industrial Medicine* 5 (1985): 147–53.

[12] M. Blanusa, V. Varnai, M. Piasek and K. Kostial, "Chelators as Antidotes of Metal Toxicity: Therapeutic and Experimental Aspects," *Current Medical Chemistry* 12 (2005): 2771–94; H. Aposhian, R. Maiorino, D. Gonzalez-Ramirez, M. Zuniga-Charles, Z. Xu, K. Hurlbut, P. Junco-Munoz, R. Dart and M. Aposhian, "Mobilization of Heavy Metals by Newer, Therapeutically Useful Chelating Agents," *Toxicology* 97 (1995): 23–38.

[13] D. Kennedy, K. Cooley, T. Einarson and D. Seely, "Objective Assessment of an Ionic Footbath (IonCleanse): Testing Its Ability to Remove Potentially Toxic Elements from the Body," *Journal of Environmental and Public Health* 2012 (2012): 1–13.

[14] S. Horne, "Colon Cleansing: A Popular, but Misunderstood Natural Therapy," *Journal of Herbal Pharmacotherapy* 6 (2006): 93-100; R. Acosta and B. Cash, "Clinical Effects of Colonic Cleansing for General Health Promotion: A Systematic Review," *American Journal of Gastroenterology* 104 (2009): 2830–36.

[15] V. Nadeau, G. Truchon, M. Brochu and R. Tardif, "Effect of Physical Exertion on the Biological Monitoring of Exposure to Various Solvents following Exposure by Inhalation in Human Volunteers: I. Toluene," *Journal of Occupational Environmental Hygiene* 3 (2006): 481–89; R. Tardif, V. Nadeau, G. Truchon and M. Brochu, "Effect of Physical Exertion on the Biological Monitoring of Exposure to Various Solvents following Exposure by Inhalation in Human Volunteers: II. N-Hexane," *Journal of Occupational Environmental Hygiene* 4 (2007): 502–508; quiz D568-569.

[16] F. Ibrahim, T. Halttunen, R. Tahvonen and S. Salminen, "Probiotic Bacteria as Potential Detoxification Tools: Assessing Their Heavy Metal Binding Isotherms," *Canadian Journal of Microbiology* 52 (2006): 877–85.

[17] A. Barnes, M. Smith, S. Kacinko, E. Schwilke, E. Cone, E. Moolchan and M. Huestis, "Excretion of Methamphetamine and Amphetamine in Human Sweat following Controlled Oral Methamphetamine Administration," *Clinical Chemistry* 54 (2008): 172–80; N. Fucci, N. de Giovanni and S. Scarlata, "Sweat Testing in Addicts under Methadone Treatment: An Italian Experience," *Forensic Science International* 174 (2008): 107–10.

[18] J. Domingo, M. Gomez, J. Llobet and J. Corbella, "Comparative Effects of Several Chelating Agents on the Toxicity, Distribution and Excretion of Aluminum," *Human Toxicology* 7 (1998): 259–62; Z. Zhao, L. Liang, X. Fan et al. "The Role of Modified Citrus Pectin as an Effective Chelator of Lead in Children Hospitalized with Toxic Lead Levels," *Alternative Therapeutic Health Medicine* 14 (2008): 34–38.

[19] For an excellent account of the contamination of human breasts, see F. Williams, *Breasts: A Natural and Unnatural History* (New York: W. W. Norton, 2012).

[20] U.S. Department of Veterans Affairs, "Camp Lejeune: Past Water Contamination" (https://www.publichealth.va.gov/exposures/camp-lejeune/; accessed March 14, 2018).

[21] "Camp Lejeune Lawsuit Goes Forward," *Veterans Today Military and Foreign Affairs Journal*, February 4, 2011 (http://www.veteranstoday.com/2011/02/04/camp-lejeune-lawsuit-goes-forward/; accessed March 14, 2018).

[22] For the full story, watch the documentary film *Semper Fi: Always Faithful*, directed by R. Libert and T. Hardmon (Wilder Film Projects, 2011).

[23] U.S. National Cancer Institute, "Cancer Stats Fact Sheet" (https://seer.cancer.gov/statfacts/; accessed March 14, 2018).

[24] American Cancer Society, "Cancer Facts and Figures 2010" (https://www.cancer.org/content/dam/cancer-org/research/cancer-facts-and-statistics/annual-cancer-facts-and-figures/2010/cancer-facts-and-figures-2010.pdf; accessed April 2013). The American Cancer Society expects 609,640 Americans to die of cancer in 2018. See "Cancer Facts & Figures 2018," 2018 (https://www.cancer.org/content/dam/cancer-org/research/cancer-facts-and-statistics/annual-cancer-facts-and-figures/2018/cancer-facts-and-figures-2018.pdf; accessed March 27, 2018).

[25] Canadian Cancer Society, "Canadian Cancer Statistics 2012"

(https://www.cancer.ca/~/media/cancer.ca/CW/cancer%20information/cancer%20101/Canadian%20cancer%20statistics/Canadian-Cancer-Statistics-2012-EN.pdf?la=en; accessed March 14, 2018). The Canadian Cancer Society expected 80,800 Canadians to die of cancer in 2017. See "Canadian Cancer Statistics 2017" (http://www.cancer.ca/~/media/cancer.ca/CW/publications/Canadian%20Cancer%20Statistics/Canadian-Cancer-Statistics-2017-EN.pdf; accessed March 14, 2018).

[26] Australian Institute of Health and Welfare, Canberra, "Cancer in Australia 2010: An Overview" (http://www.aihw.gov.au/publication-detail/?id=6442472459; accessed March 14, 2018). Cancer Australia expected 48,586 Australians to die of cancer in 2018. See "Cancer in Australia Statistics," 2018 (https://canceraustralia.gov.au/affected-cancer/what-cancer/cancer-australia-statistics; accessed March 27, 2018).

[27] See Getting to Know Cancer, "The Halifax Project," http://www.gettingtoknowcancer.org (accessed July 22, 2018).

[28] See Centers for Disease Control and Prevention, "Colorectal Cancer Statistics" (http://www.cdc.gov/cancer/colorectal/statistics/; accessed April 1, 2013) and Canadian Cancer Society, "Colorectal Cancer Statistics" (http://www.cancer.ca/en/cancer-information/cancer-type/colorectal/statistics/?region=on; accessed April 1, 2013).

[29] Dr. Stephen Genuis mentioned the presence of birth control drugs in exhaled breath in an interview with the author in August 2012.

[30] G. Lamas, C. Goertz, R. Boineau, D. Mark, T. Rozema, R. Nahin, L. Lindlblad et al., "Effect of Disodium EDTA Chelation Regimen on Cardiovascular Events in Patients with Previous Myocardial Infarction: The TACT Randomized Trial," *Journal of the American Medical Association* 309 (2013): 1241–50.

Ten: Sweat the Small Stuff

[1] Choice Online, "Tempter by Detox-in-a-Box?" October, http://www.choice.com.au/reviews-and-tests/food-and-health/general-health/therapies/detox-kits-review-and-compare/page.aspx (originally accessed April 1, 2013).

[2] G. E. Mullin, "Popular Diets Prescribed by Alternative Practitioners: Part 1," *Nutrition in Clinical Practice* 25, no. 2 (2010): 212–14.

[3] D. Valle and T. Manolio, "Applying Genomics to Clinical Problems – Diagnostics, Preventive Medicine, Pharmacogenomics: A White Paper for the National Human Genome Research Institute," National Institutes of Health, 2008 (http://www.genome.gov/27529204; accessed June 27, 2013).

[4] Stanford Medicine Cancer Institute, "Hereditary Breast Ovarian Cancer Syndrome (BRCA1/BRCA2)," 2013 (http://cancer.stanford.edu/information /geneticsAndCancer/types/herbocs.html; accessed June 4, 2013).

[5] A. Jolie, "My Medical Choice," *New York Times*, May 14, 2013 (http://www.nytimes.com/2013/05/14/opinion/my-medical-choice.html; accessed June 4, 2013).

[6] Breastcancer.org, U.S. Breast Cancer Statistics, 2012 (http://www .breastcancer.org/symptoms/understand_bc/statistics; accessed June 4, 2013).

[7] T. Doshi, S. S. Mehta, V. Dighe, N. Balasinor and G. Vanage, "Hyper-methylation of Estrogen Receptor Promoter Region in Adult Testis of Rats Exposed Neonatally to Bisphenol A," *Toxicology* (2011), http://dx.doi.org/10.1016 /j.tox.2011.07.011.

[8] H. Roberts, "Vitamin C: Linus Pauling Was Right All Along – A Doctor's Opinion," August 17, 2004 (http://www.medicalnewstoday.com/releases /12154.php; accessed April 1, 2013).

[9] R. J. Reiter, D. X. Tan, L. C. Manchester, S. Lopez-Burillo, R. M. Sainz and J. C. Mayo, "Melatonin: Detoxification of Oxygen and Nitrogen-Based Toxic Reactants," *Advances in Experimental Medicine and Biology* 527 (2003): 539–48.

[10] S. J. James, W. Slikker III, S. Melnyk, E. New, M. Pogribna and S. Jernigan, "Thimerosal Neurotoxicity Is Associated with Glutathione Depletion: Protection with Glutathione Precursors," *NeuroToxicology* 26, no. 1 (2005): 1–8.

[11] National Fire Protection Association, "Number of Fires by Type of Fire" (https://www.nfpa.org/News-and-Research/Fire-statistics-and-reports /Fire-statistics/Fires-in-the-US/Overall-fire-problem/Number-of-fires -by-type-of-fire; accessed March 15, 2018).

[12] C. C. Austin, D. Wang, D. J. Ecobichon and G. Dussault, "Characterization of Volatile Organic Compounds in Smoke at Environmental Fires," *Journal of Toxicology and Environmental Health* 63 (2001): 437–58.

[13] "September 11th Terror Attacks Fast Facts", CNN, August 24, 2017

(https://www.cnn.com/2013/07/27/us/september-11-anniversary-fast-facts/index.html; accessed July 12, 2018).

[14] M. Webber, J. Gustave, R. Lee, J. K. Niles, K. Kelly, H. W. Cohen and D. Prezant, "Trends in Respiratory Symptoms of Firefighters Exposed to the World Trade Center Disaster: 2001–2005," *Environmental Health Perspectives* 117 (2009): 975–80.

[15] J. Li, J. Cone, A. Kahn, R. Brackbill, M. Farfel, C. Greene, J. Hadler et al., "Association Between World Trade Center Exposure and Excess Cancer Risk," *Journal of the American Medical Association* 308 (2012): 2479–88.

[16] World Trade Center Health Program, "Program Statistics" (https://www.cdc.gov/wtc/ataglance.html; accessed July 13, 2018).

[17] New Hampshire Department of Environmental Services, "Environmental Health Program: Cancer and the Environment" (http://des.nh.gov/organization/commissioner/pip/publications/co/documents/cancer_environment.pdf; accessed March 1, 2013).

[18] J. Shatki, "Wellness Education: Ayurveda," 2010 (https://www.jivanshakti.com/ayurveda.aspx; accessed March 1, 2013).

[19] J. Dahl and K. Falk, "Ayurvedic Herbal Supplements as an Antidote to 9/11 Toxicity," *Alternative Therapies in Health and Medicine* 14 (2008): 24–28.

[20] My intention is not to minimize the value of the study, but to point out that the data is survey data, not clinical data of patients' chemical body burdens. A study of declines in their chemical levels would be very helpful, however.

[21] Dahl and Falk, "Ayurvedic Herbal Supplements as an Antidote."

[22] S. Genuis, "Blood, Urine and Sweat (BUS) Study: Monitoring and Elimination of Bioaccumulated Toxic Elements," *Archives of Environmental Contamination and Toxicology* 61 (2011): 344–57.

[23] We wish to thank SGS AXYS Analytical Services of Sidney, BC, for their advice and support in undertaking the sweat analysis.

[24] S. Genuis, "Elimination of Persistent Toxicants from the Human Body," *Human and Experimental Toxicology* 30 (2010): 3–18; Genuis, "Blood, Urine and Sweat (BUS) Study."

[25] According to the claims of some infrared sauna manufacturers, it is possible to produce a litre of sweat in fifteen minutes. This is highly unlikely, but

based on my experience, it could be possible to produce that much sweat during a forty-five-minute session.

[26] See table 1 in A. Calafat, Z. Kuklenvik, J. Reidy, S. Caudill, J. Ekong and L. Needham, "Urinary Concentrations of Bisphenol A and 4-Nonylphenol in a Human Reference Population," *Environmental Health Perspectives* 113 (2004): 391–95.

[27] See table 1 in R. Stahlhut, E. van Wijngaarden, T. Dye, S. Cook and S. Swan, "Concentrations of Urinary Phthalate Metabolites Are Associated with Increased Waist Circumference and Insulin Resistance in Adult U.S. Males," *Environmental Health Perspectives* 115 (2007): 876–82.

[28] Genuis, "Blood, Urine and Sweat (BUS) Study."

Eleven: A Stationary Road Trip

[1] For example, the Little Trees Car Freshener Corporation's New Car Scent (https://www.littletrees.com/fragrances/Masculine; accessed March 15, 2018).

[2] Ecology Center, *2011/2012 Guide to New Vehicles*, 2012 (https://www.ecocenter .org/sites/default/files/2012_Cars.pdf; accessed March 15, 2018).

[3] E. Leamy, "How to Find Flame-Resistant Pajamas for Kids, Without Toxic Chemicals," *Washington Post*, November 16, 2017 (https://www.washingtonpost .com/lifestyle/on-parenting/how-to-find-flame-resistant-pajamas-for-kids -without-toxic-chemicals/2017/11/08/fe587216-c32d-11e7-afe9-4f60b5a6c4a0 _story.html?utm_term=.c51ab2b30bff; accessed April 2, 2018).

[4] Adapted from N. Klepeis, W. Nelson, J. Robinson, A. Tsang, P. Switzer, J. Behar, S. Hern et al., "The National Human Activity Pattern Survey (NHAPS): A Resource for Assessing Exposure to Environmental Pollutants," *Journal of Exposure Analysis and Environmental Epidemiology* 11 (2001): 231–52. See also U.S. EPA Indoor Air Division and Office of Research and Development, *Federal Programs Addressing Indoor Air Quality*, vol. 1, 1989, http://1.usa.gov/ XfwS7G.

[5] C. R. Kirman, L. L. Aylward, B. C. Blount, D. W. Pyatt and S. M. Hays, "Evaluation of NHANES Biomonitoring Data for Volatile Organic Compounds in Blood: Application of Chemical-Specific Screening Criteria," *Journal of Exposure Science and Epidemiology* 22 (2012): 24–34.

[6] This study found that levels of some brominated pollutants are up to ten

times the maximum level found in homes and offices: C. C. Carignan, M. D. McClean, E. M. Cooper, D. J. Watkins, A. J. Fraser, W. Heiger-Bernays, H. M. Stapleton et al., "Predictors of Tris(1,3-dichloro-2-propyl) Phosphate Metabolite in the Urine of Office Workers," *Environment International* 55 (2013): 56–61. Other studies found a myriad of chemicals in the cabin air of automobiles. See T. Yoshida, "Approach to Estimation of Absorption of Aliphatic Hydrocarbons Diffusing from Interior Materials in an Automobile Cabin by Inhalation Toxicokinetic Analysis in Rats," *Journal of Applied Toxicology* 30 (2009): 42–52; O. Geiss, S. Tirendi, J. Barrero-Moreno and D. Kotzias, "Investigation of Volatile Organic Compounds and Phthalates Present in the Cabin Air of Used Private Cars," *Environment International* 35 (2009): 1188–95.

[7] L. Sabatini, A. Barbieri, P. Indiveri, S. Mattioli and F. S. Violante, "Validations of an HPLC-MS/MS Method for the Simultaneous Determination of Phenylmercapturic Acid, Benzylmercapturic Acid and O-Methylbenzyl Mercapturic Acid in Urine as Biomarkers of Exposure to Benzene, Toluene and Xylenes," *Journal of Chromatography* 863 (2008): 115–22; J. G. Filser, G. A. Csanady, W. Dietz, W. Kessler, P. E. Krenzen, M. Richter and A. Stormer, "Comparative Estimation of the Neurotoxic Risks of N-Hexane and N-Heptane in Rats and Humans Based on Formation of Metabolites 2,5-Hexanedione and 2,5-Heptanedione," *Advances in Experimental Medicine and Biology* 387 (1996): 411–27.

[8] J. T. Brophy, M. Keith, A. Watterson, R. Park, M. Gilbertson, E. Maticka-Tyndale, M. Beck et al., "Breast Cancer Risk in Relation to Occupations with Exposure to Carcinogens and Endocrine Disruptors: A Canadian – Case-Control Study," *Environmental Health* 11 (2012). doi:10.1186/1476-069X-11–87.

[9] R. DeMatteo, M. Keith, J.T. Brophy, A. Wordsworth, A. Watterson, M. Beck, A. Ford et al., "Chemical Exposure of Women Workers in the Plastics Industry with Particular Reference to Breast Cancer and Reproductive Hazards," *New Solutions* 22 (2012): 427–48.

[10] Ibid.

[11] "Injection Molding," Wikipedia (http://en.wikipedia.org/wiki/Injection_molding#Applications; accessed March 1, 2013).

[12] Brophy et al., "Breast Cancer Risk."

[13] Ibid.

[14] C. Butt, M. Diamond, J. Truong, M. Ikonomov and A. Ter Schure, "Spatial Distribution of PBDEs in Southern Ontario as Measured in Indoor and Outdoor Window Organic Films," *Environmental Science and Technology* 38 (2004): 724–31.

[15] H. Jones-Otazo, J. Clarke, M. Diamond, J. Archbold, G. Ferguson, T. Harner, G. Richardson et al., "Is House Dust the Missing Exposure Pathway of PBDEs? An Analysis of the Urban Fate and Human Exposure to PBDEs," *Environmental Science and Technology* 39 (2005): 5121–30.

[16] M. Fang, T. Webster, D. Gooden, M. Coopers, M. McClean, C. Carignan, C. Makey et al., "Investigating a Novel Flame Retardant Known as V6: Measurements in Baby Products, House Dust and Car Dust," *Environmental Science and Technology* 47 (2013): 4449–54.

[17] Ibid.

[18] J. Herbstman, A. Sjodid, M. Kurzon, S. Lederman, R. Jones, V. Rauh, L. Needham et al., "Prenatal Exposure to PBDEs and Neurodevelopment," *Environmental Health Perspectives* 118 (2010): 712–19.

[19] C. G. Bornehag and E. Nanberg, "Phthalate Exposure and Asthma in Children," *International Journal of Andrology* (2010): 333–45; C.-G. Bornehag, J. Sundell, C. J. Weschler, T. Sigsgaard, B. Lundgren, M. Hasselgren and L. Hägerhed-Engman, "The Association Between Asthma and Allergic Symptoms in Children and Phthalates in House Dust: A Nested Case-Control Study" *Environmental Health Perspectives* 112 (2004): 1393–97; R. E. Dodson, M. Nishioka, L. J. Standley, L. J. Perovich, J. G. Brody and R. A. Rudel, "Endocrine Disruptors and Asthma-Associated Chemicals in Consumer Products," *Environmental Health Perspectives* 120 (2012): 935–43.

[20] For two recent examples of this research, see L. Robinson and R. Miller, "The Impact of Bisphenol A and Phthalates on Allergy, Asthma, and Immune Function: A Review of Latest Findings," *Current Environmental Health Reports* 2, no. 4 (December 2015): 379–87 (https://www.ncbi.nlm.nih.gov/pmc/articles/PMC4626318/; accessed June 6, 2018); and ii) M. H. Soomro, N. Baiz, C. Philippat, C. Vernet, V. Siroux, C. N. Maesano, S. Sanyal, "Prenatal Exposure to Phthalates and the Development of Eczema Phenotypes in Male Children: Results from the EDEN Mother–Child Cohort Study," *Environmental*

Health Perspectives 126, no.2 (February 2018), https://ehp.niehs.nih.gov /wp-content/uploads/2018/02/EHP1829.alt_.pdf (accessed June 6, 2018).

[21] E. Woods, U. Bhaumik, S. Sommer, S. Ziniel, A. Kessler, E. Chan, R. Wilkinson et al., "Community Asthma Initiative: Evaluation of a Quality Improvement Program for Comprehensive Asthma Care," *Pediatrics* 129 (2012): 464–572.

[22] R. Knox, "To Control Asthma, Start with the Home Instead of the Child," *NPR Health Blogs*, March 18, 2013. (http://www.npr.org/blogs/health/2013 /03/18/174393981/to-control-asthma-start-with-the-home-instead-of -the-child; accessed March 15, 2018).

[23] Ibid. For more details, read the report in Woods et al., "Community Asthma Initiative."

[24] C. J. Weschler, "Changes in Indoor Pollutants Since the 1950s," *Atmospheric Environment* 43 (2009): 156–72.

[25] C. J. Weschler and W. W. Nazaroff, "SVOC Exposure Indoors: Fresh Look at Dermal Pathways," *Indoor Air* 22 (2012): 356–77.

[26] Ibid.

[27] Canada Green Building Council, "LEED," (https://www.cagbc.org/@/CAGBC /Programs/LEED/Going_green_with_LEE?hkey=54c44792-442b-450a -a286-4aa710bf5c64; accessed March 15, 2018).

[28] U.S. Green Building Council, "LEED Is Green Building," 2018 (https://new.usgbc.org/leed; accessed June 6, 2018).

[29] Ibid.

[30] J. Kriss, "U.S. Green Building Council Certifies 20,000th LEED Commercial Project," U.S. Green Building Council, December 20, 2013 (https://www.usgbc.org/articles/us-green-building-council-certifies -20000th-leed-commercial-project; accessed March 15, 2018).

[31] U.S. Green Building Council, "Square Footage of LEED-Certified Existing Buildings Surpasses New Construction," press release, December 7, 2011 (http://www.usgbc.org/ShowFile.aspx?DocumentID=10712; accessed March 1, 2013).

[32] Living Building Challenge (http://living-future.org/lbc; accessed February 1, 2013).

[33] Canada Green Building Council, "Living Building Challenge" (https://www.cagbc.org/CAGBC/Programs/Programs_recognized_by_CaGBC_/LivingBuildingChallenge/CAGBC/Programs/Living_Building_Chal.aspx?hkey=b04e1897-c875-4520-8645-31f9d70bce91; accessed March 15, 2018).

[34] C. Bagli, "$2.4 Billion Deal for Chelsea Market Enlarges Google's New York Footprint," *New York Times*, February 7, 2018 (https://www.nytimes.com/2018/02/07/nyregion/google-chelsea-market-new-york.html; accessed June 6, 2018).

[35] J. Hiskes, "Google Drops Red List Building Materials, Vendors Listen Up," *Sustainable Industries*, May 2, 2011 (http://www.unrbep.org/dealerportal/google-drops-red-list-building-materials-vendors-listen-up/; accessed February 1, 2013).

[36] N. DiNenno, "Living Building: Year One," *Williams*, October 27, 2016 (https://www.williams.edu/feature-stories/update-on-the-living-building-challenge/; accessed June 6, 2018).

[37] Canadian Broadcasting Corporation, "Burned: Company Statements," *Marketplace*, November 23, 2012 (http://www.cbc.ca/marketplace/blog/company-statements-burned; accessed March 15, 2018).

[38] "IKEA Flame Retardants," IKEA, 2017 (https://www.ikea.com/gb/en/doc/general-document/ikea-flame-retardants-pdf_1364489404536.pdf; accessed April 15, 2018).

Twelve: Clean, Green Economic Machine

[1] Letter to the editor, "The London Pharmacopoeia," *The Water Cure Journal and Hygienic Magazine* 5 (June 1850).

[2] S. Xu, H. Zhang, P. He and L. Shao, "Leaching Behaviour of Bisphenol A from Municipal Solid Waste into Landfill Environment," *Environmental Technology* 32 (2011): 1269–77; E. Davis, S. Klosterhaus and H. Stapleton, "Measurement of Flame Retardants and Triclosan in Municipal Sewage Sludge and Biosolids," *Environment International* 40 (2012): 1–7.

[3] K. Xia, A. Bhandari, K. Das and G. Dillar, "Occurrence and Fate of Pharmaceutical and Biosolids," *Journal of Environmental Quality* 34 (2005): 91–104.

[4] D. Kolpin, E. Furlong, M. Meyer, E. Thurman, S. Zaugg, L. Barber and H. Buxton, "Pharmaceuticals, Hormones and Other Organic Wastewater

Contaminants in U.S. Lakes and Streams, 1999–2000: A National Reconnaissance," *Environmental Science and Technology* 36 (2002): 1202–11.

5 N. Nassiri Koopaei and M. Abdollahi, "Health Risks Associated with the Pharmaceuticals in Wastewater," *Daru* 25 (2017): 9; doi: 10.1186/s40199-017-0176-y.

6 R. Yang, H. Wei, J. Guo and A. Li, "Emerging Brominated Flame Retardants in the Sediment of the Great Lakes," *Environmental Science and Technology* 46 (2012): 3119–26.

7 H. Spiegelman, "Unintended Consequences: A Short History of Waste," presentation at the Coast Waste Management Association spring conference, Victoria, B.C., March 29, 2007.

8 D. Hoornweg and P. Bhada-Tata, "What a Waste: A Global Review of Solid Waste Management," World Bank, Urban Development Series Knowledge Papers, 2012, http://openknowledge.worldbacnk.org.

9 Ibid.

10 R. Geyer, J. R. Jambeck and K. Lavender Law, "Production, Use, and Fate of All Plastics Ever Made" *Science Advances* 3, no. 7, (2017) e1700782, doi: 10.1126/sciadv.1700782 (accessed April 14, 2018).

11 National Oceanic and Atmospheric Administration, "Marine Debris Program Factsheet" (https://marinedebris.noaa.gov/file/4456/download ?token=o2cqB4f_; accessed March 16, 2018).

12 "High Level of Plastics Found in Great Lakes," *Toronto Star*, March 12, 2013.

13 A. Gomm, P. O'Hara, L. Kleine, V. Bowes, L. Wilson and K. Barry, "Northern Fulmars as Biological Monitors of Trends of Plastic Pollution in the Eastern North Pacific," *Marine Pollution Bulletin* 64, no. 9 (September 2012): 1776–81.

14 G. Readfearn, "WHO Launches Health Revciew after Microplastics Found in 90% of Bottled Water," *The Guardian*, March 15, 2018 (https://www.theguardian.com/environment/2018/mar/15/microplastics-found-in-more-than-90-of-bottled-water-study-says; accessed July 22, 2018).

15 T. Cook, Keynote presentation, Goldman Sachs Technology and Internet Conference, San Francisco, CA, February 15, 2012.

16 I. Watson, *"China: The Electronic Wastebasket of the World,"* CNN, May 30, 2013

(https://www.cnn.com/2013/05/30/world/asia/china-electronic-waste-e
-waste/index.html; accessed March 16, 2018).

[17] U.S. Environmental Protection Agency, "Waste Education Resources: The
Life Cycle of a Cell Phone," 2012 (http://www.mass.gov/eea/docs/dep
/recycle/reduce/06-thru-l/life-cell.pdf; accessed March 16, 2018).

[18] "Gartner Says Worldwide Sales of Smartphones Recorded First Ever
Decline During the Fourth Quarter of 2017," press release, Gartner Inc.,
Egham, UK, February 22, 2018, https://www.gartner.com/newsroom/
id/3876865 (accessed April 15, 2018).

[19] J. Greene, "The Environmental Pitfalls at the End of an iPhone's Life,"
CNET, September 26, 2012 (http://news.cnet.com/8301-13579-3-57520123
-37/the-environmental-pitfalls-at-the-end-of-an-iphones-life/; accessed
March 1, 2013).

[20] "Lead Levels in Children Linked to Rise in E-Waste Profits," *China Daily*,
November 16, 2011 (http://www.chinadaily.com.cn/cndy/2011-11/16/con-
tent_14101761.htm; accessed March 1, 2013).

[21] P. Guo, X. Xu, B. Huang, D. Sun, J. Zhang, X. Chen, Q. Zhang et al., "Blood
Lead Levels and Associated Factors among Children in Guiyu of China: A
Population-Based Study," *PLoS One* 9, no. 8 (2014): e105470, doi: 10.1371/
journal.pone.0105470 (accessed April 18, 2018).

[22] The industry is represented by Call2Recycle Canada. The board of direc-
tors includes representation from Sony, Rayovac, Energizer Canada,
Panasonic Canada and Procter & Gamble Canada.

[23] Minnesota Pollution Control Agency, *2005–2008 Perfluorochemical
Evaluation at Solid Waste Facilities in Minnesota: Technical Evaluation and
Regulatory Management Approach*, April 14, 2010.

[24] K. Ward, Jr., "C8 Linked to Thyroid, Bowel Disease," *Charleston Gazette*,
July 30, 2012.

[25] P. Anastas and J. Warner, *Green Chemistry: Theory and Practice* (New York:
Oxford University Press, 1998). (https://www.acs.org/content/acs/en
/greenchemistry/what-is-green-chemistry/principles/12-principles-of
-green-chemistry.html; accessed July 15, 2018).

[26] Ibid.

[27] "Many Chemicals, But Limited Toxicity Data," European Environmental Agency, April 20, 2016 (https://www.eea.europa.eu/publications/NYM2/page006.html; accessed April 15, 2018).

[28] J. M. Benyus, *Biomimicry: Innovation Inspired by Nature* (New York: William Morrow, 1997).

[29] City of Toronto, "Water Quality Assurance Program: Protecting Water Quality," (http://www.toronto.ca/water/protecting_quality/quality_assurance.htm; accessed February 1, 2013).

[30] W. MacKenzie, N. Hoxie, M. Proctor, M.S. Gradus, K. Blair, D. Peterson, J. Kazmierczak et. al, "A Massive Outbreak in Milwaukee of Cryptosporidium Infection Transmitted through the Public Water Supply," *New England Journal of Medicine* 331 (1994): 161–67.

[31] Environmental Protection Agency, "Cryptosporidium: Drinking Water Health Advisory," EPA-822-R-01-009, March 2001.

[32] D. O'Connor, *Report of the Walkerton Inquiry: A Strategy for Safe Drinking Water*, 2002 (http://www.attorneygeneral.jus.gov.on.ca/english/about/pubs/walkerton/; accessed February 22, 2013).

[33] "Consumer Background: Bottled Water," *CBC News*, August 20, 2008.

[34] C. Mintz, "Stuck on the Bottle," *Globe and Mail*, March 20, 2017 (https://www.theglobeandmail.com/life/food-and-wine/food-trends/why-canadians-are-or-arent-drinking-bottledwater/article34353867/; accessed April 15, 2018).

[35] Health Canada, "Environmental and Workplace Health: Drinking Water Quality," http://www.hc-sc.gc.ca/ewh-semt/water-eau/drink-potab/index-eng.php (accessed February 22, 2013).

[36] World Health Organization, "Pharmaceuticals in Drinking Water," 2012 (http://apps.who.int/iris/bitstream/10665/44630/1/9789241502085_eng.pdf; accessed March 1, 2013).

[37] Ibid.

[38] E. Teuten, J. Saquing, D. Knappe, M. Barlaz, S. Jonsson, A. Björn, S. Rowland et al., "Transport and Release of Chemicals from Plastics to the Environment and to Wildlife," *Philosophical Transactions of the Royal Society B* 364 (2009): 2027–45.

[39] Health Canada, "Food and Nutrition: Frequently Asked Questions about Bottled Water," (www.hc-sc.gc.ca/fn-an/securit/facts-faits/faqs_bottle_water-eau_embouteillee-eng.php; accessed February 1, 2013).

[40] Ibid.

[41] A. Theen, "Ivy Colleges Shunning Bottled Water Jab at $22 Billion Industry," Bloomberg News, March 7, 2012 (http://www.bloomberg.com /news/2012-03-07/ivy-colleges-shunning-bottled-water-jab-at-22-billion -industry.html; accessed February 1, 2013).

[42] Pacific Institute, "Bottled Water and Energy Fact Sheet," February 2007 (http://pacinst.org/publication/bottled-water-and-energy-a-fact-sheet/; accessed March 16, 2018).

[43] "Bottled Water Sales Outpace Soda for First Time in U.S.," CBS, March 9, 2017 (https://www.cbsnews.com/news/bottled-water-sales-outpace-soda- for-the-first-time/; accessed April 15, 2018).

[44] V. Wong, "Almost No Plastic Bottles Get Recycled into New Bottles," CNBC, April 25, 2017 (https://www.cnbc.com/2017/04/24/almost-no-plastic-bottles -get-recycled-into-new-bottles.html; accessed April 15, 2018).

[45] R. Copes, G. Evans and S. Verhille, "Bottled vs. Tap Water," *BC Medical Journal* 51 (2009): 112–13 (http://www.bcmj.org/council-health-promotion/ bottled-vs-tap-water; accessed February 1, 2013).

[46] Consumer Reports, "Water Filter Buying Guide," July 2012 (http://www.consumerreports.org/cro/water-filters/buying-guide.htm?pn=0; accessed February 1, 2013).

[47] NSF International, "About NSF" (http://www.nsf.org/about-nsf/; accessed March 16, 2018).

[48] NSF International, "Drinking Water Treatment Standards" (http://www.nsf .org/services/by-type/standards-publications/water-wastewater-standards /drinking-water-systems-standards; accessed March 16, 2018).

[49] NSF International, "Consumer Products and Service Listing Search" (http://www.nsf.org/consumer-resources/; accessed March 1, 2018).

[50] Adapted from Natural Resources Defense Council, "Water Issues: Consumer Guide to Water Filters," http://www.nrdc.org/water/drinking /gfilters.asp (accessed February 2013).

[51] See Ellen MacArthur Foundation, "Toward the Circular Economy: Economic and Business Rationale for an Accelerated Transition," vol. 1: 2012 (http://www.ellenmacarthurfoundation.org/business/reports/ce2012; accessed July 11, 2013).

[52] T. T. Schug, R. Abagyan, B. Blumberg, T. J. Collins, D. Crews, P. L. Defur, S. M. Dickenson et al., "Designing Endocrine Disruption Out of the Next Generation of Chemicals," *Green Chemistry* 15, no.1 (January 2013): 181–90, doi: 10.1039/c2gc35055f.

[53] Tiered Protocol for Endocrine Disruption (TiPED), "What is TiPED™?," 2012, http://www.tipedinfo.com/tiped_tier/whats-tiped/ (accessed June 1, 2013).

[54] Adapted from the Ellen MacArthur Foundation's Higher Education Resources. © Graham Pritchard / Ellen MacArthur Foundation after W. McDonough and M. Braungart.

[55] "Green Chemistry Success Stories," *LANXESS Webmagazine*.

[56] S. Everts, "Better Living Through Green Chemistry: Pharmaceuticals," *New Scientist*, March 12, 2010 (http://www.newscientist.com/article/dn18641 -better-living-through-green-chemistry-pharmaceuticals.html; accessed April 1, 2013).

[57] J. Shankleman and H. Warren, "Solar Power Will Kill Coal Faster Than You Think," Bloomberg, June 15, 2017 (https://www.bloomberg.com/news/arti- cles/2017-06-15/solar-power-will-kill-coal-sooner-than-you-think; accessed April 16, 2018).

[58] I. Johnston, "World Renewable Energy Production Increases by Record Levels in 2016," *The Independent*, June 7, 2017 (https://www.independent. co.uk/environment/world-renewable-energy-production-record- increase-2016-green-power-western-europe-half-ren21-a7776646.html; accessed April 18, 2018).

[59] R. Becque, E. Mackres, J. Layke, N. Aden, S. Liu, K. Managan, C. Nesler, "Accelerating Building Efficiency: Eight Actions for Urban Leaders," *World Resources Institute*, May 2016 (publications.wri.org/buildingefficiency/; accessed April 16, 2018).

Thirteen: The "Slow Death by Rubber Duck" Top Ten

[1] L. Parlett, A. Calafat and S. Swan, "Women's Exposure to Phthalates in Relation to Use of Personal Care Products," *Journal of Exposure Science and Environmental Epidemiology* 23 (2013): 197–206.

[2] See table 5 in chapter 2.

[3] Y.-H. Chiu, P.L. Williams, M.W. Gillman, A. J. Gaskins, L. Minguez-Alarcón, I. Souter, T. L. Toth et al., "Association Between Pesticide Residue Intake from Consumption of Fruits and Vegetables and Pregnancy Outcomes among Women Undergoing Infertility Treatment with Assisted Reproductive Technology," *Journal of the American Medical Association Internal Medecine* 178 (2018):17–26 (accessed July 22, 2018).

[4] T. Roberts, "We Spend 90% of Our Time Indoors. Says Who?," BuildingGreen, December 15, 2016 (https://www.buildinggreen.com/blog/we-spend-90-our-time-indoors-says-who; accessed June 11, 2018).

[5] L. Robinson and R. Miller, "The Impact of Bisphenol A and Phthalates on Allergy, Asthma, and Immune Function: A Review of Latest Findings," *Current Environmental Health Reports* 2, no. 4 (December 2015): 379–87 (https://www.ncbi.nlm.nih.gov/pmc/articles/PMC4626318/; accessed June 11, 2018).

[6] S. Genuis, "Elimination of Persistent Toxicants from the Human Body," *Human and Experimental Toxicology* 30 (2010): 3–18.

[7] Ibid.

[8] V. Nadeau et al., "Effect of Physical Exertion 1. Toluene."

[9] "Wal-Mart Names Eight Chemicals to Be Removed From Products," Reuters, July 20, 2016 (https://www.reuters.com/article/us-walmart-chemicals/wal-mart-names-eight-chemicals-to-be-removed-from-products-idUSKCN1002IJ; accessed April 15, 2018).

ACKNOWLEDGEMENTS

We are so grateful to the many people around the world who gave generously of their time to make *Slow Death by Rubber Duck* and *Toxin Toxout* the successes they've been. Thank you all!

In crafting this tenth-anniversary edition of *Slow Death*, we want to acknowledge in particular executive publisher Louise Dennys at Knopf Canada for believing in this book from the very beginning and publisher Anne Collins for seeing the value in re-issuing it a decade later. Senior editor Craig Pyette and our editors Doris Cowan and Gillian Watts worked overtime to ensure this new edition was as tight and current as could be. Our agent Rick Broadhead, as always, kept us on track.

Thanks to Tim Gray, Muhannad Malas and Sarah Jamal at Environmental Defence Canada for once again joining us to explore the disturbing frontiers of personal pollution, to Michael McCulloch for research support, and to SGS AXYS Analytical in Sidney, British Columbia, for analyzing the urine samples from our cash register receipt experiment. We appreciate the ongoing support of our employers, the Ivey Foundation and the Broadbent Institute.

Our wives, Biz and Jen, and our kids Claire, Ellen, Zack and Owain (who are a lot taller than they were in 2009), have taken this decade-long toxic chemical journey along with us. We couldn't have done it without them.

CREDITS

Grateful acknowledgement is made to the following for the permission to reprint previously published material:

Quotation on page 1 is from "Canary in a Coal Mine," words by Sting, music by Sting and Nigel Gray, ©1980 Universal Music Corporation and Songs of Universal, Inc. and used with permission.

Reprinting of the photo on page 7, "No Yucky in My Duckie", was permitted by Genevieve K. Howe, the Ecology Center and Sara Talpos (parent of Jackson, the child in the photo).

Quotation on page 51 is from "Shimmer," *Saturday Night Live,* Episode 9, Season 1, January 10, 1976 and published by NBC Courtesy of Broadway Video Enterprises and NBC Studios, Inc. ©1976 by NBC Studios, Inc. Distributed by Broadway Video Enterprises.

Quotation on page 53 is from CBC *Marketplace*: "PFOA: What Is It, and How Did It Get Into Our Blood?", broadcast on March 20, 2005. Excerpted from the interview with Erica Johnson, *Marketplace* reporter, and Scott Mabury, environmental chemist at the University of Toronto.

Quotation on page 55 is from an interview with Della Tennant, National Public Radio, January, 2006.

Quotation on page 68 is from "Cat People (Putting Out Fire)", words by David Bowie and music by Giorgio Moroder. ©1982 by Universal Music Corp. and Songs of Universal, Inc. Used with permission.

Quotation on page 71 is from "Intentions Gone Astray: The Facts about Tris Don't Leave Much Choice" by Linda Charlton, published in the *New York Times, The Week in Review,* July 3, 1977 and reprinted with permission.

Quotation on page 72 is from the Environmental Defense Fund Petition.

Quotations on page 72 are from "Flame Retardant Sleepwear: Is There a Risk of Cancer?" by Nadine Brozan, published in *The New York Times*, April 10, 1976 and reprinted with permission.

- Quotation on page 76 is from "Safety of a New Flame Retardant Questioned" by Joan Lowy, published in Scripps Howard News Service, 2004 and reprinted with permission.

Quotations on page 92 are from "Actress Describes Mercury Poisoning Ordeal" by Liz Bordo Wright and published by ABC News Program.

Quotation on page 111 is from Donald Trump and published on the Donald Trump University website, 2006.

Quotation on page 125 is from "Nanosilver: A Threat to Soil, Water and Human Health?" by Rye

Senjen, published in *Friends of the Earth Australia*, 2007 and Reprinted with permission.

Quotation on page 135 is from *Environmental Persistence and Human Exposure*

Studies with 2,4-D and Other Turfgrass Pesticides by G.R. Stephenson, K.R. Solomon and L. Ritter and published by Centre for Toxicology at the University of Guelph.

Quotation on page 143 is from "Scientists: EPA 'Under Siege' Survey of EPA Scientists Finds Rampant Political Interference" by Suemedha Sood and published by the *Washington Independent*, 2008. Reprinted with permission.

Quotation on page 147 is from *The Graduate*, 1967, and published by Vivendi/Canal. ©1967 by Studio Canal.

Quotation on page 154 is from "Rona Brockovich?" by Terence Corcoran, published in the *National Post*, 2006 and reprinted with permission.

Photo on page 148, "BPA Rally Photo of Young Girl Holding her Baby Picket," is reprinted with permission from Monique Fabregas.

Quotation on page 161 is from "Chapel Hill Bisphenol A Expert Panel Consensus Statement: Integration of Mechanisms, Effects in Animals and Potential to Impact Human Health at Current Levels of Exposure" by F.S. vom Saal, B.T. Akingbemi, S.M. Belcher, L.S. Birnbaum, D.A. Crain, M. Eriksen, F. Farabollini, L.J. Guillette, R. Hauser, J.J. Heindel, S.M. Ho, P.A. Hunt, T. Iguchi, S. Jobling, J.

Kanno, R.A. Keri, K.E. Knudsen, H. Laufer, G.A. LeBlanc, M. Marcus, J.A. McLachlan, J.P. Myers, A. Nadal, R.R. Newbold, N. Olea, G.S. Prins, C.A. Richter, B.S. Rubin, C. Sonnenschein, A.M. Soto, C.E. Talsness, J.G. Vandenbergh, L.N. Vandenberg, D.R. Walser-Kuntz, C.S. Watson, W.V. Welshons, Y. Wetherill and R.T. Zoeller, published by *Reproductive Toxicology* (2007). ©2007 and published by Elsevier, Inc. Reprinted with permission.

Quotation on page 192 is from the "Rehab (Remix)" by Amy Winehouse, Jay-Z and Mark Ronson, ©2007 Islands Records, Universal Music Corporation and Songs of Universal, Inc. Used by permission, courtesy of the Hal Leonard Corporation.

Quotation on page 234 is from "Smoke Gets in Your Eyes," *Mad Men*, Episode 1, Season 1 (July 19, 2007) and provided courtesy of LionsGate.

Figure 17 on page 238 is adapted from "The National Human Activity Pattern Survey (NHAPS): A Resource for Assessing Exposure to Environmental Pollutants" by N. Klepeis, W. Nelson, J. Robinson, A. Tsang, P. Switzer, J. Behar, S. Hern and W. Engelman, published in the *Journal of Exposure Analysis and Environmental Epidemiology* 11 (2001): 231–52 and reproduced with permission from Nature Publishing Group (License No.: 3171361345710).

Figure 21 on page 282 is reproduced with permission from the Ellen MacArthur Foundation.

Every effort has been made to contact the relevant copyright holders; in the event of an inadvertent omission or error, please notify the publisher.

RICK SMITH is a Canadian author, environmentalist and non-profit leader and Executive Director of the Broadbent Institute. From 2003 to 2012 he served as Executive Director of Environmental Defence, where he was the driving force behind making Canada the first country in the world to ban BPA in baby bottles. He is the co-author of two bestselling books on the health effects of pollution: *Slow Death by Rubber Duck* (2009) and *Toxin Toxout* (2013).

BRUCE LOURIE is an environmental thought leader in Canada and an acknowledged global expert on pollution and sustainable energy. He has founded many important environmental organizations such as the Clean Economy Fund, the Canadian Environmental Grantmakers Network, the Sustainability Network and the Canadian Energy Efficiency Alliance. Bruce is President of the Ivey Foundation, one of the largest private foundations supporting sustainability in the country, and is an advisor to Canada's Ecofiscal Commission.